Fourth Edition

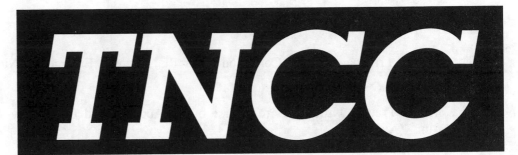

TNCC

Trauma

Nursing

Core

Course

Provider Manual

Copyright© 1995
Emergency Nurses Association

The official Trauma Nursing Core Course of the National Emergency Nurses' Affiliation (NENA) (Canada)

The official Trauma Nursing Core Course of the Accident and Emergency Association of New South Wales Inc. (Australia)

The official Trauma Nursing Core Course of the Accident and Emergency Association of New Zealand

The official Trauma Nursing Core Course of the Royal College of Nursing Accident and Emergency Association Committee of Trauma Nursing (United Kingdom)

TRAUMA NURSING CORE COURSE

Sample Questions

1. The correct sequence for the initial assessment of the trauma patient is:

   a. airway, breathing, circulation, cervical spine stabilization, disability, secondary assessment.

   b. circulation, airway, breathing, cervical spine stabilization, disability, secondary assessment.

   c. airway, cervical spine stabilization, breathing, circulation, disability, secondary assessment.

   d. secondary assessment, disability, airway, cervical spine stabilization, breathing.

   Reference: Initial Assessment chapter – page 44.

2. The position that best optimizes the microcirculation to an extremity with a suspected compartment syndrome is:

   a. elevating the extremity above the level of the heart.

   b. turning the patient to the unaffected side.

   c. elevating the extremity to the level of the heart.

   d. placing the patient in Trendelenburg position.

   Reference: Musculoskeletal Trauma chapter – page 249.

3. A gastric tube is inserted in a trauma patient primarily to:

   a. administer medication until intravenous access is established.

   b. decompress the stomach to prevent vomiting and aspiration.

   c. test the patient's gag reflex.

   d. test the gastric aspirate for suspected toxic substances.

   Reference: Initial Assessment chapter – page 55; Abdominal Trauma chapter – page 186.

QUESTIONS 4 AND 5 REFER TO THE FOLLOWING SCENARIO:

An unrestrained driver involved in a front-end collision arrives restless with pale, cold, and clammy skin. Vital signs are blood pressure 90/70 mmHg, pulse 120 beats/minute, respirations 24 breaths/minute. The patient's airway is patent, oxygen via nonrebreather mask at 15 L/minute is being administered, and two large-bore intravenous catheters with lactated Ringer's solution have been initiated. Initial assessment reveals equal and bilateral breath sounds and a rigid abdomen with absent bowel sounds.

4. Based on the assessment findings, the emergency nurse should suspect a:

   a. ruptured spleen.

   b. contused kidney.

   c. pericardial tamponade.

   d. tension pneumothorax.

   Reference: Abdominal Trauma chapter – page 178.

5. The patient suddenly becomes more restless and complains of increased difficulty breathing. The patient now has a blood pressure of 90/76 mmHg, pulse 140 beats/minute, respirations 32 breaths/minute. The priority nursing intervention is:

   a. obtaining baseline laboratory and radiologic studies.

   b. reassessing the patient's breathing status.

   c. preparing the patient for diagnostic peritoneal lavage.

   d. inserting a nasogastric tube.

   Reference: Initial Assessment chapter – pages 44 and 50.

6. The basis for the physiologic response of the body to hypovolemic shock is:

   a. ventilation/perfusion abnormalities.

   b. pump or left ventricular failure.

   c. anaerobic cellular metabolism due to inadequate tissue perfusion.

   d. vasodilatation and clotting abnormalities.

   Reference: Shock chapter – page 79.

7. Assessment of breathing effectiveness includes:

   a. skin color, respiratory rate and depth.

   b. edema, chest rise and fall.

   c. tachycardia, use of accessory muscles.

   d. heart sounds, bilateral breath sounds.

   Reference: Initial Assessment chapter – pages 48 and 49.

8. The most common injury to a pregnant female that results in fetal death is:

   a. tension pneumothorax.

   b. lacerated liver.

   c. pelvic fracture.

   d. subdural hematoma.

   Reference: Trauma and Pregnancy chapter – page 286.

9. Hemoptysis and subcutaneous emphysema of the neck would be indicative of a:

   a. tension pneumothorax.

   b. tracheobronchial injury.

   c. ruptured diaphragm.

   d. pulmonary contusion.

   Reference: Thoracic and Neck Trauma chapter – page 161.

10. A construction worker sustains significant facial trauma after falling two stories. The patient is transported to the emergency department by coworkers. On arrival, the patient develops respiratory arrest. The most immediate intervention is:

   a. preparing for cricothyrotomy.

   b. applying a nonrebreather mask at 15 L/minute.

   c. inserting an oral airway.

   d. performing a jaw thrust maneuver with cervical spine stabilization.

   Reference: Initial Assessment chapter – page 46.

11. Interventions for a patient in neurogenic shock include:

   a.   administering intravenous fluid calculated by the patient's weight.

   b.   administering decreasing doses of steroids.

   c.   infusing fluids judiciously.

   d.   lowering the room temperature.

   Reference: Shock chapter – page 96;
               Spinal Cord and Vertebral Column chapter – page 222.

12. A 23-year-old is transported to the emergency department after being involved in a motor vehicle crash. The patient is alert and oriented but anxious. Initial vital signs are blood pressure 100/60 mmHg, pulse 124 beats/minute, respirations 28 breaths/minute. Secondary assessment reveals abrasions of the right lower leg and ecchymosis of the right pelvic area. The patient complains of pain when gentle pressure is applied to the iliac crests. The emergency nurse should be most concerned about:

   a.   fat embolism.

   b.   sepsis.

   c.   hypovolemic shock.

   d.   spleen laceration.

   Reference: Musculoskeletal Trauma chapter – page 242.

QUESTIONS 13 AND 14 REFER TO THE FOLLOWING SCENARIO:

A five-year-old child hit a curb while riding her bicycle. A bystander states she fell against the handlebars of the bicycle before falling to the ground. She is awake, alert, and oriented on arrival to the emergency department.

13. Common injuries that may occur when a child is thrown against bicycle handlebars include:

   a.   head and liver injuries.

   b.   duodenal and pancreatic injuries.

   c.   aorta and rib injuries.

   d.   lung and spleen injuries.

   Reference: Pediatric Trauma chapter – page 306.

14. Normal urinary output for a five-year-old child is:

    a.   0.5 ml/kg/hr.

    b.   1.0 ml/kg/hr.

    c.   2.0 ml/kg/hr.

    d.   3.0 ml/kg/hr.

    Reference: Pediatric Trauma chapter – page 320.

15. Tissue damage caused by a stabbing object is related to:

    a.   fragmentation, length of the instrument, and shape of the instrument.

    b.   length of the instrument, angle of entry, and striking velocity.

    c.   type of tissue struck, mass, and range.

    d.   shape of the instrument, range, and angle of entry.

    Reference: Biomechanics and Mechanisms of Injury chapter – page 33.

16. A major cause of death in a patient with brain or craniofacial trauma is:

    a.   hypovolemia.

    b.   airway obstruction.

    c.   respiratory compromise.

    d.   increased intracranial pressure.

    Reference: Brain and Craniofacial Trauma chapter – page 108.

17. What immediate action should be taken if a chest tube becomes dislodged from the patient's chest?

    a.   Notify the physician and apply supplemental oxygen

    b.   Cover the wound with a petroleum impregnated, occlusive dressing, taped on three sides

    c.   Reinsert the chest tube and notify the physician

    d.   Cover the wound with a sterile gauze, taped on three sides

    Reference: Chest Trauma Interventions skill station – page 434.

18. Which of the following is the proper sequence for spinal immobilization?

    a. Apply a rigid cervical collar, position the patient on a backboard, place the back-board straps, place the head support devices and tape

    b. Apply a rigid cervical collar, position the patient on a backboard, place the head support devices and tape, place the backboard straps

    c. Position the patient on a backboard, apply a rigid cervical collar, place the backboard straps, place the head support devices and tape

    d. Position the patient on a backboard, apply a rigid cervical collar, place the head support devices and tape, place the backboard straps

    Reference: Spinal Immobilization skill station – page 428.

19. Which of the following interventions is the highest priority for a patient with a suspected cervical spine injury?

    a. Initiating intravenous fluid for volume replacement

    b. Administering supplemental oxygen

    c. Stabilizing the cervical spine

    d. Inserting a nasogastric tube

    Reference: Spinal Cord and Vertebral Column Trauma chapter – pages 215 and 216.

20. The priority nursing intervention for a patient with facial trauma is:

    a. applying a dressing to uncontrolled facial bleeding.

    b. stabilizing the cervical spine.

    c. clearing the airway of debris.

    d. administering intravenous fluids.

    Reference: Brain and Craniofacial Trauma chapter – pages 120 to 123.

21. Hypotension in head injury patients may result in:

    a. increased cerebral perfusion and amnesia.

    b. decreased cerebral perfusion and secondary brain injury.

    c. primary brain injury and hypoxia.

    d. decreased intracranial pressure and increased cerebral perfusion.

    Reference: Brain and Craniofacial Trauma chapter – pages 104 and 105.

22. A 32-year-old who fell from a roof is admitted to the emergency department with absent motor and sensory function in his arms and legs. His cervical spine radiographs demonstrate C-4 and C-5 dislocations. The priority nursing diagnosis for this patient is:

    a. breathing pattern, ineffective.

    b. skin integrity, impaired.

    c. self-concept, disturbance in.

    d. infection, potential for.

    Reference: Spinal Cord and Vertebral Column Trauma chapter – pages 214 and 215.

23. When assessing a patient with an electrical burn, it is important to determine the:

    a. entrance wound site, presence of extremity injury, exit wound site.

    b. duration of contact, type of electrical equipment, entrance wound site.

    c. voltage, type of current, duration of contact.

    d. patient location at time of injury, type of current, entrance wound site.

    Reference: Burn Trauma chapter – page 278.

24. A 50 kg patient sustained deep partial thickness burns covering 40% of the body surface area at 10 pm. By 6 am the patient should receive how many milliliters of fluid? (Use 4 ml/kg/% BSA to calculate the intravenous fluid replacement).

    a. 4000 ml

    b. 2000 ml

    c. 8000 ml

    d. 500 ml

    Reference: Burn Trauma chapter – page 274.

25. In dealing with a family following a death, all of the following may be helpful **except:**

    a. allowing the family to see the patient.

    b. suggesting that the family hold or touch the patient.

    c. using terms such as expired or passed away.

    d. discussing organ donation.

    Reference: Psychosocial Aspects of Trauma Care chapter – page 337.

TNCC SAMPLE QUESTIONS
ANSWER KEY

1.	C	14.	B
2.	C	15.	B
3.	B	16.	B
4.	A	17.	B
5.	B	18.	A
6.	C	19.	C
7.	A	20.	C
8.	C	21.	B
9.	B	22.	A
10.	D	23.	C
11.	C	24.	A
12.	C	25.	C
13.	B		

TABLE OF CONTENTS

TABLE OF CONTENTS (Continued)

Appendixes

Optional Chapters

TABLES

TABLES (Continued)

TABLES (Continued)

FIGURES

ACKNOWLEDGMENTS

The Emergency Nurses Association (ENA) would like to extend its appreciation to the 1993-1994 TNCC Revision Task Force for the development and implementation of the Trauma Nursing Core Course (TNCC).

EDITORS
Barbara Bennett Jacobs, RN, MPH, MS
Faculty, St Joseph College Division of
  Nursing
Clinical Instructor in Surgery
University of Connecticut School of
  Medicine
West Hartford, CT

Pam Baker, RN, BSN, CCRN, CEN
Director, Trauma and Pediatric Services
Emergency Nurses Association
Park Ridge, IL

SECTION EDITORS
Peggy Hollingsworth-Fridlund, RN, BSN
Trauma Coordinator
UC San Diego Medical Center
San Diego, CA

Ginger Morse, RN, MN, CEN, CCRN
Clinical Nurse Specialist/Program Director
Trauma Services
Truman Medical Center-West
Kansas City, MO

Vicki Patrick, RN, MS, CEN
Director, Emergency Trauma Services
Methodist Hospital of Dallas
Dallas, TX

BOARD LIAISON
Jean Proehl, RN, MN, CEN, CCRN
Emergency Clinical Nurse Specialist
Dartmouth-Hitchcock Medical Center
Lebanon, NH

CONTRIBUTING AUTHORS
Kathi Ayers, RN, MSN, CFNP
Trauma Program Manager
Sharp Memorial Hospital
San Diego, CA

Pam Baker, RN, BSN, CCRN, CEN
Director, Trauma and Pediatric Services
Emergency Nurses Association
Park Ridge, IL

Barbara Bennett Jacobs, RN, MPH, MS
Faculty, St Joseph College Division of
  Nursing
Clinical Instructor in Surgery
University of Connecticut School of
  Medicine
West Hartford, CT

Susan Cox, RN, MSN
Trauma Program Director
Childrens Hospital and Health Center
San Diego, CA

Peggy Hollingsworth-Fridlund, RN, BSN
Trauma Coordinator
UC San Diego Medical Center
San Diego, CA

Sue Moore, RN, MS, CCRN, CEN
Staff Nurse
Emergency Department
Washoe Medical Center
Reno, NV

Ginger Morse, RN, MN, CEN, CCRN
Clinical Nurse Specialist/Program Director
Trauma Services
Truman Medical Center-West
Kansas City, MO

Margie A. Murdock, RN, MSN, CEN
Consultant, Trauma and Emergency
  Nursing
Orange, CA

Connie Pardee, RN, MSN
Emergency Clinical Nurse Specialist
Borgess Medical Center
Kalamazoo, MI

Mark Parshall, RN, MSN, CS, CEN
Santa Fe, NM

Jean Proehl, RN, MN, CEN, CCRN
Emergency Clinical Nurse Specialist
Dartmouth-Hitchcock Medical Center
Lebanon, NH

Vicki Patrick, RN, MS, CEN
Director, Emergency Trauma Services
Methodist Hospital of Dallas
Dallas, TX

Judi Roling, RN, MSN, CEN
Trauma Nurse Coordinator
Saint Joseph Health Center
Kansas City, MO

Judy Selfridge-Thomas, RN, MSN, CEN
General Partner
Selfridge, Sparger, Shea & Associates
Ventura, CA

Reneé Semonin-Holleran, RN, PhD, CEN,
  CCRN, CFRN
Chief Flight Nurse/Clinical Nurse
  Specialist
University of Cincinnati Medical Center
Cincinnati, OH

Mindy Spinella, RN, BSN, CEN
Staff Nurse-Emergency Department
Harris Methodist-Fort Worth
Fort Worth, TX

Denise R. Turner, RN, BSN, CCRN,
  CEN
Assistant Trauma Nurse Coordinator
Trauma Services
Truman Medical Center-West
Kansas City, MO

Steven A. Weinman, RN, CEN
Clinical Nurse II/Educator
Department of Emergency Medicine
Truman Medical Center-West
Kansas City, MO

REVIEWERS
Barbara A. Bires, RN, MSN, CEN
Assistant Clinical Professor
Critical Care/Trauma Graduate Program
School of Nursing
University of California
San Francisco, CA

Joseph S. Blansfield, RN, MS, CS, CEN
Trauma Nurse Coordinator, Surgery
Boston City Hospital
Boston, MA

Val A. Catanzarite, MD, PhD
Associate Director Maternal Fetal
  Medicine
Mary Birch Hospital for Women
Sharp Memorial Hospital
San Diego, CA

Liz Cloughessy, RN
President, Accident and Emergency
  Association of New South Wales
Paramatta, Australia

Emilie B.K. Crown, RN, CEN
Staff Nurse
Shady Grove Adventist Hospital
Rockville, MD

Elizabeth C. Denwalt, RN, CEN
Charge Nurse, Emergency Department
University Medical Center
Oklahoma City, OK

Joan Garcia, RN, BSN, CCRC
Trauma Research Coordinator
UC San Diego Medical Center
San Diego, CA

Yolanda Otero Inman, RN, BS, CEN
Trauma Nurse Coordinator
University of New Mexico Hospital
Albuquerque, NM

Linell M. Jones, RN, BSN, CCRN
Assistant Nurse Manager
Valley Medical Center
Renton, WA

Sandra B. Knight, RN, BS, CEN
Emergency Clinician/Educator
Naples Community Hospital
Naples, FL

Crela L. Landreth, RN, BSN, CEN,
  MICN
Trauma Services Coordinator
Memorial Mission Hospital
Asheville, NC

Louise LeBlanc, RN, BSCN
Manager, Emergency Department
Scarborough General Hospital
Scarborough, Ontario, Canada

Cynthia Maroun, RN
San Antonio, TX

John Trickett, RN, CEN (UK), CC CERT.
Trauma Coordinator
Ottawa General Hospital
Ottawa
Ontario, Canada

Deloris Welken, RN, CEN
Emergency Room/Hospital Supervisor
Mercy Hospital
Valley City, ND

David W. Unkle, RN, MSN, CEN,
  CCRN, FCCM
Nurse Manager, Emergency Department
West Jersey Hospital
Camden, NJ

Darlene S. Whitlock, RN, MA, CEN
Trauma Coordinator
Stormont Vail Regional Medical Center
Topeka, KS

Eugene Williamson, RN, CEN
Clinical Nurse Educator
Salem Hospital
Salem, OR

Jill Windle, RN
Turton, Lancashire, England

STAFF SUPPORT
Pam Baker, RN, BSN, CCRN, CEN
Director, Trauma and Pediatric Services
Emergency Nurses Association
Park Ridge, IL

Larry Hamsing
Publication Specialist
Emergency Nurses Association
Park Ridge, IL

Sharon Tarnoff
Group Director, Association Resource
  Development and Promotion
Emergency Nurses Association
Park Ridge, IL

SPECIAL
ACKNOWLEDGMENT

The TNCC Revision Task Force, TNCC National Faculty, and the ENA Board of Directors would like to extend a special appreciation to Barbara Bennett Jacobs, RN, MPH, MS for serving as editor for this project. This revision could not have been completed without Barbara's expert guidance, persistence, and strong committment to trauma nursing.

PREFACE

The Emergency Nurses Association (ENA) recognizes that trauma victims need comprehensive nursing care provided by knowledgeable professional registered nurses. ENA's dedicated Board of Directors, members, and professional staff developed the Trauma Nursing Core Course (TNCC) as a means for standardizing the principles of nursing care, improving the quality of care, and ultimately maximizing patient outcomes.

The first Trauma Nursing Core Course was held in Honolulu, Hawaii in 1986. Since then, thousands of nurses have been verified as TNCC-Providers in the United States, United Kingdom, Canada, Australia, and New Zealand. With the publication of this new fourth edition, the TNCC Revision Task Force was fortunate to have suggestions from TNCC Instructors and "learners" who over the past eight years had the opportunity to participate in programs across four countries. With these suggestions and with a commitment to improving the course, the Task Force began the revision process.

Two conceptual underpinnings of the new TNCC are that the information, both in terms of cognitive knowledge and psychomotor skills, is core-level knowledge and secondly, the six-phase nursing process is the standard of trauma nursing. All the nursing care principles presented in the clinical chapters as well as the new skill station, termed the Trauma Nursing Process, follow the six phases. Recognizing that patients present with problems which require collaborative intervention from other trauma disciplines, the TNCC serves as the standard for the discipline of nursing.

As violence escalates and the number of patients with intentional injuries increases, the tragedy of trauma has profound effects on the victims and their families. Many sectors of society including public health, business and industry, and government are also influenced. Injury prevention programs, strategies, and legislation are spanning many of these sectors. However, emergency nurses are responsible for engaging in nurse-patient relationships on a daily basis when patients' physiologic and psychologic criticality are at their peak. The information in the TNCC is for all emergency nurses whether practicing in a Level I trauma center or in a remote rural clinic. The principles of care remain the same and the patient's ultimate outcome will be affected by the actions of caring, compassionate, and competent trauma nurses. It is the intent of the Emergency Nurses Association that participants in the TNCC be given the opportunity to enhance their knowledge, refine skills, and build a firm foundation in trauma nursing.

Barbara Bennett Jacobs, RN, MPH, MS
TNCC Revision Task Force, Chairperson

CHAPTER ONE

THE TRAUMA NURSING CORE COURSE AND TRAUMA NURSING

OBJECTIVES

Upon completion of this chapter/lecture, the learner should be able to:

1. Describe the purpose of the *Trauma Nursing Core Course*.
2. Describe the seven concepts of the discipline of nursing.
3. Define the six phases of the nursing process.
4. Identify three additional roles, other than those related to the nursing process, associated with trauma nursing.

INTRODUCTION

Trauma is a major threat to the immediate and often long-term health of individuals. The Emergency Nurses Association has responded to the needs of trauma patients by developing the *Trauma Nursing Core Course* (TNCC). This chapter describes the TNCC and the trauma nursing process, which serves as a basis for a standardized approach to initial trauma care.

BELIEF STATEMENTS

After analyzing the impact of trauma in the United States and the potential for positive contributions by professional nurses in the care of the trauma patient, the Emergency Nurses Association has formulated the following belief statements:

1. The optimal care of the trauma patient is best accomplished within a framework in which all members of the trauma team use a systematic, standardized approach to the care of the injured patient.

2. Emergency nurses are essential members of the trauma team. Morbidity and mortality of trauma patients can be significantly reduced by educating nurses to provide competent trauma care.

3. The Emergency Nurses Association and its constituents have the responsibility to facilitate trauma-related, continuing education opportunities for nurses who provide care to trauma patients.

TRAUMA NURSING CORE COURSE

In response to the third belief statement, the Emergency Nurses Association developed the *Trauma Nursing Core Course* (TNCC) for national and international dissemination as a means for identifying standards of nursing care based on current knowledge related to trauma. The first TNCC was presented in 1986. Courses are currently offered in the United States, Canada, United Kingdom, Australia, and New Zealand.

Course Description

The *Trauma Nursing Core Course* (TNCC) is a 16- or 20-hour course designed to provide the learner with cognitive knowledge and psychomotor skills. The trauma nursing process is used to standardize the approach to trauma care and is reflected in the chapters and in the psychomotor skill stations in the manual. Participants receive 18 CECHs for attending the 16-hour course or 22.2 CECHs for attending the 20-hour course.

Lectures and psychomotor skill stations are presented by verified TNCC Instructors and TNCC Instructor Candidates. The lecture content is organized to provide the learner with substantive knowledge for use in the psychomotor skill stations. Evaluation of learners includes (1) a written multiple choice examination designed to assess their acquisition of content presented in the manual and during the lectures and (2) performance at psychomotor skill stations designed to evaluate acquisition of important skills. To successfully complete the TNCC, the learner must achieve a minimum of 80% on the written examination and demonstrate 70% of all steps in each skill station.

A learner may repeat the written examination (if score is between 70 to 78%), only if successful in all psychomotor skill stations. A learner may repeat only one psychomotor skill station as long as he or she successfully completes the multiple choice examination the first time.

Purpose

The purpose of the TNCC is to present core-level knowledge and psychomotor skills associated with implementing the trauma nursing process. The psychomotor skill stations facilitate initial integration of psychomotor abilities in a setting that simulates trauma patient situations. It is the intent of the TNCC to enhance the nurse's ability to assess, rapidly and accurately, the patient's responses to the trauma event. It is anticipated that the use of the knowledge and skills learned in the TNCC will ultimately contribute to a decrease in the morbidity and mortality associated with trauma.

Course Participants

It is recommended that the course participants in a TNCC have at least six months of clinical nursing experience in an emergency care setting prior to taking the course. It is assumed that the course participant has an understanding of emergency trauma care terminology and is familiar with standard emergency trauma equipment. If the participant is a novice in trauma nursing, then the course content and psycho-motor skill stations will provide valuable information and practice within a supportive learning environment.

The TNCC may be officially attended only by Registered Nurses (RNs). It is recognized that nurses in other clinical areas besides those associated with emergency settings may desire to take the TNCC. Auditing the course is permitted; however, those who do audit, e.g., EMT-paramedics and/or licensed practical nurses (LPNs), are not eligible for evaluation or verification.

TRAUMA NURSING DEFINED

Trauma nursing as a discipline refers to the process and content of all the different roles nurses have in the care of the trauma patient. Knowledge is the core of any discipline. Nursing knowledge is derived from nursing theory and from clinical experiences. Additional knowledge is derived from other disciplines.[1] In conjunction with this knowledge, seven concepts can be considered central to the discipline of nursing. They are patient, environment, interaction, nursing process, interventions, transition, and health. Trauma nursing is the active interaction between the trauma nurse and a patient who are both influenced by their own internal and external environments. A trauma nurse utilizes the focused nursing process and plans interventions to help the patient in his or her transition to optimal preinjury health.

THE NURSING PROCESS

The *Standards of Clinical Nursing Practice* developed by the American Nurses Association and the *Standards of Emergency Nursing Practice* developed by the Emergency Nurses Association are the standards that describe the implementation of the nursing process.[2,3] "The nursing process encompasses all significant actions taken by nurses in providing care to all clients, and forms the foundation of clinical decision-making."[2]

The nursing process involves six phases: assessment, nursing diagnosis, outcome identification, planning, implementation, and evaluation. As an important member of the trauma team, the professional nurse may provide trauma care in a variety of settings, ranging from prehospital to hospital environments. The nursing process can be implemented in all environments in which care is provided. Nursing care activities follow the sequential phases of the nursing process:

1. Performs an organized, initial assessment of the trauma patient to identify the extent and severity of injuries.

    In some settings, the nurse is the first health professional to interact with the patient and may be solely responsible for patient assessment. In other settings, the nurse may function as a member of a trauma team with predefined responsibilities, one of which may be patient evaluation.

2. Determines appropriate nursing diagnoses based on assessment findings.

    Nursing diagnoses are the basis of a classification system that labels or conceptualizes the patient's current health status and identifies problems that may develop. To arrive at a nursing diagnosis, the nurse must make judgments based on the patient's condition and assessment findings. The North American Nursing Diagnosis Association (NANDA) currently has approximately 100 labels that can be used to summarize a patient's health status[4] (see Appendix 1). In critical and/or life-threatening circumstances, assessment and determination of nursing diagnoses may occur simultaneously and spontaneously. Actual nursing diagnoses are differentiated from risk diagnoses. The formulation of actual nursing diagnoses are based on the patient's signs and symptoms. The formulation of risk diagnoses are based on whether the patient is vulnerable to certain problems because of risk factors or other contributing factors.

3.   Identifies specific outcomes as patient-centered goals based on nursing diagnoses.

Specific patient outcomes are often determined simultaneously when nursing diagnoses are being formulated. For example, the nurse caring for a patient who is having difficulty breathing may simultaneously identify the nursing diagnosis as being an altered breathing pattern and one outcome of intervention as being the return of the patient's respiratory rate to normal. In the *TNCC*, nursing diagnoses and expected outcomes are listed together.

4.   Develops a plan for achieving identified patient outcomes.

In the settings associated with care of critical trauma patients, the planning phase of the nursing process may occur simultaneously with the intervention phase.[5] Ideally, the nursing care plan should be written to document the nursing diagnoses, expected outcomes, and interventions. The nursing care plan, developed in consultation with the patient and family, should address discharge plans if indicated. Standardized care plans for specific types of trauma patients may serve as a basis for developing an individual plan. In the *TNCC*, the planning and implementation phases are presented together.

5.   Implements interventions according to priorities based on threats to airway patency, breathing, circulation, and/or any other compromises to the function of body systems.

Interventions are conducted according to a sequence whereby airway, breathing, and circulatory problems are addressed first. The degree of independent or interdependent nursing interventions is a function of state nurse practice acts, institutional policies, and educational background. In some settings, the development of trauma protocols has enabled the professional nurse to function with a greater degree of autonomy in providing care to the trauma patient.

6.   Evaluates and monitors the patient's responses to interventions.

An analysis of the trends in the patient's responses to the injury event and interventions will assist all the members of the trauma team to adjust their care in order to achieve optimal patient outcomes.

ADDITIONAL TRAUMA NURSING ROLES

A collaborative nursing model utilizes the nursing process for inter-action and recognizes the role trauma nurses have within the organization where they practice. Additional trauma nursing responsibilities other than those directly associated with the nursing process include:

1. Communicates with other team members.

    In the emergency care setting, the professional nurse is responsible for the clinical leadership and direction of nursing activities with respect to the trauma patient. The professional nurse may also be responsible for communicating with health care members outside the emergency setting, e.g., the intensive care unit, operating room, labor and delivery and/or nursing staff located in other facilities where a trauma patient may be transferred. The trauma nurse is often the team coordinator responsible for organizing, through effective use of communication skills, the care of the trauma victim.

2. Engages in and promotes a professional nurse-patient relationship.

    A model that reflected the need for nurses to be patient advocates was introduced in the 1970s and gained more recognition in the early 1980s.[6] The advocacy model was developed to guide nurses in the protection of patients from unethical or incompetent care. A professional nurse-patient relationship is one that means more than just advocacy.[7] It is an opportunity for nurses to consult with other health care team members and to utilize a team approach to resolve the patient's problems.

    The professional nurse-patient relationship suggests that the "professional power" the relationship generates for the nurse is actually being given by the patient in exchange for knowledgeable and safe care.[7] Utilizing this model, trauma nurses can be viewed as more than just advocates. They are collaborators with other trauma team members who all share a common interest in ethical, safe, and appropriate patient care.

3. Documents the care of the trauma patient.

    The nurse's documentation of care provides an important source of data to evaluate the extent, appropriateness, quality, and timeliness of care. Analysis of the trauma team's performance serves as an important resource for identifying educational needs of the staff and may contribute to a database, such as a trauma registry, which is used to monitor and evaluate trauma care.

ORGANIZATION OF THE *TNCC MANUAL*

The TNCC manual is designed to reinforce and supplement lectures and psychomotor skill content. The book has been organized to facilitate note-taking. Readers may either make annotations in the left margin or highlight important concepts. To enhance learning, each chapter is presented in a consistent format throughout the manual as follows:

- Anatomy and Physiology – A brief review of relevant anatomy and physiologic concepts are presented to enhance the understanding of the injury process for specific injuries described in each chapter. This section of each chapter will not be discussed during lectures nor will the material be evaluated in the multiple choice examination.

- Introduction – Within this section, information regarding epidemiology, mechanisms of injury, and biomechanics are presented. Types of injuries are categorized as blunt or penetrating. Usual concurrent injuries associated with the injury of the specific body system are described.

- Pathophysiology as a Basis for Signs and Symptoms – Pathophysiologic concepts are presented to explain the body's physiologic responses to injury and to provide a pathophysiologic basis for signs and symptoms.

- Nursing Process – The nursing process is used to organize the nursing care principles. The process is divided into the following phases:

  - Assessment – Appropriate history and physical assessment principles are described. Only the usual assessment procedures or findings are described within each chapter.

Within the history section, it is recognized that life-saving interventions must begin prior to obtaining a relevant history from the patient, family, bystanders, or prehospital emergency medical service (EMS) personnel. Once the patient's condition permits, historical data provide valuable information regarding the presence of more subtle and potentially life-threatening injuries. Data from the pre-hospital personnel are discussed along with data related to the victim's past medical history.

Within the physical assessment section, the content is organized using the assessment skills of inspection, auscultation, percussion, and palpation. Only those skills appropriate for specific body system injuries are presented.

In the diagnostic procedures section, appropriate radiographic studies and laboratory studies are listed for the specific body system injured.

- Nursing Diagnoses and Outcome Identification – As in the *Emergency Nursing Core Curriculum*,[8] nursing diagnoses, developed by the North American Nursing Diagnosis Association (NANDA), are used to categorize the patient's responses to the trauma event.[4] The expected outcomes associated with each nursing diagnosis are listed.

- Planning and Implementation – In the planning and implementation section, interventions are listed in a descending order of priority. This classification of interventions is designed to stress the need to set priorities for trauma patient care, based on correcting life-threatening conditions first.

- Evaluation – Specific areas requiring ongoing assessment are highlighted in those chapters dealing with specific body system injuries. While the trauma nurse may not always observe a positive patient response to a specific intervention, ongoing evaluation of the patient is necessary to determine the patient's status and to determine any lack or change in response. Based on the ongoing evaluation, the nursing interventions can be adjusted to meet the changing needs of the patient.

- Selected Injuries – In this section, the most frequently occurring or life-threatening injuries associated with a particular body system are presented. A brief description of the selected injury is followed by a discussion of specific signs and symptoms. Only interventions that vary from those presented earlier in each chapter are described.

- Skill Stations – The content related to the psychomotor skill stations is presented in a separate chapter. Each psychomotor skill station uses the following format: equipment, preparation, introduction, principles, steps in the skill performance, and summary.

- Appendixes – Nursing Diagnoses, Epidemiology of Trauma, Universal Precautions, Pharmacologic Adjuncts for Endotracheal Intubation, Pain Assessment and Control, Tetanus Prophylaxis, and Injury Severity Indices.

- Glossary – Definitions of over 300 terms and phrases used in the TNCC manual.

- Optional Chapters – Two optional chapters, "Eye Trauma" and "Geriatric Trauma," are included as supplemental reading but will not be presented during a TNCC.

SUMMARY

The impact of trauma in the United States and other countries requires an immediate and coordinated action to control this health threat. The Emergency Nurses Association believes that the knowledge and psychomotor skills as identified in the *Trauma Nursing Core Course* will assist professional nurses to systematically assess the trauma patient and to intervene or to assist with interventions in a manner that will decrease the current mortality and morbidity associated with trauma.

The six phases of the trauma nursing process are: assessment, nursing diagnosis, outcome identification, planning, implementation, and evaluation. Through adherence to standards of clinical nursing practice, trauma nurses can demonstrate their role in achieving this goal in an objective and measurable manner.

REFERENCES

1. Meleis AL. *Theoretical Nursing Development and Progress.* 2nd ed. Philadelphia, Pa: JB Lippincott Co; 1991.

2. American Nurses Association. *Standards of Clinical Practice.* Kansas City, Mo: Author; 1991:3.

3. Emergency Nurses Association. *Standards of Emergency Nursing Practice.* 3rd ed. St. Louis, Mo: Mosby-Year Book; 1994.

4. North American Nursing Diagnosis Association. *Nursing Diagnoses: Definitions and Classification, 1995-1996.* Philadelphia, Pa: Author; 1994.

5. Emergency Nurses Association. *Emergency Nurses Guide to Nursing Diagnosis.* Chicago, Ill: Author; 1992.

6. Miller BK, Mansen TJ, Lee H. Patient advocacy: do nurses have the power and authority to act as a patient advocate? *Nurse Leadership.* 1983;6:56-60.

7. Bernal EW. The nurse as patient advocate. *Hastings Center Report.* 1992;22:8-23.

8. Emergency Nurses Association. *Emergency Nursing Core Curriculum.* 4th ed. Philadelphia, Pa: WB Saunders Co; 1994.

CHAPTER TWO

BIOMECHANICS AND MECHANISMS OF INJURY

OBJECTIVES

Upon completion of this chapter/lecture, the learner should be able to:

1. Define the term "trauma."
2. Identify five characteristics associated with trauma.
3. Describe the body's response to energy transfer from the environment and the effects on human tissues.
4. Identify potential injuries that may occur from specific mechanisms and patterns of injury.

INTRODUCTION

Trauma is defined as injury to human tissues and organs resulting from the transfer of energy from the environment. Injuries are caused by some form of energy that is beyond the body's resilience to tolerate.[1,2] Trauma epidemiology is the study of the distribution of trauma in populations, the determinants of injury, and the associated causes and risk factors.[1]

The term "accident" is obsolete since it has a tendency to mean an injury occurred without intent, and it implies focus on the behavior of the injured victim. For example, the phrase "motor vehicle accident" has been substituted by the phrase "motor vehicle crash or collision (MVC)" and injuries are now classified as intentional (suicide or homicide) or unintentional (motor vehicle crashes or falls).

EPIDEMIOLOGY OF TRAUMA

It is suggested that the learner focus on the particular country in which the TNCC is being conducted. For a more complete description of the epidemiology of trauma, injury prevention, and the injury epidemiology model, please see Appendix 2. No information on this epidemiology section will be evaluated.

UNITED STATES (For presentation in the US only)

Incidence

Trauma is the third leading cause of death for all ages combined in the United States and the first leading cause of death for those persons between the ages of one and 44.[3-9] Annually, approximately 146,000 deaths are due to trauma caused by:

- Motor vehicle crashes (28%)

- Suicide (21%)

- Homicides and legal intervention (17.5%)

- Other trauma events and their adverse effects (33.5)

Approximately 2.7 million persons are hospitalized each year as a result of injuries and/or poisonings.[10]

Human Characteristics

The Subcommittee on Epidemiology of the American Trauma Society has guidelines for trauma that are used to use to monitor the epidemiology of trauma. They suggest that demographic data elements such as age, gender, and ethnicity be collected in order to link particular populations with specific mechanisms of injury. These data can be used for planning injury prevention programs.

Age

Injuries result in the death of more persons between the ages of 25 and 34 than in any other age group. Although the actual number of persons who die from injuries is highest in the age group from 25 to 34, those over the age of 85 have a greater likelihood of dying.[9] The leading cause of death for every age from six years to 33 years of age is motor vehicle crashes.[11]

Gender

There are differences in the ratio of male to female injury death rates depending on the cause of the injury. The overall death rate from injuries is twice more for males than females.[9,12] Exposure to injury-producing events, the amount of risk involved, occupation, and cultural norms have been considered reasons for the gender difference.

Race

The causes of death from injury and subsequent death rates vary by race. The overall injury death rate (per 100,000 population of each group) by race is as follows[9]:

- Whites – 54.0

- Blacks – 84.9

- All others – 73.4

Alcohol

Approximately 36% of those drivers involved in a fatal motor vehicle crash were considered intoxicated (BAC 0.10% or greater).[11] The estimate of fatal motor vehicle crashes related to alcohol (blood alcohol concentration, BAC 0.01% or greater) dropped from 1982 to 1993 (from 56.8% to 44%).[11,13]

Violence

It is estimated that assaultive violence leads to the death of 19,000 to 23,000 persons a year in the United States.[14] In 1991 seven states had more deaths due to firearms than motor vehicles.[15] Assault and handguns are indicative of the violence in our society, but they are particularly alarming in the teenage population. The use of firearms is related to both violence and suicide. The firearm death rate for teenagers (15 to 19 years of age) rose at the alarming rate of 77% from 1985 to 1990.[16]

Assaults on women in the United States are another manifestation of the violence in society today. Research shows that approximately 1.8 million women a year were assaulted by their partners.[17]

Injury Prevention/Control

Injury prevention focuses on reducing the incidence of injury events. Injury control is a broader concept to include not only reducing the incidence but also reducing the severity.[1] The Centers for Disease Control and Prevention (CDC) has officially designated the National Center for Injury Prevention and Control a "center" within the CDC. The Center identified five areas of injury control where funds may be awarded: injury epidemiology, prevention, biomechanics, acute care, and rehabilitation. Most injury control strategies can be classified as one of the following:

- Engineering and technologic interventions, e.g., high-mounted rear brake lights.

- Legislative and enforcement interventions, e.g., seat belt laws.

- Education and behavioral interventions, e.g., school-based injury prevention programs.

Altering the engineering and technologic aspects of injury-producing products and objects is the most effective strategy to reduce injuries. Regulating peoples' behavior through laws and regulations is the second most effective. Educational programs are the least effective.

PROCEED TO PAGE 28

UNITED KINGDOM (For presentation in the UK only)

Incidence

In the United Kingdom, a national data system for auditing trauma is being implemented. Similar to the Major Trauma Outcome Study done in the United States, the system aims to improve the quality of information being collected regarding trauma patients and the care they receive. Data elements being collected are related to physiologic and anatomic manifestations of injuries on scene, during transportation, and during all stages of the hospital stay. The system contains provisions for research into specific aspects of initial trauma care and will use data for purposes of statistical analysis.

Trauma is the fourth leading cause of death for all ages combined in the United Kingdom and the first leading cause of death for those persons between the ages of one and 44. Annually, approximately 16,676 deaths are due to trauma caused by:

- Motor vehicle crashes (26%)

- Suicide (24%)

- Homicides and legal intervention (0.75%)

- All other trauma events and their adverse effects (49.9%)

In 1993, the Office of Population Censuses and Surveys reported that those deaths attributed to all other trauma causes included all environmental and industrial accidents and overdoses.

Human Characteristics

Age

Injuries result in the death of more persons between the ages of 25 and 34 years than in any other age group. Although the actual incidence is greatest in this age group, the death rate from trauma is greatest for those over the age of 85. The leading cause of death for every age from six to 33 years of age is motor vehicle crashes.

Gender

There are differences in the ratio of male to female injury death rates depending on the cause of the injury. The overall death rate for injuries is twice more for males than females. Exposure to the injury-producing event, the amount of risk involved, the occupation, and cultural norms are possible reasons for the gender differences.

Alcohol

The relationship of alcohol to fatal motor vehicle crashes is well studied. In the past 10 years, the incidence of fatal motor vehicle crashes related to illegal alcohol levels (blood alcohol concentration, BAC, 80 mg/100 ml or greater) has dropped. In the United States, a similar trend is noted.

Violence

In British society the presence of violence is becoming increasingly more common. Violent incidents can be classified as assaults (with or without weapons), rape, and sexual assault. Assaultive violence "includes both nonfatal and fatal inter-personal violence where physical force or other means is used by one person with the intent of causing harm, injury, or death to another."[1] In the United States, the use of firearms is related to both violence and suicide. The firearm death rate for US teenagers (15 to 19 years of age) rose at the alarming rate of 77% from 1985 to 1990.[2] As a comparison, in 1992 0.3% of total deaths of persons in the UK between one and 64 years of age were due to firearms.

The increasing incidence of violence as a public health problem in the UK is raising the awareness of the public and government. The risks and predetermining factors that need to be investigated include gang culture, lack of nonviolent male role models, drug culture, and unemployment.

REFERENCES

1. Rosenberg ML, Fenley MA. *Violence in America: A Public Health Approach*. New York, NY: Oxford University Press; 1991.

2. Fingerhut LA. Firearm mortality among children, youth, and young adults 1-34 years of age, trends and current status: United States 1985-90. *Advance Data from Vital and Health Statistics*. Hyattsville, Md: National Center for Health Statistics; 1993;231:1-20.

PROCEED TO PAGE 28

AUSTRALIA (For presentation in Australia only)

Incidence

In Australia, mortality figures over recent years indicate that trauma is the fourth leading cause of death for all ages (73 deaths per 100,000) behind cancer, ischemic heart disease and cerebrovascular deaths.[1] There were 23,127 injury deaths in Australia between 1990 and 1992.[2]

The leading causes of fatal injury were motor vehicle crashes, which accounted for 31% of both male and female injury deaths, and suicide, which accounted for 31% of male injury deaths and 18% of female injury deaths.[3]

By 1991, suicide deaths continued to increase in number, overtaking deaths from motor vehicle crashes (which continue to decline).[1] Other injury-related deaths are caused by incidents involving trains, boats and aircraft. A significant number of deaths and injuries result from industrial accidents, sporting, and leisure activities.

Human Characteristics

Age

Deaths from the external causes of accidents, poisonings, and violence are a major cause of premature death representing 6.3% of deaths of people of all ages and 19% of deaths in the 15 to 64 year age group. Injuries accounted for 50.1% of those between the ages of one and 44 years.[1] The age group with the highest injury deaths is 15 to 24 years of age. Those between 25 and 44 years form the second largest group of injury deaths.

Gender

Males predominate in the number of deaths from accidents, poisonings, and violence, accounting for 70.3%.[4] Exposure to the injury-producing event, the amount of risk involved, the occupation, and cultural norms are possible reasons for the gender differences.

Race

Aboriginal people have the highest death rate in Australia. The Aboriginal male has a 3.5 times greater death rate from accidents, poisoning, or violence than nonAboriginal males. The Aboriginal female death rate is 3.8 times greater than the nonAboriginal death rate.[3] The increased death rate among Aboriginal people is due to many factors including the fact that many people travel in open vehicles, such as trucks, which do not have safety restraints.

Alcohol

The use and especially the abuse of alcohol has been linked to accidents, injuries, and death. Therefore, it is expected that a reduction in alcohol use will lead to a reduction in injury and death. A report in New South Wales (NSW) claims that random blood testing (RBT) produced an average annual savings of 274 lives.[1] There has been a decline in alcohol-related motorcycle deaths.

Violence

The homicide rate of just over 4% is relatively small compared to that of other countries. While this figure is small, it should be noted that the amount of severe injury from personal violence and terrorism is rising.[5] The incidence of violent acts such as rape, physical assault, child abuse, and violence against women is increasing in our society despite awareness, help, and prevention programs.

There were 1,860 firearm deaths during the three-year period from 1990 to 1992, with 84% of these due to suicide, 14% due to interpersonal violence, and 5% due to unintentional personal injury.[2] At present, laws restricting the ownership of guns and, especially handguns, may play a significant role in limiting the amount of gun-related violence in Australia. The Sporting Shooters Association of Australia estimates that there are up to four million firearms in Australia.[6]

Suicide

Suicide accounted for 5,392 male deaths and 1,412 female deaths between 1990 and 1992. The crude rate of male deaths attributed to suicide has been fairly steady in the most recent years after a sharp increase in the mid-1980s to a peak in 1987. The rate for females has slightly declined since 1987.

In 1991, the suicide rate for males increased and has now become the leading cause of injury related deaths in males 15 to 24 years.[1] Reasons for this rise have been attributed to the socioeconomic situation of widespread unemployment for youth and also the lessening of the social stigma that was once attached to suicide.

Prevention

The number of deaths and injuries from motor vehicle crashes has shown a steady decrease over the past 20 years. Between 1960 and the late 1970s, the annual fatality rate fluctuated around 25 deaths per 100,000, but has since declined by 5% per year to 13.6 deaths per 100,000 in 1990.[3] Bicyclist fatalities dropped 27.5%, which may have been due to greater publicity or widespread adoption of protective headgear.[1] The reason for the decrease in road vehicular mortality is largely due to continuous and aggressive prevention programs in each state. These programs include mandatory seatbelt legislation and drink-driving laws.[1]

REFERENCES

1. Grant C, Lapsley HM. *The Australian Health Care System*. Sydney, Australia: University of New South Wales; 1992.

2. Moller J. The spatial distribution of injury deaths in Australia: urban, rural and remote areas. *Australian Injury Prevention Bulletin*. Bedford Park, South Australia: Australian Institute of Health and Welfare; 1994;8:1-8.

3. *Third Biennial Report of the Australian Institute of Health and Welfare. Australia's Health*. Canberra, Australia: Australian Government Publishing Service; 1992.

4. Glover J, Woollacott T. *A Social Health Atlas of Australia*. Adelaide, Australia: South Australian Health Commission; 1992.

5. National Health and Medical Research Council. *Discussion Paper on the Management of Severe Injuries*. Canberra, Australia: Australian Government Publishing Service; 1988.

6. Harford S. *Sydney Morning Herald*. February 5 1994:29. Newspaper article.

PROCEED TO PAGE 28

CANADA (For presentation in Canada only)

Introduction

The Canadian Institute for Health Information (CIHI), created in 1994, is a national agency responsible for coordinating the development and maintenance of a comprehensive and integrated health information system. CIHI receives information related to 78% of all acute care discharges. The database utilizes "E codes" from the International Classification of Diseases (ICD) ninth edition. "E codes" relate to the external cause of injury, e.g., motor vehicle crashes, poisoning, homicide. Information from the database can be used to quantify both the financial and human costs of injuries.

Provincial trauma registries are also currently being established across the country. These provincial registries focus on data related to both fatal and nonfatal injuries. The data elements collected include comprehensive information from the prehospital through inpatient visit, and postdischarge.

Injuries due to motor vehicle collision are the leading cause of death for people less than 35 years of age.[1] Deaths due to motor vehicle collisions have steadily declined since 1970. In 1974, there were 6,290 MVC deaths compared to 3,601 in 1993, representing a 57% decline over the last 19 years.[2] The advances in medical care and improved restraining devices are likely to have contributed to this trend. The significant reduction in the number of motor vehicle deaths has not been matched by a reduction in the overall injury rate. The number of persons injured has remained essentially unchanged during this time, while the number of licensed drivers has almost doubled during this 19-year period.[2]

Human Characteristics

Age

Injuries claim the lives of more Canadian children annually than all other causes of death combined.[3] Injuries are the leading cause of death for persons between one and 44 years.[4] In 1993, 61% of the total deaths due to motor vehicle collisions (3,601) were in the 15 to 44-year age group.[2] Seven out of 10 teenagers who died in Canada died as a result of a preventable injury.[3]

Falls are the leading cause of injury for those in the over-65 age group, and the sixth leading cause of death in persons over 65.[5] One third to one half of those over 65 years of age are prone to falling, with falls being more common in older females.

Gender

In the province of Ontario, male drivers account for 54% of the driving population, and account for 79% of the drivers involved in fatal motor vehicle crashes. Among drivers fatally injured in Ontario, 53% of male drivers had been drinking alcohol compared to only 27% of the female fatalities.[6] The teenage male is at the greatest risk of injury and traumatic death. Males under the age of 24 accounted for 15% of the driving population of Ontario, and comprised 24% of drivers involved in collisions.[7,8] The suicide rate in Canada in 1992 was three times greater for males than females.[9] The homicide rate was twice as high for males.

Race and Geographical Considerations

Native Canadian children have a consistently higher death rate due to injuries in comparison to the total number of children in Canada. In one reported year, the injury death rate of Native Canadian children was six times higher for ages one to four, and four times higher for ages 15 to 19 years than for nonnatives.[10] There is a larger population of Native Canadians in the northern communities.

Snowmobiles are a leading cause of injury and death in the north, as this is a common form of transport, particularly during the long winters. Faster machines and more widespread use of snowmobiles for recreation have lead to an increase in the incidence of injury.[11] Only one work-related snowmobile injury was identified in a population of 132 injured patients, spanning a five-year period.[12]

Alcohol

In a survey of 32 industrialized countries, Canada ranked 21st in terms of alcohol sales (liters) per person over 15 years of age. Between 1978 and 1985 there was some indication of a shift toward more moderate drinking habits among Canadians; this trend seems to be continuing.[6] A national survey on alcohol and drugs found that 20% of current drinkers admitted to driving at least once in the last 12 months after consuming more than two drinks. Additionally, 43% of people who consumed more than eight drinks per week admitted to driving after consuming more than two drinks. Men are three times more likely to report such drinking and driving activities.[13] The results of the Ontario road safety report indicated a definite downward trend in alcohol involvement and vehicular fatalities.[14] Of those killed in motor vehicle crashes, 40% had positive alcohol readings, as compared to 50% 10 years ago.[8]

There is evidence that alcohol, drugs, and medical impairment contribute to highway crashes. Injuries caused by snowmobiles are even more directly influenced by drugs and alcohol.[12]

Prevention

Injuries account for more years of potential lost life than heart disease, stroke, and cancer combined.[15] Canada has many groups working both nationally and internationally towards the prevention of injuries. The Canadian Institute of Child Health has recently published a directory which lists the current national and provincial child/youth/teenage injury prevention programs and research initiatives. Nationally, there are more than 36 programs available to the public, from agencies such as St. John Ambulance (advanced first aid), Health Canada (Kids Care Program), Canadian Injury Prevention Foundation (Heroes Program), Canadian Bike Helmet Coalition, Canadian Red Cross Society (water safety services), and the Canada Safety Council (ATV Riders Course).

Examples of provincial programs are:

- Prevent Alcohol and Risk-related Trauma in Youth (PARTY) – presented in Alberta and Ontario

- Water Smart and Kiwanis Safety City – presented in British Columbia

- Traffic Safety Program – presented in Saskatchewan

- Nobody's Perfect – presented in Quebec

- On Your Own – presented in New Brunswick

- Hi-Line Hazards – presented in Newfoundland and Labrador

- Right Rider Program – presented in Prince Edward Island

In Ontario, there is a movement to mobilize community agencies and members-at-large to become involved in injury prevention. This initiative has resulted in the formation of many community coalitions addressing the issues in their communities. They are currently developing plans to market social change and ultimately decrease the numbers of preventable injuries and deaths.

Costs

It has been estimated that injuries cost approximately $13.2 billion per year in medical costs alone. This figure does not include the lost income or the cost in human terms.[15] An Ontario provincial report published in 1994 estimates that motor vehicle crashes in Ontario alone (30% of Canada's population) cost individuals, organizations, and governments in Ontario $9 billion.[16]

REFERENCES

1. Traffic deaths hit 39-year low. *Ottawa Citizen*. December 1994. Newspaper article.

2. *Canadian Motor Vehicle Traffic Collision Statistics*. Transport Canada; 1993:TP 3322.

3. *The Health of Canada's Children; A CIHI Profile*. Canadian Institute of Child Health; 1989:39.

4. *Health Reports*. Quarterly Canadian Centre for Health Information; 1989:82-003.

5. Ontario Medical Association. *Falls in the Elderly – A Report of the OMA Committee on Accidental Injuries*. Toronto, Canada: Author; 1992.

6. King AJC, Coles B. *The Health of Canada's Youth*. Health and Welfare Canada; 1992:H39-239/1992E.

7. Ministry of Health. *Ontario Health Survey*. Ontario, Canada: Author; 1990.

8. Mehew DR, Simpson HM, Brown SW. *Alcohol Use Among Person's Fatally Injured in Motor Vehicle Accidents*. Ottawa, Ontario: Traffic Injury Research Foundation of Canada; 1993:13-15.

9. *Causes of Death*. Ottawa, Canada: Statistics Canada; 1992:84-208.

10. *Injury Prevention Projects with Native Populations; A Review of the Literature.* Ottawa, Canada: Health Canada; 1993.

11. Addiction Research Foundation. *Snowmobilers in a Northeastern Community.* Ontario, Canada: Author; 1994:7.

12. Rowe B, Bota G. Serious snowmobile trauma in Northern Ontario: a case series. *Ann RCPS (Canada).* 1991;24:501-505.

13. *National Alcohol and Other Drugs Survey.* Canada: Health and Welfare Canada; 1989;30-31:H39-175/1990E.

14. Safety Research Office, Ministry of Transportation. *Ontario Road Safety Annual Report.* Ontario, Canada: Author; 1992.

15. *Accidents in Canada – General Social Survey Analysis Series.* Ottawa, Canada: Statistics Canada; 1991;1:11-62E.

16. Ontario Ministry of Transportation, Safety Research Office, Safety Policy Branch, Research Development Branch. *The Social Cost of Motor Vehicle Crashes in Ontario 1994.* Ontario, Canada: Author; 1994;5:SRO-94-101.

BIOMECHANICS AND MECHANISMS OF INJURY

The terms "biomechanics," "kinematics," and "mechanism of injury" are often used interchangeably although they really have different meanings. The broadest term, biomechanics, refers to the "study of the principles of the action of forces and their effects."[18] Kinematics is a branch of mechanics (energy transfer), which refers to motion and does not consider the concepts of force and mass of the object or body.[19]

Mechanism of injury refers to the mechanisms whereby the energy is transferred from the environment to the person, i.e., mechanical energy from a motor vehicle crash, electrical energy from a wall socket, or chemical energy from contact with hydrofluoric acid. The agent that causes physical injury is energy. Energy sources are mechanical/kinetic, thermal, chemical, electrical, and radiant. Drowning is a special circumstance whereby the agent or cause of the injury and/or death is lack of oxygenation (see Table 1 and Figure 1). Mechanical energy is given the most attention in this chapter since it is the most common agent of injury in motor vehicle crashes, motorcycle crashes, falls, stabbings, and bullet-inflicted wounds.

Table 1

ENERGY SOURCES AND MECHANISMS OF INJURY	
Energy Agent	**Mechanism of Injury**
Mechanical or kinetic energy	• Motor vehicle crashes • Motorcycle crashes • Firearms, falls, assaults
Thermal energy	• Heat, steam, fire
Chemical energy	• Plant and animal toxins • Chemical substances
Electrical energy	• Lightning • Exposure to wires, sockets, plugs
Radiant energy	• Rays of light (sun rays) • Sound waves (explosions) • Electromagnetic waves (x-ray exposure) • Radioactive emissions (nuclear leak)
Oxygen deprivation	• Drowning • Asphyxiation from inhalation of toxic substances, e.g., carbon monoxide, heat, soot

Figure 1
Energy Sources

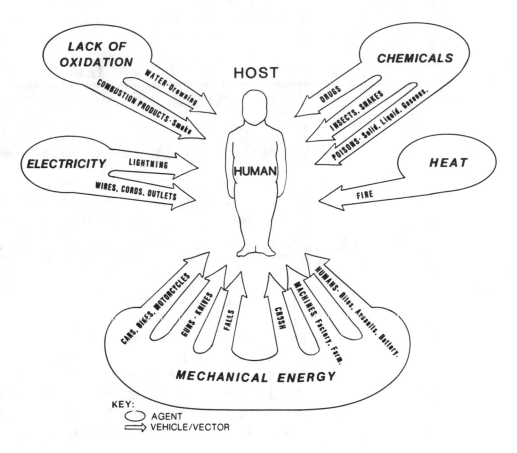

Mechanical Energy

Injuries sustained from motor vehicle crashes, falls, gunshots, or any other moving source result from the mechanical energy that is loaded onto the victim and the body's response to that energy. Energy that is beyond the body's resistance to tolerate may cause injury to one of the four types of body tissues. The type of tissue injured is important since certain tissues and structures have different responses and tolerances to the energy load. The four types of tissues are epithelial, connective, muscle, and nerve tissue. Examples are listed in Table 2.[20]

External Forces Associated with Mechanical Energy and Moving Objects

Mechanical energy from a crash or fall affects the body with either deceleration forces, acceleration forces, or a combination of both. The amount of force an object or body has depends on the mass of the object or body and the velocity at which it is moving. Both animate objects, e.g., occupants of a moving motor vehicle, and inanimate objects, e.g., a motor vehicle or motorcycle traveling at any speed, have energy. Although both mass and velocity contribute to the amount of energy a moving object has, velocity has the greatest influence. If the mass of an object is doubled, the energy is doubled. However, if the velocity is doubled, the energy is quadrupled; therefore, the faster the victim or object is moving (velocity), the greater the energy on impact.

Table 2

TYPES AND EXAMPLES OF BODY TISSUES	
Type	**Example**
Epithelial tissue	• Skin, trachea, mucous membranes, linings of blood vessels and body cavities
Connective tissue	• Cartilage, bone, and joint structures
Muscle tissue	• Cardiac, skeletal, and smooth (blood vessels, viscera)
Nerve tissue	• Neurons and supporting (glial) cells

DECELERATION FORCES

The force that stops or decreases the velocity of a moving victim is termed deceleration or drag.[21] When a moving object decelerates or decreases its velocity to zero, the energy on impact is dissipated and absorbed around the impact site. When a person falls from a height and strikes the ground, body tissues partially absorb the sudden change in velocity (deceleration) on impact.

When the body in motion comes to a stop, e.g., fall, motor vehicle crash, the energy load on human tissue can cause injuries mainly due to deceleration forces. The motor vehicle decelerates and comes to a complete stop as a result of the vehicle's impact. Once in contact with some immovable surface, e.g., the steering column or windshield, the victim will also come to a stop, dissipating additional energy. During a crash or fall the body decelerates, yet not all anatomical structures decelerate at the same time. The relative fixation of certain anatomical structures predisposes them to deceleration-type injuries.

It is possible that there are differences in the rate of deceleration between the body as a whole and certain specific body parts. Two anatomic locations susceptible to injury from this type of force are the descending thoracic aorta and the duodenum. The aorta, just distal to the take-off of the left subclavian artery, near the ligamentum arteriosum, may be partially or completely transected as a result of deceleration force. This area of the aorta is more firmly fixed than other areas because the ligamentum, a cord which is the remnant of the fetal ductus arteriosus, extends from the pulmonary artery to the aorta.

Similar forces may cause injury to the retroperitoneal duodenum (portion of the second section, third and fourth sections), or the jejunum near the ligament of Treitz (a fibrous band at the duodenojejunal flexure). If the ligament of Treitz is stressed at the same time the pylorus of the stomach closes, the C-loop of the duodenum (the area where the duodenum leaves the stomach) may sustain an increase in its intraluminal pressure resulting in perforation of the small bowel.[22]

ACCELERATION FORCES

A stationary or slow moving pedestrian who is struck by a car or an occupant of a slow moving car who is struck from the rear by another faster moving car, may sustain injuries from the acceleration of his or her body. Acceleration is an increase in speed. Some injury events, like certain motor vehicle collisions, may lead to injuries that result from a combination of acceleration and deceleration forces.

OTHER FORCES

Bullets, fists, and stabbing instruments are all examples of objects in motion with varying amounts of energy. The amount of energy is dependent upon the velocity at which the object strikes the victim and the object's mass. Blasts and/or explosions are another force that cause human tissue damage. The injuries are a result of contact with light, heat, and/or pressure.[22] Blast forces may lead to either blunt or penetrating wounds.

Internal Forces Associated with Mechanical Energy and Moving Objects

As energy is loaded onto the body, internal forces, e.g., stress and strain, are exerted within the body as the body tissues change their dimensions.[23] Stresses are defined as "the forces applied to deform the body or the equal and opposite forces with which the body resists."[19] The degree to which specific tissues are injured is dependent on the resistance of the tissues to energy loads. Stress can be:

- Tensile stress whereby the tissue cells are separated, e.g., stretch on the splenic capsule.

- Compressive stress whereby they are pressed together, e.g., comminuted bone fracture.

- Shearing stress whereby the stress resulted from a tangential force, e.g., tearing of the aorta.[1]

31

Strain is the tissue damage or deformation that results from the stress.[19] Strain, among other things, is dependent on the properties of the particular tissue involved. For example, because of their elastic fibers, muscles may be stretched and deformed as a result of energy loads. The spleen and liver have minimal elastic ability and may rupture.[21]

Certain bones can resist energy loads and forces better than others. The femur, sternum, scapula, and the first and second ribs, fall into this category. The contents of the cranium are somewhat protected by the meninges and the bony skull. However, the rigidity and internal bony protuberances of the skull may injure the cortex or surface of the brain. This is especially true during injury events that cause the brain to rebound in the cranial vault in a contrecoup fashion.[23] A blow to the back of the head may cause frontal contusions as the brain strikes the anterior portion of the skull.

Types of Injuries

One method to categorize injuries resulting from the transfer of mechanical energy is determining whether the energy causes disruption of the skin. Penetrating or open injuries disrupt the skin, while in blunt or closed injuries the skin surface is intact. The energy associated with blunt trauma is more widespread around the impact point but can be absorbed by the underlying structures.

A second method to categorize injuries is determining whether the insult to the body tissues was direct or indirect. Injury resulting from a dynamic energy load leading to contusion or concussion of brain cells is considered a direct injury. The patient may also have indirect injuries resulting from cerebral ischemia, cerebral edema, or bleeding.[23] These indirect insults are often referred to as secondary insults.

Blunt Trauma

Most injuries associated with motor vehicle crashes, motorcycle crashes, and falls are blunt. As a result of a motor vehicle crash, the injuries to occupants may vary depending on the victim's location in the vehicle, speed at impact, stopping distance, and many other environmental factors, e.g., type of vehicle, point of impact, protective barriers.

Penetrating Trauma

STAB WOUNDS

A variety of objects can produce a penetrating injury. Damage to underlying tissues occurs as structures in the path of the wounding instrument are punctured. Wounds are commonly caused by knives, but other impaling objects may also cause stab-type injuries. Tissue injury is related to the length of the instrument, the velocity at which the force was applied, and the angle of entry. Although the puncture site may apparently follow a straight path, this is not always true. Tissues may be disrupted and pushed aside by the penetrating instrument, thus causing damage to adjacent structures.

FIREARM INJURIES

Firearms are categorized as handguns, rifles, and shotguns. Handguns are classified as revolvers or autoloading pistols and are mostly low-velocity weapons. Rifles are high-velocity weapons, which can release a single shot or can be semiautomatic or fully automatic (holding down the trigger releases more than one bullet). Shotguns, classified by the gauge (diameter of the barrel), release multiple pellets. The tissue damage inflicted by bullets is related to the projectile, mass, shape, fragmentation, type of tissue struck, and striking velocity.[24,25] The range, or the distance between the barrel of the weapon and the victim, affects the velocity at which the bullet strikes the body tissues. The impact velocity at which the bullet strikes the victim more closely approximates the actual bullet velocity the closer the range.[22] The wound that a penetrating projectile causes is characterized by the amount and location of crushed and stretched tissue.

The penetrating projectile crushes the tissue it strikes and causes a permanent cavity. In addition, tissue surrounding the bullet path is stretched and displaced from the temporary cavity that is formed. Predicting potential tissue disruptions is based on the "penetration depth of the projectile, the size of the hole it makes, and any unusual deviations in course direction through tissue."[24]

The size of the permanent cavity can be increased by three mechanisms: yaw, bullet deformation, and bullet fragmentation. Yaw refers to the deviation of the bullet from a straight path, within the tissue, up to a 90-degree angle. This deviation of the bullet causes more tissue to come in contact with the bullet and, therefore, more tissue damage. Bullet deformation refers to an increase in bullet diameter as a result of mushrooming or flattening of the bullet tip. This can cause a four-to-six times greater amount of tissue contact and, therefore, damage. Bullet fragmentation causes tremendous increases in the amount of

33

tissue disruption. Fragmentation causes the tissue to be perforated multiple times before being subjected to the stretch of temporary cavitation.

The temporary cavity refers to a localized area of trauma along the bullet path. This stretch phenomenon is better tolerated by the relatively elastic tissues (lung, muscle, bowel wall) than by the nonelastic solid organs. In fact, most muscle stretched by temporary cavitation survives. Temporary cavitation can also disrupt blood vessels or break bones at some distance from the bullet track.

Patterns of Injury

Motor Vehicle-Related

The pattern of injury for each trauma patient is different. The pattern of injury is a combination of the patient's age, mechanism of injury, anatomic structures involved, and pre-existing factors, e.g., alcohol ingestion, restraint systems.[22] Knowing the pattern of injury can guide the trauma nurse to predict and be prepared for the manifestations of certain injuries. The history of the injury event may reveal information leading to early identification and treatment of injuries.

Factors contributing to the pattern of injury sustained by persons involved in motor vehicle crashes include the use or nonuse of restraint systems, the position of the victim in the vehicle, and the type of collision or impact. The five types of collisions are frontal or head-on, rear impact, lateral or side impact, rotational impact, and a rollover.[26] Table 3 describes patterns of motor vehicle crashes and their predicted injuries.[21,27]

Table 3

PATTERNS OF INJURY IN UNRESTRAINED OCCUPANTS	
Type of Impact	**Predicted Injuries**
Frontal impact (down-and-under trajectory)	• Point of impact, e.g., knee, femur, ankle • Posterior dislocation of hip • Chest (heart and aorta most vulnerable) • Abdomen (liver and spleen most vulnerable)
Frontal impact (up-and-over trajectory)	• Head and neck • Chest and upper abdomen
Lateral impact (T-bone impact)	• Cervical spine • Same side shoulder, clavicle • Lateral abdomen (liver of right-side occupant, spleen of left-side occupant) • Head and face if thrust forward
Rear impact	• Head and neck

Table 4 describes injuries that may occur when pedestrians or motorcyclists are struck by motor vehicles.[21] When a pedestrian or motorcyclist is struck, different injuries may be sustained: during impact, when thrown on top of the vehicle, when sliding from the vehicle to the ground, or when dragged under the vehicle.

Table 4

PATTERNS OF INJURY RELATED TO PEDESTRIANS AND MOTORCYCLISTS STRUCK BY MOTOR VEHICLES	
Mechanism of Injury	**Possible Injuries**
Adult pedestrian struck by a motor vehicle • When struck	• Knees • Tibia, fibula, femur • Pelvis
• When thrown on top of vehicle (hood or windshield)	• Depends on victim's position when struck • If struck from the front, truncal injury, e.g., ribs, spleen • If struck from the back, vertebral column injury
• When sliding from vehicle to ground	• Cranial and spinal injuries
• When dragged under the vehicle	• Pelvis
Motorcyclist • Head-on collision	• Ejected over the motorcycle • May strike face and chest on handlebars
• Angular collision	• Lower legs may become trapped
• Ejection	• Cranial injuries and cervical injuries
• Lay bike down on side	• Inside leg fractures and soft tissue injuries

Table 5 reflects percentages of injuries sustained by unrestrained occupants and drivers of actual nonfatal motor vehicle crashes.[28]

Table 5

INJURIES (PERCENT) OF OCCUPANTS AND DRIVERS INJURED IN NONFATAL MOTOR VEHICLE CRASHES	
Position in Vehicle	**Injuries**
Unrestrained front seat passenger (right side of car)	• Pelvic fractures (46%) • Femur fractures (41%) • Cranial injuries (24%) • Abdominal injuries (13%)
Unrestrained driver (left side of car)	• Femur fracture (65%) • Pelvic fracture (46%) • Chest injury (46%) • Ankle fractures (39%) • Facial bone fractures (37%) • Cranial injuries (16%)

Research demonstrated that, of those drivers fatally injured in a motor vehicle crash, the following three body areas were the most frequently injured (percents in each category represent the percent of all victims studied)[28]:

- 33.7% – head injury

- 25.2% – chest injury

- 25.1% – abdominal injury

Falls and Jumps

Falling or jumping from a height that results in the victim landing on his or her feet or head is termed axial loading because the energy on impact is applied to the axial skeleton. Fractures of the lower extremities and vertebral column are associated with victims who land on their feet. Head and cervical spine injuries can result from axial loading onto the head, e.g., diving into a pool.

The pattern of injury related to falls or jumps from heights is a consequence of the:

- Age of the victim

- Distance from which the victim fell or jumped

- Energy-absorbency of the surface on which the victim fell

- Pre-existing conditions of the victim

- Pre-existing conditions of the environment

- Anatomic point of impact

- Energy (deceleration) loaded onto the victim at the time of impact

Vehicular Occupant Protection

Some familiarity with occupant protection technology will also contribute information to the trauma nurse's understanding of patterns of injury. Vehicle crash worthiness, friendly interiors, and restraint systems are the three main occupant protection concepts.[29] An example of increased crash worthiness is improved construction of the vehicle's front end so that during an impact intrusion into the occupant's compartment is minimized. Examples of friendly interiors are cars equipped with energy-absorbing steering systems or high-penetration-resistant windshields.

Restraint systems used in modern cars are safety belt restraints, car seats for infants and children, and inflatable restraints, i.e., air bags. The rapid inflation of the air bag (which uses a pyrotechnic technique to fill the bag with nitrogen) and occasional debris from the air bag pose some risk to the occupant. The air bag is a passive restraint system, meaning the occupant does not have to engage the system for it to be effective. It provides protection that does not have to rely on the occupant's behavior. Air bags do not replace safety belts. Since the air bag immediately deflates, safety belt restraints should be worn to protect the occupant from vehicular ejection. In general, air bags have prevented serious and fatal injuries, and the injuries that may result from air bag inflation are mostly limited to minor abrasions and ocular irritation.[30] The use of lap and shoulder safety belts reduces the risk of fatal injury to front seat passengers by 45% and reduces the risk of moderate to critical injury by 50%.[11]

There are many varieties of car seats for infants and children. Some car manufacturers are constructing back seats that can be converted into a car seat for children. The use of different styles of infant and child car seats is based on the weight and age of the occupant. Rear-facing child car seats should not be used in front passenger seats equipped with air bags.[31]

All 50 states and the District of Columbia have some form of child restraint law.[13] It is estimated that there is a 69% reduction in fatalities to infants less than one year of age and a 47% reduction in fatalities to toddlers between the ages of one and four because of the use of child safety seats.

SUMMARY

Epidemiology defines the scope of injuries in terms of their incidence, and identifies associated factors and determinants of specific types of injury. Statistics and quantitative data are only a portion of the epidemiologic view of the injury problem. The epidemiologic foundation can, however, help direct program planners to form injury prevention and control programs.

Energy is the agent of injury. The type and severity of injuries that result from the transfer of energy from the environment to the human host depend on the types of forces applied, the internal forces, the characteristics of the anatomic structures affected, and the pattern of injury (see Figure 2). Even though a certain pattern of injury may be predictable of specific injuries, every trauma victim must be assessed according to the principles outlined in the primary and secondary assessment to be sure that all injuries are identified.

Figure 2
Biomechanics in Trauma

1 **PHASES OF INJURY**   **EXAMPLES**

MECHANISMS OF INJURY Vehicle of transfer of energy from environment to human host	• Falls • Motor Vehicle Crashes • Bullets • Stabbing Instruments • Blasts/Bombs

2   **EXTERNAL FORCES**

DECELERATION FORCES Decrease in speed of a moving object or person	• Victim strikes steering column • Victim impacts ground
ACCELERATION FORCES Increase in speed of a moving object or person	• Pedestrian thrown when struck by moving vehicle
BLAST FORCES Heat, light, pressure	• Bomb explosion
LOW AND HIGH VELOCITY MISSILES	• Bullets • Stabbing instruments

3   **INTERNAL FORCES**

Human Body's Response to Kinetic Energy Load	*STRESS* • Cells separate, stretch, compress, or shear *STRAIN* • Tissue damage or deformation from stress

4   **TYPES OF INJURIES**

Description for clinical and diagnostic purposes	Blunt vs Penetrating Closed vs Open Primary vs Secondary Direct vs Indirect

REFERENCES

1. Robertson L. *Injury Epidemiology*. New York, NY: Oxford University Press; 1993.

2. Robertson L. *Injuries: Causes, Control Strategies, and Public Policy*. Lexington, Mass: Lexington Books; 1983.

3. Advance report of final mortality statistics, 1986. *Monthly Vital Statistics Report*. National Center for Health Statistics, Hyattsville, Md: 1988;37:1-55.

4. Advance report of final mortality statistics, 1987. *Monthly Vital Statistics Report*. National Center for Health Statistics, Hyattsville, Md: 1989;38:1-48.

5. Advance report of final mortality statistics, 1988. *Monthly Vital Statistics Report*. National Center for Health Statistics, Hyattsville, Md: 1990;39:1-48.

6. Advance report of final mortality statistics, 1989. *Monthly Vital Statistics Report*. National Center for Health Statistics, Hyattsville, Md: 1991;40:1-52.

7. Advance report of final mortality statistics, 1990. *Monthly Vital Statistics Report*. National Center for Health Statistics, Hyattsville, Md: 1992;41:1-52.

8. Advance report of final mortality statistics, 1991. *Monthly Vital Statistics Report*. National Center for Health Statistics, Hyattsville, Md: 1993;42:1-64.

9. Advance report of final mortality statistics, 1992. *Monthly Vital Statistics Report*. National Center for Health Statistics, Hyattsville, Md: 1994;43:1-76.

10. 1990 summary: national hospital discharge survey. *Vital and Health Statistics*. National Center for Health Statistics, Hyattsville, Md: 1992;210:1-12.

11. National Highway Traffic Safety Administration. *Traffic Safety Facts 1992*. US Department of Transportation, National Center for Statistics and Analysis: Washington, DC; 1993:DOT HS 808 022.

12. Baker SP, O'Neill B, Ginsburg MJ, Guohua LM. *The Injury Fact Book*. 2nd ed. New York, NY: Oxford University Press; 1992.

13. National Highway Traffic Safety Administration. *Traffic Safety Facts 1993*. US Department of Transportation, National Center for Health Statistics and Analysis: Washington, DC; 1994:DOT HS 808 169.

14. Rosenberg ML, Fenley MA. *Violence in America: A Public Health Approach*. New York, NY: Oxford University Press; 1991.

15. Death resulting from firearm-and motor-vehicle related injuries, United States, 1968-1991. *MMWR*. Atlanta, Ga: Centers for Disease Control; 1994;43:1-42.

16. Fingerhut LA. Firearm mortality among children, youth, and young adults 1-34 years of age, trends and current status: United States 1985-90. *Advance Data from Vital and Health Statistics*. Hyattsville, Md: National Center for Health Statistics; 1993;231:1-20.

17. Strauss MA, Gelles RJ. How violent are American families? In: Strauss MA, Gelles RJ, eds. *Physical Violence in American Families: Risk Factors and Adaptations to Violence in 8,145 Families*. New Brunswick, NJ: Transaction Publishers; 1990:95-112.

18. Nahum AM, Melvin J. *The Biomechanics of Trauma*. Norwalk, Conn: Appleton-Century-Crofts; 1985.

19. Illingworth V, ed. *The Penguin Dictionary of Physics*. 2nd ed. London, England: Penguin Books; 1991.

20. Porth CM. *Pathophysiology Concepts of Altered Health States*. 4th ed. Philadelphia, Pa: JB Lippincott Co; 1994.

21. Jones SA, McSwain NE. Kinematics of trauma. In: Jones SA, Weigel A, White RD, McSwain NE, Breiter M, eds. *Advanced Emergency Care for Paramedic Practice*. Philadelphia, Pa: JB Lippincott Co; 1992;262-283.

22. Feliciano DV, Wall M. Patterns of injury. In: Moore EE, Mattox KL, Feliciano DV, eds. *Trauma*. 2nd ed. Norwalk, Conn: Appleton & Lange; 1991;81-96.

23. Ommaya AK. Biomechanics of head injury: Experimental aspects. In: Nahum AM, Melvin J, eds. *The Biomechanics of Trauma*. Norwalk, Conn: Appleton-Century-Crofts; 1985;245-270.

24. Fackler M. Wound ballistics: a review of common misconceptions. *JAMA*. 1988;259:2730-2736.

25. Fackler M, Bellamy R, Malinowksi J. The wound profile: illustration of the missile-tissue interaction. *J Trauma*. 1988; 28(suppl):S21-29.

26. Martinez R, Gardner J. Mechanisms of blunt trauma in motor vehicle accidents. *Emerg Care Q*. 1988;4:1-9.

27. McSwain NE, Kerstein MD. *Evaluation and Management of Trauma*. Norwalk, Conn: Appleton-Century-Crofts; 1987.

28. Daffner RH, Lupetin AR. Patterns of high-speed impact injuries in motor vehicle occupants. *J Trauma*. 1988;28:498-501.

29. Viano DC. Cause and control of automotive trauma. *Bulletin of the New York Academy of Medicine*. 1988;64:376-421.

30. Insurance Institute for Highway Safety. *Special Issue: Air Bags in Perspective*. Washington, DC; 1993.

31. American Public Health Association. *The Nation's Health*. Washington, DC; July 1993:6.

CHAPTER THREE

INITIAL ASSESSMENT

OBJECTIVES

Upon completion of this chapter/lecture, the learner should be able to:

1. Describe the components of the primary assessment.
2. Correlate life-threatening conditions with the specific component of the primary assessment.
3. Identify interventions to manage life-threatening conditions assessed during the initial assessment.
4. Identify the components of the secondary assessment.
5. Describe how to conduct a complete head-to-toe assessment.

INTRODUCTION

A systematic process for initial assessment of the trauma patient is essential for recognizing life-threatening conditions, identifying injuries, and for determining priorities of care based on assessment findings.[1] The initial assessment is divided into two phases, primary and secondary assessments. Both phases can be completed within several minutes unless resuscitative measures are required. Within an organized team approach to trauma care, this first step of the nursing process (assessment) is often simultaneously conducted with the identification of nursing diagnoses that require immediate intervention. Utilizing an organized, systematic approach when assessing each trauma patient also helps to ensure that injuries will not be missed and that priorities can be set for each intervention based on the life-threatening potential of each injury.

Adherence to universal precautions (see Appendix 3) and the use of lead aprons by the trauma team are necessary and can often be initiated prior to the patient's arrival.

A Guide to Initial Assessment

The following mnemonic may assist nurses during the initial assessment of a trauma patient:

- **Primary Assessment**

  - A Airway with simultaneous cervical spine stabilization and/or immobilization

  - B Breathing

  - C Circulation

  - D Disability (neurologic status)

- **Secondary Assessment**

  - E Expose (remove clothing)

  - F Fahrenheit (keep patient warm)

  - G Get a complete set of vital signs

  - H History and head-to-toe assessment

  - I Inspect posterior surfaces

PRIMARY ASSESSMENT AND RESUSCITATION

Airway, with simultaneous cervical spine stabilization and/or immobilization, breathing, circulation, and disability (neurologic status) are the A-B-C-Ds of the primary assessment. Remove only those clothes necessary to expose the patient in order to conduct the primary assessment. If any life-threatening compromises or injuries are determined, implement interventions to correct them immediately. Additional assessment steps are not taken until measures to ensure an adequate airway, effective breathing, and effective circulation have been instituted.

In the presence of potentially life-threatening injuries, begin assessment immediately on the patient's arrival to collect objective assessment information. The extent and timing of obtaining information related to both the injury event and the patient's past medical history depend on the severity of the patient's condition. Subjective information from prehospital personnel, family, or the patient at this point of the assessment process is limited to a brief statement comprised of the patient's major injuries or chief complaints and the mechanism of injury. A more detailed history is obtained during the secondary assessment.

Airway

Assessment

Inspect the patient's airway while maintaining cervical spine stabilization or immobilization. Since partial or total airway obstruction may threaten the patency of the upper airway, observe for the following:

- Vocalization

- Tongue obstructing airway in an unresponsive patient

- Loose teeth or foreign objects

- Bleeding

- Vomitus or other secretions

- Edema

Interventions

AIRWAY PATENT

- Maintain cervical spine stabilization and/or immobilization

    - Stabilization includes holding the head in a neutral position or placing bilateral head support devices and using tape to secure the head and the devices. If immediately available, apply a rigid cervical collar before applying the head supports and tape. The tape should extend to the backboard, if present, or to the stretcher, if not.

    - Spinal immobilization includes stabilization as defined and the application of a backboard and straps.

    - Any patient whose mechanism of injury, symptoms, or physical findings suggest a spinal injury should be stabilized or immobilized.

- If the patient is awake and breathing, he or she may have assumed a position that maximizes the ability to breathe. Before proceeding with cervical spine stabilization be sure interventions do NOT compromise the patient's breathing status.

AIRWAY TOTALLY OBSTRUCTED OR PARTIALLY OBSTRUCTED

- Position the patient

    Position the patient in a supine position. If the patient is not already supine, logroll the patient onto his or her back while maintaining cervical spine stabilization. Remove any head gear to allow access to the airway and cervical spine.

- Open and clear the airway

    - Techniques to open or clear an obstructed airway during the primary assessment include:

        - Jaw thrust

        - Chin lift

        - Removal of loose objects or foreign debris

        - Suctioning

    - Suctioning and other manipulation of the oropharynx must be done gently to prevent stimulation of the gag reflex and subsequent vomiting and/or aspiration.

    - Maintain the cervical spine in a neutral position. Do not hyperextend, flex, or rotate the neck during these maneuvers.

- Insert an oropharyngeal or nasopharyngeal airway

- Stabilize the cervical spine

    - If the patient has not been stabilized, manually stabilize the head. Stabilization includes holding the head in a neutral position or placing bilateral head support devices and using tape to secure the head and the devices.

    - If the patient is already in a rigid cervical collar and strapped to a backboard, do NOT remove any devices. Check that the devices are placed appropriately.

- ■ Complete spinal immobilization with a backboard and straps should be done at the completion of the secondary assessment, depending on the degree of resuscitation required and the availability of team members.

- ● Consider endotracheal intubation (oral or nasal route)

  Ventilate the patient with a bag-valve-mask device prior to endotracheal intubation. For those patients requiring control of the airway with an endotracheal tube, the decision must be made to use the oral versus the nasal route.

  - ■ Oral endotracheal intubation is done with the patient's cervical spine in a neutral position and without any extension or flexion of the cervical spine. This requires a second person to hold the patient's head in this position.

  - ■ Blind nasotracheal intubation is NOT indicated when the following are present:

    - ◆ Apnea

    - ◆ Signs of major mid-face fractures, e.g., maxillary fractures

    - ◆ Signs of a basilar skull fracture

      A relative contraindication is the presence of signs indicating a fracture of the posterior fossa. An absolute contraindication is the presence of signs indicating a fracture of the anterior fossa.[2]

    - ◆ Leakage of cerebrospinal fluid through the nares

    - ◆ Age less than six years

  - ■ The use of neuromuscular blocking agents alone or in combination with other drugs administered before intubation is usually dictated by institutional protocols (see Appendix 4).

- Consider needle or surgical cricothyroidotomy

Ventilate the patient with a bag-valve-mask device prior to these procedures. In rare circumstances, the patient's condition may restrict passage of an endotracheal tube. To establish an airway, a needle cricothyroidotomy may be performed with an over-the-needle catheter placed into the trachea through the cricothyroid membrane. Another method is a surgical crico-thyroidotomy. An incision is made in the cricothyroid membrane, and a tube is placed into the trachea.[2] Both of these approaches to a cricothyroidotomy should be performed by skilled physicians. In some settings, advanced life support (ALS) personnel, e.g., flight nurses, or advanced practice nurses, may also be trained and qualified to perform cricothyroidotomies.

If there are any life-threatening compromises in airway status, stop and intervene to correct the problem before proceeding to breathing assessment. Examples of life-threatening airway conditions are partial or complete obstruction of the airway from foreign bodies or debris (blood, mucus, vomitus) and/or obstruction by the tongue. Penetrating wounds may cause disruption of the integrity of the airway, and blunt trauma may lead to injury of the larynx and/or other upper airway structures.

Breathing

Assessment

Life-threatening compromises in breathing may occur with a history of any of the following:

- Blunt or penetrating injuries of the thorax

- Patient striking the steering column or wheel

- Acceleration, deceleration, or a combination of both types of forces, e.g., motor vehicle crashes, falls, crush injuries

Once the patency of the airway is assured, assess for the following:

- Spontaneous breathing

- Chest rise and fall (depth and symmetry)

- Skin color

- General respiratory rate and depth, i.e., normal, slow, or fast

- Integrity of the soft tissue and bony structures of the chest wall

- Use of accessory and/or abdominal muscles

- Bilateral breath sounds

  Auscultate the lungs bilaterally at the second intercostal space midclavicular line and at the fifth intercostal space anterior axillary line bilaterally.

- Jugular veins and position of trachea

Interventions

BREATHING PRESENT: EFFECTIVE

Administer oxygen via a nonrebreather mask at a flow rate sufficient to keep the reservoir bag inflated; usually requires 12 to 15 L/minute.

BREATHING PRESENT: INEFFECTIVE

When spontaneous breathing is present but ineffective, the following may indicate a life-threatening condition related to breathing:

- Altered mental status, i.e., restless, agitated

- Cyanosis, especially around the mouth

- Asymmetrical expansion of the chest wall

- Use of accessory and/or abdominal muscles

- Sucking chest wounds

- Paradoxical movement of chest wall during inspiration and expiration

- Tracheal shift from the midline position

- Distended external jugular veins

- Absent or diminished breath sounds

Removal of the anterior portion of the cervical collar may be necessary to inspect and palpate the anterior neck region, i.e., jugular veins and trachea. Another team member must hold the patient's head while the collar is being removed and replaced.

- If respiratory distress is present, auscultate breath sounds to determine if they are present, diminished, or absent

- Administer oxygen via a nonrebreather mask or assist ventilations with a bag-valve-mask device, as indicated

- Assist with endotracheal intubation as previously described

BREATHING ABSENT

- Ventilate the patient with 100% oxygen via a bag-valve-mask device with an attached reservoir system

- Assist with endotracheal intubation; attach bag-valve device to endotracheal tube

If there are any life-threatening injuries that compromise breathing, stop and intervene before proceeding to circulation assessment. Examples of life-threatening injuries which may compromise breathing are tension pneumothorax, sucking chest wound, flail chest with pulmonary contusion, and hemothorax. These conditions may require simultaneous assessment and intervention.

Circulation

Assessment

- Palpate the pulse for quality, i.e., normal, weak, or strong; and rate, i.e., normal, slow, or fast. Palpate a central pulse, e.g., femoral or carotid, initially if there is any question as to whether the patient has adequate circulation.

- Inspect and palpate the skin for color, temperature, and degree of diaphoresis

- Inspect for any obvious signs of external bleeding

- Auscultate blood pressure

    If there are other members of the trauma team available, auscultate the blood pressure. If not, proceed with the primary assessment and auscultate the blood pressure at the beginning of the secondary assessment.

Interventions

CIRCULATION: EFFECTIVE

If the circulation is effective, proceed with assessment and intervene according to interventions for ineffective circulation, as indicated.

CIRCULATION PRESENT: INEFFECTIVE

Although the pulse is present, other signs may indicate inadequacy of the circulation such as:

- Tachycardia

- Decreased level of consciousness

- Uncontrolled external bleeding

- Distended external jugular veins

- Pale, cool, diaphoretic skin

- Distant heart sounds

CIRCULATION: EFFECTIVE OR INEFFECTIVE

- Control any uncontrolled external bleeding by:

  - Applying direct pressure over the bleeding site

  - Elevating the extremity

  - Applying pressure over arterial pressure points

  - The use of a tourniquet is rarely indicated. However, if the above interventions do not control the bleeding and operative bleeding control is not readily available, a tourniquet may be the last resort.

- Cannulate two veins with large-bore, 14- or 16-gauge catheters, and initiate infusions of lactated Ringer's solution

  - Use warmed solutions

  - Use plastic bags to facilitate pressurized infusion

- Use "Y" tubing for possible administration of blood

- Use rapid infusor device, as indicated

- Use normal saline (0.9%) in intravenous tubing through which blood is administered

- Venous cannulation may require a surgical cutdown and/or central vein venipuncture

- Consider use of a pneumatic antishock garment (PASG) for intra-abdominal and/or pelvic bleeding with hypotension

- Obtain a blood sample for typing to determine the ABO and Rh group

CIRCULATION: ABSENT

If a patient does not have a pulse, cardiopulmonary resuscitation (CPR) is indicated. If, at this point in the assessment, the patient's electrocardiographic rhythm is being monitored and if the patient is hypovolemic, it is possible to have some electrocardiographic activity without an auscultatable blood pressure or pulse. The term electro-mechanical dissociation (EMD) refers to one example of pulseless electrical activity (PEA) whereby the patient has no pulse but has narrow complexes indicating depolarization of the myocardium with no mechanical contraction. Pseudo-EMD, another form of PEA, is usually seen when a patient has no blood pressure by auscultation but may have some degree of myocardial muscle contraction, albeit too weak to generate a blood pressure.[3] If there is no palpable carotid pulse:

- Initiate cardiopulmonary resuscitation (CPR)

- Initiate advanced life support measures

- Administer blood, as prescribed

- Prepare for and assist with an emergency thoracotomy in the emergency department or resuscitation area. Open thoracotomies should only be done in facilities with the resources to manage postthoracotomy patients.

- Prepare patient for definitive operative care after thoracotomy, if indicated

If there are any life-threatening conditions compromising circulation, stop and intervene before proceeding to the neurologic assessment. Examples of life-threatening conditions that may compromise circulation are: uncontrolled external bleeding, shock due to hemorrhage or massive burns, pericardial tamponade, or direct cardiac injury.

Disability-Brief Neurologic Assessment

Assessment

After the primary assessment of airway, breathing, and circulation, conduct a brief neurologic assessment to determine the degree of disability (D) as measured by the patient's level of consciousness.[2]

- Determine the patient's level of consciousness by assessing the patient's response to verbal and/or painful stimuli using the **AVPU** mnemonic as follows:

    - **A** Speak to the patient. The patient who is alert, awake, responsive to voice, and oriented to person, time, and place is considered **A** for **Alert**.

    - **V** The patient who responds to voice but not fully oriented to person, time, or place is considered **V** for **Verbal**.

    - **P** Apply a painful stimulus, e.g., squeeze the patient's hand. The patient who does not respond to voice but does respond to painful stimulus is considered **P** for **Pain**.

    - **U** The patient who does not respond to painful stimulus is considered **U** for **Unresponsive**.

- Assess pupils for size, shape, equality, and reactivity to light

Interventions

- If the disability assessment indicated a decreased level of consciousness, conduct further investigation during the secondary focused assessments.

- If the patient is not alert or verbal, consider the need for hyperventilation.

SECONDARY ASSESSMENT

After each component of the A-B-C-D of the primary assessment has been addressed and life-saving interventions initiated, start the secondary assessment. This assessment is a brief, systematic process to identify **ALL** injuries. **Exposure (E)** of the patient is necessary to assess the patient adequately. It may be necessary to cut away clothing in certain circumstances. Timing of the removal of clothing will depend on the number of trauma team members available. Once clothing has been removed, it is important to prevent heat loss by using overhead warmers, light blankets, and warmed intravenous fluids. The **F** of the assessment mnemonic stands for **fahrenheit** and reminds the trauma nurse to keep the patient warm.

Prior to initiating the head-to-toe assessment to identify other injuries, obtain a complete set of vital signs, including blood pressure, pulse rate, respiratory rate, and temperature. The **G** of the assessment mnemonic is a reminder to the trauma nurse to **get a complete set of vital signs**. If chest trauma is suspected, auscultate the blood pressure in both arms.

Additional Assessments and Interventions
Before the History

After completing the A-B-C-D-E-F-G of the assessment and intervening for life-threatening conditions, critical decision-making will determine whether to proceed with the secondary assessment or to perform additional interventions. The availability of other trauma members to perform these interventions will influence the decision. If the patient sustained significant trauma and required life-saving interventions during the primary assessment, perform the following interventions before proceeding with the secondary assessment:

- Assign another trauma team member to attach leads and monitor the patient's cardiac rate and rhythm

- Assign another trauma team member to attach a pulse oximeter, if available, to monitor the patient's arterial oxygen saturation (SpO_2). The normal SpO_2 is 98%, meaning hemoglobin is 98% saturated with oxygen. SpO_2 readings may not be accurate if the patient has inconsistent blood flow, vasoconstriction, or carboxyhemoglobin. Even if the patient has only a slight change in SpO_2 readings, the change in arterial partial pressure of oxygen (PaO_2) is significant.[4] Oxygen saturation measurements can also be calculated from an arterial blood sample (SaO_2).

- Insert an indwelling urinary catheter to monitor urinary output. Suspected injury to the urethra is a contraindication to catheterization through the urethra. Indications of possible urethral injury are:

- Blood at the urethral meatus

- Palpation of a displaced prostate gland during a rectal examination

- Blood in the scrotum

- Suspicion of an anterior pelvic fracture

● Insert a gastric tube. If a fracture of the cribriform plate is suspected, insert the gastric tube through the patient's mouth. Gastric decompression and emptying of gastric contents will reduce the risk of aspiration, reduce the risk of respiratory compromise, reduce the risk of vagal stimulation and bradycardia, and prepare the patient for possible operative intervention. Test gastric contents for blood. The tube must be passed carefully while:

- Maintaining cervical spine stabilization or immobilization

- Minimizing the stimulation of the patient's gag reflex

- Having suction equipment available

● Facilitate laboratory studies

- Blood typing is the highest priority. Depending on the severity of the patient's condition, blood typing studies may also include screening and crossmatching.

- Frequently-ordered studies are: blood typing, hematocrit (Hct), hemoglobin (Hgb), blood urea nitrogen (BUN), creatinine, blood alcohol, toxicology screen, arterial partial pressure of oxygen (PaO_2), arterial partial pressure of carbon dioxide ($PaCO_2$), pH, electrolytes, glucose and clotting profile (platelets, prothrombin time [PT], partial thromboplastin time [PTT]), and beta human chorionic gonadatropin for pregnancy.

History

- Prehospital information

  Obtain information from prehospital personnel as indicated by the circumstances of the injury event. The mnemonic, **MIVT**, which stands for **M**echanism of injury, **I**njuries sustained, **V**ital signs, and **T**reatment, can be used as a guide to obtaining prehospital information.[5]

  - Mechanism and pattern of injury

    Knowledge of the mechanism of injury and specific injury patterns, e.g., type of motor vehicle impact, will help to predict certain injuries. If the patient was transported by prehospital personnel, have them describe pertinent on-scene information to the trauma team. Such information includes the location of the patient on their arrival, length of time since the injury event, and extent of extrication or reasons for extended on-scene time.

  - Injuries suspected

    Ask prehospital personnel to describe the patient's general condition, level of consciousness, and apparent injuries.

  - Vital signs

  - Treatment initiated and patient responses

- Patient-generated information

  If the patient is responsive, ask questions in order to evaluate the patient's level of consciousness and for the patient to describe discomforts or other complaints. Elicit patient's description of pain, i.e., location, duration, intensity, and character. Talking to the patient provides reassurance and emotional support and provides the patient with information regarding upcoming procedures.

- Past medical history

  Gather information from the patient or family regarding:

  - Age

  - Pre-existing medical conditions

- Current medications

- Allergies

- Tetanus immunization history

- Previous hospitalizations and surgeries

- Recent use of drugs or alcohol

- Last menstrual period

Assessment

Head-to-Toe Assessment

Information from this assessment is collected primarily through inspection, auscultation, and palpation. While systematically moving from the patient's head to the lower extremities, complete the assessment as described on the following pages.

General Appearance

Note the patient's body position, posture, and any guarding or self-protection movements. Observe for stiffness, rigidity, or flaccidity of muscles. Characteristic positions of limbs (flexion or extension), trunk, or head may indicate specific injuries. Note and document any unusual odors such as alcohol, gasoline, chemicals, vomitus, urine, or feces.

HEAD AND FACE

- Soft tissue injuries

  - Inspect for lacerations, abrasions, contusions, avulsions, puncture wounds, impaled objects, ecchymosis, and edema

  - Palpate for crackling associated with subcutaneous emphysema

  - Palpate for areas of tenderness

- Bony deformities

  - Inspect for exposed bone

  - Inspect for loose teeth or other material in the mouth that may compromise the airway

- Inspect and palpate for depressions, angulation, or areas of tenderness

- Inspect and palpate for facial fractures resulting in loss of maxillary and/or mandibular or structural integrity

- Observe for asymmetry of facial expressions. Also inspect the area for any exposed tissue that may indicate disruption of the central nervous system (CNS), i.e., CNS tissue from open wounds.

- Eyes

  - Determine gross visual acuity by asking the patient to identify how many of your fingers you are holding up

  - Inspect for periorbital ecchymosis (raccoon's eyes), subconjunctival hemorrhage, and/or edema. Determine whether the patient is wearing contact lenses.

  - Assess pupils for size, shape, equality, and reactivity to light

  - Assess eye muscles by asking the patient to follow your moving finger in six directions to determine extraocular eye movements (EOMs)

- Ears

  Inspect for ecchymosis behind the ear (Battle's sign), skin avulsion, or unusual drainage, such as blood or clear fluid from the external ear canal. Do **NOT** pack ear to stop drainage as it may be cerebrospinal fluid (CSF).

- Nose

  - Inspect for any unusual drainage, such as blood or clear fluid. Do **NOT** pack nose to stop clear fluid drainage as it may be CSF. If CSF or drainage is present, notify the physician and do not insert a gastric tube through the nose.

  - Inspect position of nasal septum

- Neck

  - Inspect for signs of penetrating or surface trauma, including presence of impaled objects, ecchymosis, edema, or any open wounds

  - Observe position of trachea and appearance of external jugular veins

  - Palpate trachea to determine position, i.e., midline, deviated

  - Palpate neck area for signs of subcutaneous emphysema and/or areas of tenderness

CHEST

- Inspection

  - Observe breathing for rate, depth, degree of effort required, use of accessory and/or abdominal muscles, and any paradoxical chest wall movement

  - Inspect the anterior and lateral chest walls, including the axillae for lacerations, abrasions, contusions, avulsions, puncture wounds, impaled objects, ecchymosis, edema, and scars

  - Inspect the expansion of the chest and excursion during ventilation

  - Observe for expressions or reactions that may indicate the presence of pain

- Auscultation

  - Auscultate lungs for breath sounds and note presence of any adventitious sounds, such as wheezes, rales, or rhonchi

  - Auscultate heart sounds for presence of murmurs, friction rubs, and/or muffled sounds

- Palpation

  - Palpate for signs of subcutaneous emphysema

  - Palpate the clavicles, sternum, and the ribs for bony crepitus or deformities, e.g., step-off, areas of tenderness

ABDOMEN/FLANKS

- Inspection

    - Inspect for lacerations, abrasions, contusions, avulsions, puncture wounds, impaled objects, ecchymosis, edema, and scars

    - Observe for evisceration, distension, and scars

- Auscultation

    Auscultate for presence or absence of bowel sounds. Auscultate before palpating because palpation may change the frequency of bowel sounds.[6]

- Palpation

    Gently palpate all four quadrants for rigidity, guarding, masses, and areas of tenderness

PELVIS/PERINEUM

- Inspect for lacerations, abrasions, contusions, avulsions, puncture wounds, impaled objects, ecchymosis, edema, and scars

- Bony deformities

    - Inspect for exposed bone

    - Palpate for instability and tenderness over the iliac crests and the symphysis pubis

- Inspect for blood at the urethral meatus (more common in males than females due to length of urethra), vagina, and rectum

- Altered neurologic function

    - Inspect penis for priapism (persistent abnormal erection)

    - Palpate anal sphincter for presence or absence of tone (this may also be done in the posterior assessment)

- Note pain and/or the urge, but inability, to void

EXTREMITIES

- Inspect previously applied splints and do **NOT** remove if applied appropriately and if neurovascular function is intact

- Circulation

  - Inspect color

  - Palpate skin temperature

  - Palpate pulses

    In lower extremities palpate femoral, popliteal, dorsalis pedis and, in upper extremities, palpate the brachial and radial pulses.

- Soft tissue injuries

  - Inspect for bleeding

  - Inspect for lacerations, abrasions, contusions, avulsions, puncture wounds, impaled objects, ecchymosis, edema, angulations, deformity, and any open wounds

- Bony injuries

  - Inspect for angulation, deformity, open wounds with evidence of protruding bone fragments, edema, and ecchymosis

  - Note bony crepitus

  - Palpate for deformity and areas of tenderness

- Motor function

  - Inspect for spontaneous movement of extremities

  - Determine motor strength and range of motion in all four extremities

- Determine patient's ability to sense touch in all four extremities

Inspect Posterior Surfaces

- Maintain cervical spine stabilization

- Support extremities with suspected injuries

- Logroll patient with the assistance of members of the trauma team. This maneuver keeps the vertebral column in alignment during the turning process. Do not logroll the patient onto the side with an injured extremity. Logroll away from you (if possible) to inspect the back, flanks, buttocks, and posterior thighs for: lacerations, abrasions, contusions, avulsions, puncture wounds, impaled objects, ecchymosis, edema, or scars.

- Palpate the vertebral column including the costovertebral angles (CVA) for deformity and areas of tenderness

- Palpate all posterior surfaces for deformity and areas of tenderness

- Palpate anal sphincter for presence or absence of tone, if not already done during the assessment of the pelvis and perineum

FOCUSED SURVEY

After the primary and secondary assessments and any simultaneous interventions are completed, a more detailed, focused assessment will be necessary for each area or system injured. This will further direct the priorities of care.

Frequently-ordered radiographic studies are of the cervical spine, chest, and pelvis. C-1 through T-1 must be visualized. Follow cervical spine clearance procedures, as indicated by individual hospital protocols. These x-rays may be performed during any phase of the primary or secondary assessment, depending on the patient's condition, and the availability of resources.

PAIN MANAGEMENT

The patient's perception of pain may originate from a number of sources due to injury, e.g., the actual injury, procedures, the environment. There are various assessment techniques and a number of treatment methods including use of analgesics, conscious sedation, cutaneous stimulation, therapeutic touch, and general comfort measures. For a detailed description of pain management, see Appendix 5.

TETANUS PROPHYLAXIS

Determination of the need for tetanus prophylaxis following trauma depends on:

- Condition of the wound

- Patient's past vaccination history

First determine whether the patient has ever received primary vaccination. See Appendix 6 for specific guidelines for tetanus prophylaxis.

SEVERITY INDICES

The Glasgow Coma Scale (see Table 6) and the Revised Trauma Score (see Table 7) are two scoring systems that measure the acuity and severity of the patient's physiologic response to injury. The Revised Trauma Score may be used by prehospital personnel and emergency staff as a triage tool. Changes in both scores will reflect the patient's ongoing response to the injury event. During the TNCC and in actual clinical practice, scores can be calculated using a preprinted source indicating the points for each area. Data from the primary and secondary assessments can be used to determine the severity of the patient's condition and provide a baseline for ongoing evaluation of the patient's responses to the injury event and treatment.

Glasgow Coma Scale

The Glasgow Coma Scale (GCS) ranges from 3 to 15 and is a gross measure of the patient's level of consciousness.[7,8] It is not a measure of total neurologic function. Points on the scale correspond with specific responses in three areas: eye opening, verbal response to pain, and motor response to pain. The patient's **BEST** response in each of three areas is noted. For example, if a patient presents with paralysis of the lower extremities but can move an upper extremity, the BEST motor response is based on the patient's ability to move the upper extremity.

The patient's eye opening response cannot be measured if the eyes are so swollen that the patient cannot open them. Patients who have been given a drug for neuromuscular blockade cannot be evaluated for motor response. Patients who have been intubated or who cannot speak due to maxillofacial trauma cannot be evaluated for verbal response. If any of the these circumstances are present, the Glasgow Coma Scale total score should not be calculated, and the unusual circumstances should be noted.

Table 6

GLASGOW COMA SCALE	
Areas of Response	**Points**
Eye Opening	
Eyes open spontaneously	4
Eyes open in response to voice	3
Eyes open in response to pain	2
No eye opening response	1
Best Verbal Response	
Oriented, e.g., to person, place, time	5
Confused, speaks but is disoriented	4
Inappropriate, but comprehensible words	3
Incomprehensible sounds but no words are spoken	2
None	1
Best Motor Response	
Obeys command to move	6
Localizes painful stimulus	5
Withdraws from painful stimulus	4
Flexion, abnormal decorticate posturing	3
Extension, abnormal decerebrate posturing	2
No movement or posturing	1
Total Possible Points	**3-15**
Major Head Injury	**≤8**
Moderate Head Injury	**9-12**
Minor Head Injury	**13-15**

Revised Trauma Score

The Revised Trauma Score measures the patient's physiologic response to injuries.[9] Measurements used to calculate the score, which ranges from 0 to 12, are the Glasgow Coma Scale Score, systolic blood pressure, and the patient's respiratory rate. Coded values are used to represent ranges in each of the three measured areas.

Table 7

REVISED TRAUMA SCORE	
Area of Measurement	**Coded Value**
Systolic Blood Pressure (mmHg)	
>89	4
76-89	3
50-75	2
1-49	1
0	0
Respiratory Rate (spontaneous inspirations/minute)*	
10-29	4
>29	3
6-9	2
1-5	1
0	0
*patient initiated, not artificial ventilations	
Glasgow Coma Scale Score	
13-15	4
9-12	3
6-8	2
4-5	1
3	0
Total Possible Points	**0-12**

The probabilities of survival for patients with various revised trauma scores are the following:

Score	Survivors (Percent)
12	99.5%
11	96.9%
10	87.9%
9	76.6%
8	66.7%
7	63.6%
6	63.0%
5	45.5%
3 to 4	33.3%
2	28.6%
1	25.0%
0	3.7%

The recommendation by the developers of the Revised Trauma Score and the American College of Surgeons Committee on Trauma, is that patients with a GCS less than 13, a systolic blood pressure less than 90, a respiratory rate greater than 29 or less than 10, or a total Revised Trauma Score of 11 or less should be triaged to a trauma center.[2,9]

Nursing Diagnoses and Outcome Identification

The primary assessment will reveal information the nurse uses to analyze the patient's responses to the injury event and to determine specific nursing diagnoses. Each nursing diagnosis is derived by diagnostic reasoning, which determines the priorities of intervention. Each diagnosis represents an actual or risk health problem or one that may develop as a result of a patient being vulnerable to risk factors.[10] The problems may be corrected by the nurse or may require a collaborative intervention with other trauma team members. The identification of specific outcomes corresponds to the goals generated by the team for the patient to correct each diagnosis or health problem.[11]

POSSIBLE NURSING DIAGNOSES AND EXPECTED OUTCOMES	
Nursing Diagnosis	**Expected Outcome**
Airway clearance, ineffective related to: • Edema of the airway, vocal cords, epiglottis, and upper airway • Irritation of the respiratory tract • Laryngeal spasm • Altered level of consciousness secondary to hypoxia • Pain	The patient will maintain a patent airway as evidenced by: • Regular rate, depth, and pattern of breathing • Bilateral chest expansion • Effective cough/gag reflex • Absence of signs and symptoms of airway obstruction: stridor, dyspnea, hoarse voice • Clear sputum of normal amount without abnormal color or odor • Absence of signs and symptoms of retained secretions: fever, tachycardia, tachypnea

POSSIBLE NURSING DIAGNOSES AND EXPECTED OUTCOMES

Nursing Diagnosis	Expected Outcome

Aspiration, risk related to:
• Reduced level consciousness secondary to injury or concomitant substance abuse
• Impaired cough and gag reflex
• Structural defect to head, face and/or neck
• Secretions and debris in airway
	The patient will not experience aspiration as evidenced by:
	• A patent airway
	• Clear and equal bilateral breath sounds
	• Regular rate, depth, and pattern of breathing
	• Arterial blood gas (ABG) values within normal limits
	  ■ PaO_2 80 - 100 mmHg (10.0 - 13.3 KPa)
	  ■ SaO_2 >95%
	  ■ $PaCO_2$ 35 - 45 mmHg (4.7 - 6.0 KPa)
	  ■ pH between 7.35 - 7.45
	• Clear chest x-ray (CXR) without evidence of infiltrates
	• Ability to handle secretions independently

Gas exchange, impaired related to:
• Ineffective breathing pattern: Loss of integrity of thoracic cage and impaired chest wall movement secondary to injury, deterioration of ventilatory efforts
• Ineffective airway clearance
• Aspiration
• Shock
	The patient will experience adequate gas exchange as evidenced by:
	• ABG values within normal limits
	  ■ PaO_2 80 - 100 mmHg (10.0 - 13.3 KPa)
	  ■ SaO_2 >95%
	  ■ $PaCO_2$ 35 - 45 mmHg (4.7 - 6.0 KPa)
	  ■ pH between 7.35 - 7.45
	• Skin normal color, warm, and dry
	• Improved level of consciousness
	• Regular rate, depth, and pattern of breathing

Fluid volume deficit related to: • Hemorrhage • Fluid shifts • Alteration in capillary permeability • Alteration in vascular tone • Myocardial compromise	The patient will have an effective circulating volume as evidenced by: • Stable vital signs appropriate for developmental age • Urinary output of 1 ml/kg/hr • Strong, palpable peripheral pulses • Improved level of consciousness • Skin normal color, warm, and dry • Maintains HCT = 30 ml/dl or Hgb = 12 - 14 g/dl or greater • Central venous pressure (CVP) reading of 5 - 10 cm H_2O • External hemorrhage is controlled

POSSIBLE NURSING DIAGNOSES AND EXPECTED OUTCOMES

Nursing Diagnosis	Expected Outcome
Cardiac output, decreased related to: • Decreased venous return secondary to acute blood loss or massive peripheral vasodilation	The patient will maintain adequate circulatory function as evidenced by: • Strong, palpable peripheral pulses • Apical pulse rate of 60 - 100 beats/minute • ECG with normal sinus rhythm, absence of dysrythmias • Skin normal color, warm, dry • Improved level of consciousness • CVP reading 5 - 10 cm H_2O • Urinary output of 1 ml/kg/hr
Hypothermia related to: • Rapid infusion of intravenous fluids • Decreased tissue perfusion • Exposure	The patient will maintain a normal core body temperature as evidenced by: • Core temperature measurement of 36° - 37.5°C (98° - 99.5°F) • Absence of shivering, cool skin, pallor • Skin normal color, warm, and dry
Pain related to: • Soft tissue injury and edema • Fractures • Pleural irritation • Stimulation of nerve fibers • Invasive procedures	The patient will experience relief of pain as evidenced by: • Diminishing or absent level of pain through patient's self-report using an objective measurement tool • Absence of physiologic indicators of pain, which include: tachypnea, pallor, diaphoretic skin, increasing blood pressure • Absence of nonverbal cues of pain: crying, grimacing, inability to assume position of comfort, and/or guarding • Ability to cooperate with care as appropriate
Anxiety/Fear (patient, family) related to: • Unfamiliar environment • Unpredictable nature of condition • Invasive procedures • Possible disfigurement, scarring	The patient/family will experience decreasing anxiety/fear as evidenced by: • Oriented to surroundings • Ability to describe reasons for equipment and procedures used in treatment • Ability to verbalize concerns and ask questions to health care team • Utilize effective coping skills

POSSIBLE NURSING DIAGNOSES AND EXPECTED OUTCOMES	
Nursing Diagnosis	**Expected Outcome**
Powerlessness (individual, family) related to: • Loss of function • Uncontrolled pain • Lack of privacy • Lack of knowledge	The patient/family will experience an increasing feeling of control over the situational crisis as evidenced by: • Participation in decision-making activities • Ask questions regarding treatment and course of care • Accept appropriate referrals and resources for support • Utilize medical/nursing staff for support and assistance

Evaluation and Ongoing Assessment

The evaluation of a trauma patient is that phase of the nursing process when the nurse evaluates the patient's responses to the injury event and the effect of all interventions. The achievement of the expected outcomes is evaluated and the treatment/intervention plan is adjusted to enhance these outcomes. To evaluate the patient's progress, monitor the following:

- Airway patency

- Effectiveness of breathing

- Arterial pH, PaO_2, and $PaCO_2$

- Oxygen saturation (SpO_2 or SaO_2)

- Level of consciousness

- Skin temperature and color

- Pulse rate and quality

- Blood pressure

- Urinary output

Written documentation of all information generated during the trauma nursing process is an essential responsibility of the trauma nurse.

SUMMARY

The initial assessment of the trauma patient, the first step of the trauma nursing process, includes primary and secondary assessments. If life-threatening conditions are present, the nurse must stop the assessment and intervene to correct these problems before proceeding with the assessment. Care of the seriously injured trauma victim is best accomplished through a team approach. The A through I mnemonic is:

- **A**   Airway with simultaneous cervical spine stabilization and/or immobilization

- **B**   Breathing

- **C**   Circulation

- **D**   Disability

- **E**   Expose

- **F**   Fahrenheit

- **G**   Get a complete set of vital signs

- **H**   History and head-to-toe assessment

- **I**   Inspect posterior surfaces

In the following chapters dealing with specific injuries, pertinent assessments and interventions outlined in this chapter will not be repeated. Refer to this chapter for the information regarding a description of:

- General information related to history, which should be collected regarding every trauma victim

- The assessment of the patient's airway and effectiveness of breathing and circulation

- Frequently-ordered radiographic and laboratory studies

- Specific nursing interventions for patients with compromises to airway, breathing, and/or circulation

- Ongoing evaluation of the patient's airway and effectiveness of breathing and circulation

REFERENCES

1. Emergency Nurses Association. *Emergency Nursing Core Curriculum*. 4th ed. Philadelphia, Pa: WB Saunders Co; 1994.

2. American College of Surgeons Committee on Trauma. *Advanced Trauma Life Support® Course for Physicians (Instructor Manual)*. 5th ed. Chicago, Ill: Author; 1993.

3. Emergency Cardiac Care Committee and Subcommittees, American Heart Association. Adult advanced cardiac life support, Part III. *JAMA*. 1992;268:16:2199-2241.

4. Schneider S. Acute respiratory insufficiency. In: Schwartz GR, Cayton CG, Mangelsen MA, Mayer TA, Hanke BK, eds. *Principles and Practice of Emergency Medicine*. 3rd ed. Philadelphia, Pa: Lea & Febiger; 1992:43-72.

5. Looper P. Aeromedical mnemonics a reporting model that works. *AMJ*. 1987;25-26.

6. Bates B. *A Guide to Physical Examination*. 5th ed. Philadelphia, Pa: JB Lippincott Co; 1991.

7. Teasdale G, Jennett B. Glasgow coma scale. *Lancet*. 1974;2:81-84.

8. Jennett B, Teasdale G. *Management of Head Injuries*. Philadelphia, Pa: FA Davis; 1982.

9. Champion HR, Sacco WJ, Copes WS, Gann DS, Gennarelli TA, Flanagan ME. A revision of the trauma score. *J Trauma*. 1989;29:623-629.

10. North American Nursing Diagnosis Association. *Nursing Diagnoses: Definitions and Classification, 1995-1996*. Philadelphia, Pa: Author; 1994.

11. Emergency Nurses Association. *Emergency Nurses Guide to Nursing Diagnosis*. Chicago, Ill: Author; 1992.

CHAPTER FOUR

SHOCK

LECTURE BEGINS ON PAGE 79.

Preface

Prior to reading this chapter, it is strongly suggested that the learner read the following section entitled "Anatomy and Physiology." Specific anatomy and physiologic concepts are presented to enhance the learner's ability to correlate such concepts with specific injuries. This material related to anatomy and physiology will not be covered during lectures, nor will it be evaluated by testing. However, knowledge of normal anatomy and physiology serves as the foundation for understanding the anatomic derangements and pathophysiologic compromises that may ensue as a result of trauma.

ANATOMY AND PHYSIOLOGY

Cell Structure and Metabolism

The body's 75 to 100 trillion cells require oxygen and nutrients to sustain function. Each cell's semipermeable membrane takes part in complex processes which regulate both the intra- and extracellular environments. The cell's protoplasm is composed of 70 to 85% water with the remaining 15 to 30% made up of lipids, carbohydrates (glucose), proteins, and electrolytes such as potassium, magnesium, and phosphate. The extracellular fluid contains more sodium, chloride, and bicarbonate than intracellular fluid. The cell's primary nutrients, fatty acids, oxygen, and amino acids are also in the extracellular fluid. Through active and passive transport systems, these substances can enter the cell to participate in metabolism and the production of energy.

Structurally, the cell contains lysosomes and mitochondria, which have important roles. Lysosomes contain enzymes that are responsible for ridding the cell of foreign substances such as bacteria. Mitochondria, through an oxidative process that utilizes stored enzymes, can extract energy from nutrients and use it to produce adenosine triphosphate (ATP). Once released from the mitochondria into the cell, ATP is the energy substance that sustains cellular metabolism.[1]

Cardiovascular System

The four-chambered heart is responsible for pumping blood into both the systemic circulation via the aorta and into the pulmonary circulation via the pulmonary artery. Effective circulation depends on the fact that the flow of blood is unidirectional, that the output from the left and right ventricles is equal, and that blood flows on a pressure gradient from the arterial (high-pressure) system to the venous (low-pressure) system.[2]

The thick-walled arteries are composed of smooth muscle and an abundance of elastic fibers. The arterioles, because of their function in blood pressure control, have a predominant smooth muscle layer. The thin-walled veins are considered capacitance vessels, which are very distensible as well as collapsible. The single-cell thick capillary is where the exchange of nutrients, gases, and byproducts of cellular metabolism occurs.

The term microcirculation refers to the capillaries, venules, arterioles, metarterioles (channels from arterioles to capillaries), and the arteriovenous anastomoses (see Figure 3). Not only does the microcirculation function in the exchange of gases, nutrients, and byproducts of metabolism, it also controls total peripheral resistance (TPR). Total peripheral resistance refers to the resistance in blood vessels in the entire systemic circulation. TPR is a reflection of the rate of blood flow in the vessels (which is related to the hematocrit and viscosity of the blood) and the differences in pressure inside the vessels (the length, width, and radius of the vessels). The capillaries have precapillary sphincters which, under the control of the sympathetic nervous system, influence vasoconstriction and vasodilation to regulate blood flow into the capillary.

Figure 3
Microcirculation

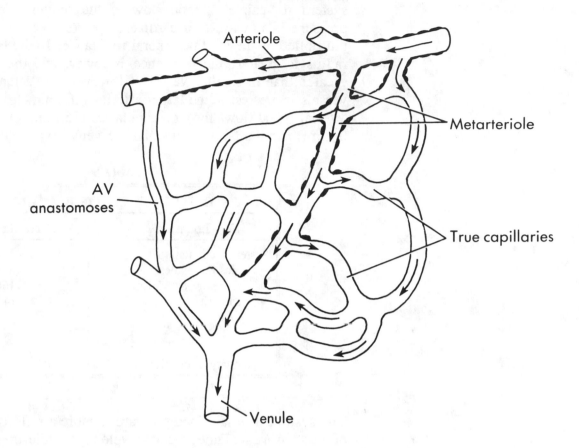

The total blood volume is approximately 5 liters (in an average 70 kg person) with 3 liters of plasma (extracellular) and 2 liters of red blood cell volume (intracellular). There are another 12 liters of extracellular fluid and another 23 liters of intracellular fluid for a total body fluid volume of 40 liters (see Table 8).

Table 8

DISTRIBUTION OF TOTAL BODY FLUIDS	
Fluid Compartment	**Liters**
Extracellular fluid (ECF) • Plasma • Interstitial fluid and other ECF compartments	15 liters (37.5%) • 3 liters • 12 liters
Intracellular fluid (ICF) • Red blood cells • All other cells	25 liters (62.5%) • 2 liters • 23 liters

The majority of blood volume (64%) is in the venous capacitance system (see Table 9). The arterial system functions as a pressure system to maintain blood flow to the tissues. The arterial blood pressure is a measure of cardiac output (stroke volume x heart rate) multiplied by the total peripheral resistance. In the larger vessels, the radius is greater, the resistance is lower, and the flow of blood is greater than in smaller vessels. However, the actual pressure inside vessels is greatest in the larger arteries (100 mmHg), decreases as the arterial blood flows through capillaries (35 mmHg), and is eventually 0 mmHg in the larger veins and the vena cavae.

Table 9

DISTRIBUTION OF BLOOD	
Location	**Percentage**
Systemic circulation • Veins & venules • Arteries & arterioles • Capillaries	84% • (64%) • (16%) • (4%)
Heart	7%
Pulmonary circulation	9%

The systolic arterial blood pressure is more a reflection of the cardiac output (stroke volume, ejection velocity) while the diastolic arterial blood pressure reflects the TPR. In shock, tissue perfusion is compromised. The mean arterial blood pressure (MAP) will reflect the degree of tissue hypoperfusion. To calculate an estimate of the MAP, take one third of the pulse pressure (the difference between the systolic and diastolic pressures) and add it to the diastolic pressure. The normal MAP (considering 120/80 mmHg as a normal blood pressure) is 93 mmHg. If the patient's blood pressure is only 90/60 mmHg, the MAP is 70 mmHg, and tissue perfusion is lower.

Calculation of Mean Arterial Blood Pressure Example 90/60 mmHg
90 mmHg – 60 mmHg = 30 mmHg 1/3 of 30 mmHg = 10 mmHg 60 mmHg + 10 mmHg = 70 mmHg

Nervous Control of the Circulatory System

In general, the autonomic nervous system (ANS) is responsible for the nervous control of smooth muscle, cardiac muscle, and glands. The ANS controls the body's visceral motor functions. The ANS is divided into the sympathetic and parasympathetic divisions. The differences in these two subdivisions stem from the location of their nerve cell bodies, their effects on various organs, and their chemical mediators.

The sympathetic nervous system (SNS) is of importance in the shock syndrome since many of the signs the patient demonstrates are a result of SNS stimulation. The SNS fibers originate in spinal cord segments T-1 through L-2. Because it is predominantly a motor system, the sympathetic nerves travel through the anterior (motor) root of the particular spinal nerves. It is the postganglionic fibers that eventually innervate receptor organs such as the heart, lungs, bronchi, stomach, adrenal glands, intestines, systemic blood vessels, and sweat glands. With some exceptions, the postganglionic fibers of the SNS are adrenergic, meaning the chemical mediator they release is norepinephrine, which is a catecholamine, neurotransmitter, and powerful vasoconstrictor.

Some of the effects of increased SNS stimulation are listed in Table 10. In general, when the body needs to respond to stress, e.g., shock, the SNS is stimulated.

Table 10

EFFECTS OF SYMPATHETIC NERVOUS SYSTEM STIMULATION	
Organ	**Effect**
Heart (muscle)	• Increased force of contraction (positive inotropy)
Heart (rate)	• Increased heart rate (positive chronotropy)
Peripheral vessels	• Vasoconstriction
Pupil	• Dilation
Sweat glands (cholinergic)	• Increased secretion
Adrenal glands	• Increased cortical and medullary secretion
Bronchi	• Dilation
Kidneys	• Renin secretion increased
Liver	• Glycogenolysis (breakdown of stored glycogen)

Special pressure sensitive receptors in the body's major arteries are innervated by ANS fibers. In the carotid sinus (wall of the internal carotid artery above the bifurcation of the common carotid artery) and in the wall of the aortic arch, there are more of these pressure sensitive sites termed baroreceptors. When the systolic blood pressure drops below 60 mmHg, the baroreceptors are no longer stretched, causing fewer inhibitory impulses to the vasomotor center in the brainstem. The lack of such impulses causes increased vasomotor activity, resulting in vasoconstriction and a rise in blood pressure.

SHOCK

OBJECTIVES

Upon completion of this chapter/lecture, the learner should be able to:

1. Define the four types of shock.
2. Analyze the pathophysiologic changes as a basis for the signs and symptoms of shock.
3. Discuss the nursing assessment of the patient in shock.
4. Based on assessment data, recall appropriate nursing diagnoses and expected outcomes associated with patients in shock.
5. Plan appropriate interventions for the patient in shock.
6. Evaluate the effectiveness of nursing interventions for patients in shock.

INTRODUCTION

Classification and Etiology

Shock is a syndrome resulting from inadequate perfusion of tissues, leading to a decrease in the supply of oxygen and nutrients required to maintain the metabolic needs of cells. When the supply of oxygen and nutrients cannot meet the demand to sustain normal cellular metabolism, the body responds initially by activating intrinsic compensatory mechanisms to improve perfusion, especially in areas of high demand such as the brain, heart, and lungs. When compensatory mechanisms fail to restore adequate perfusion, a cascade of cellular abnormalities can result in total organ dysfunction and, eventually, death.

Numerous classification systems have been used to define shock either by causes or by the underlying pathophysiologic effects. One such system classifies shock syndromes according to the underlying pathology[2,3] (see Table 11).

- Hypovolemic

- Cardiogenic

- Obstructive

- Distributive

Hypovolemic Shock

The most common shock syndrome to affect a trauma patient is shock due to hypovolemia. Hypovolemia, a decrease in the amount of circulating blood volume, may result from a significant loss of whole blood due to hemorrhage or a loss of the semipermeable integrity of the cellular membrane, leading to leakage of plasma and protein from the intravascular space to the interstitial space, as may occur with a burn.[2]

Cardiogenic Shock

Cardiogenic shock is a syndrome that results from ineffective perfusion caused by inadequate contractility of the cardiac muscle. Some of the causes of cardiogenic shock are myocardial infarction, myocardial contusion, mitral valve insufficiency, dysrhythmias, and cardiac failure. Some authors use the term cardiogenic shock to refer to the shock syndrome that is actually trauma-induced cardiac insufficiency resulting from cardiac tamponade or a tension pneumothorax.[4] Since these two injuries do not cause primary damage to the myocardium, a more descriptive classification for the shock syndrome that is trauma-induced and causes secondary cardiac insufficiency is obstructive shock.

Obstructive Shock

Obstructive shock results from an inadequate circulating blood volume due to an obstruction or compression of the great veins, aorta, pulmonary arteries, or the heart itself.[3] Cardiac tamponade may so compress the heart during diastole that the atria cannot adequately fill, leading to a decrease in stroke volume. A tension pneumothorax may also lead to an inadequate stroke volume by displacing the inferior vena cava and obstructing venous return to the right atrium. An air embolus may lead to obstruction of the pulmonary artery and subsequent obstruction to right ventricular outflow during systole with resulting obstructive shock.

Distributive Shock

The fourth category of shock is distributive shock, which is a shock syndrome resulting from either poor distribution of blood flow or blood volume. Examples of shock due to a change in the distribution of blood volume are neurogenic and anaphylactic shock. Neurogenic shock may occur as a result of injury to the spinal cord in the cervical or upper thoracic region. Autonomic sympathetic functions are lost, resulting in:

- Loss of vasomotor tone regulated by the sympathetic nervous system, which results in peripheral vasodilation and maldistribution of blood volume in the peripheral vessels, especially the veins

- Loss of cutaneous control of sweat glands, resulting in an inability to sweat

- Increased parasympathetic control of heart rate, resulting in bradycardia

Septic shock from bacteremia is an example of distributive shock whereby the blood flow is poorly distributed due to shunting in the microcirculation and venous dilation.

Table 11

CLASSIFICATION OF SHOCK ETIOLOGY AND UNDERLYING DEFECT		
Classification	**Etiology**	**Underlying Pathology**
Hypovolemic	• Hemorrhage • Burns	• Whole blood loss • Plasma loss
Cardiogenic	• Myocardial Infarction • Dysrhythmias • Myocardial Contusion	• Loss of cardiac contractility • Reduced cardiac output • Loss of cardiac contractility
Obstructive	• Cardiac Tamponade • Tension Pneumothorax • Tension Hemothorax	• Compression of heart with obstruction to atrial filling • Mediastinal shift with obstruction to atrial filling
Distributive	• Neurogenic Shock • Anaphylactic Shock • Septic Shock	• Venous pooling • Shunting in microcirculation and in later stages – decrease in venous resistance

Usual Concurrent Injuries

Hypovolemic shock due to hemorrhage can accompany a number of injuries, which are discussed in greater detail in other chapters. Injuries that involve the chest, abdomen, and/or certain bones may result in the loss of varying degrees of circulating blood volume. Injuries to the liver, spleen, major vessels in the chest, femur, multiple long bones, and the pelvis may lead to significant hypovolemia. Additionally, a combination of relatively minor injuries may also cause shock.

PATHOPHYSIOLOGY AS A BASIS FOR SIGNS AND SYMPTOMS

Shock is a syndrome that involves all cells and their chemical and metabolic balance. The consequences of inadequate tissue perfusion can be described organ by organ. The body responds to shock by initiating compensatory mechanisms as specific organ systems are affected. Untreated, shock can progress to irreversible stages as the body's own compensatory mechanisms fail to restore perfusion and as organ systems become unable to maintain homeostasis. Some of the compensatory mechanisms and their responses follow.

Vascular Response

As blood volume decreases, the peripheral blood vessels vasoconstrict as a result of sympathetic stimulation via inhibition of the baroreceptors (see Figure 4). The arterioles constrict to increase total peripheral resistance and, ultimately, blood pressure. The venous capacitance system vasoconstricts to improve venous return to the right atrium.

Figure 4
Baroreceptor Response

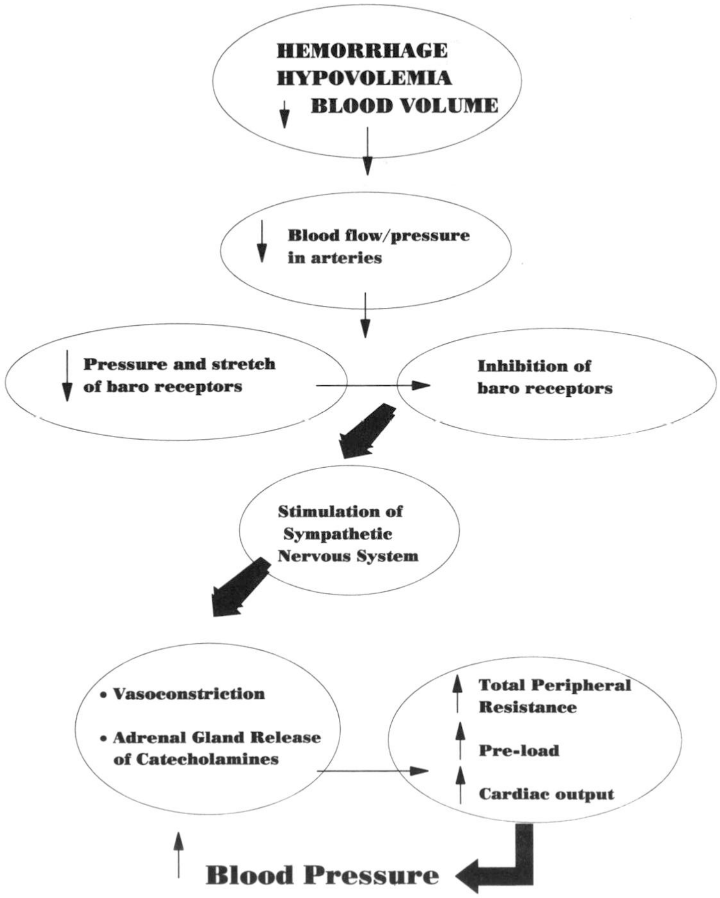

82

The carotid bodies, located at the bifurcations of the common carotid arteries, and the aortic bodies near the aorta have chemoreceptors that are sensitive to low levels of oxygen and excess levels of carbon dioxide in arterial blood. If the blood pressure is low enough, the arterial flow through the artery that supplies the chemoreceptors becomes diminished and the low oxygen and increased carbon dioxide levels stimulate the receptors. Consequently, the vasomotor center is stimulated by impulses along the same pathways as the baroreceptors. The result of this chemoreceptor response is vasoconstriction. Arterial blood pressure must be below 80 mmHg to activate the chemoreceptor response which, like the baroreceptor response, is initiated within seconds of the change in blood pressure. The vascular response may be detected by a rise in the patient's diastolic blood pressure.

Cerebral Response

As shock progresses, the primary goal of the body is to maintain perfusion of the brain, heart, and lungs. Consequently, blood flow to these centers is preserved while blood flow to other organs, such as the liver, bowel, skin, and to some extent, the kidneys, may be compromised. Sympathetic stimulation (compensatory vasoconstriction) has little effect on cerebral and coronary vessels, but the brain and heart can autoregulate blood flow based on the needs of the tissues.[1] Therefore, the brain and heart are preferentially perfused during early and intermediate stages of shock. If the blood pressure drops below 50 mmHg and cerebral ischemia ensues, the collection of carbon dioxide in the brain's vasomotor center will stimulate the central nervous system ischemic response.[1] This response yields further stimulation of the sympathetic nervous system. Alterations in level of consciousness may indicate cerebral ischemia.

Renal Response

Renal ischemia activates the release of renin, an enzyme stored in the kidneys' juxtaglomerular cells of the arterioles. When the kidneys do not receive an adequate blood supply, renin is released into the circulation. Renin causes angiotensinogen, a normal plasma protein, to release angiotensin I. Angiotensin II is then formed from angiotensin I; the conversion to angiotensin II is enhanced by the angiotensin-converting enzyme (ACE) from the lung where the majority of the conversion takes place (see Figure 5). The effects of angiotensin II are:

- Vasoconstriction of arterioles and some veins

- Stimulation of the SNS

- Retention of water by the kidneys

83

- Stimulation of the release of aldosterone from the adrenal cortex (sodium retention hormone)

Figure 5
Renin-Angiotensin-Aldosterone System

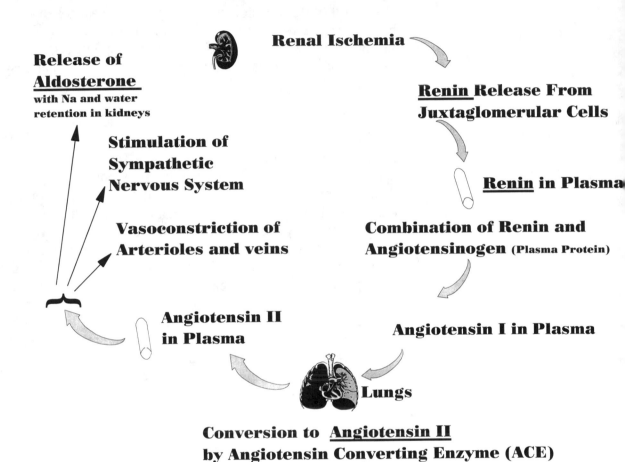

As powerful as the renin-angiotensin mechanism is, it does take approximately 20 minutes to fully activate.[1] Decreased urinary output may be a sign of renal hypoperfusion.

Adrenal Gland Response

When the adrenal glands are stimulated by the sympathetic nervous system, there will be an increase in the release of catecholamines (epinephrine and norepinephrine) from the adrenal medulla. The epinephrine stimulates receptors in the heart to increase the force of cardiac contraction (positive inotropy) and increase the heart rate (positive chronotropy) in order to improve cardiac output and, ultimately, improve blood pressure and tissue perfusion. Epinephrine also causes vasoconstriction. Norepinephrine promotes vasoconstriction to increase total peripheral resistance and, ultimately, increase blood pressure and perfusion. The signs of shock resulting from adrenal gland release of catecholamines are tachycardia, increased anxiety, and a compensatory rise in diastolic blood pressure.

Hepatic Response

The liver can store the body's excess glucose as glycogen. As shock progresses, glycogenolysis is activated by epinephrine to break down glycogen into glucose. In a compensatory response to shock, hepatic vessels constrict to redirect blood flow to other vital areas. If, however, hepatic ischemia is too profound, the function of the liver is compromised.

Pulmonary Response

The patient in shock may have tachypnea for two reasons: (1) to maintain acid-base balance, and (2) to maintain an increased supply of oxygen. For cells to produce energy, it is essential that they have enough oxygen for oxidative processes, which use the hydrogen ions produced by glucose metabolism to generate energy. When oxygen to the tissues is depleted, this oxidative phase of energy production is hampered. Since the breakdown of the glucose molecule to pyruvic acid is normally an anaerobic process, this process continues, leading to a buildup of pyruvic acid, which is converted to lactic acid. The resulting metabolic acidosis from anaerobic metabolism will be a stimulus for the lungs to increase the rate of ventilation. The increased respiratory rate is an attempt to correct the acidosis and also augments oxygen supply to maximize oxygen delivery to the alveoli.

Irreversible Shock

Untreated shock, or shock in progressive and/or irreversible stages, will eventually cause compromises in most body systems. For example, prolonged hypovolemia will cause a decrease in arterial pressure since there is inadequate venous return, inadequate cardiac filling, and decreased coronary artery perfusion. Since coronary arteries are perfused during diastole and diastolic pressure eventually falls, there will be a decrease in coronary artery perfusion with a subsequent decrease in myocardial contractility.

The membranes of the lysosomes break down within cells and release digestive enzymes that cause intracellular damage. Other chemicals in the body like histamine, serotonin, and prostaglandins are also activated. The byproducts of protein metabolism, uric acid, urea, and creatinine, are not cleared through the kidneys but reabsorbed into the circulation. As compensatory mechanisms continue to fail, thrombi develop in the microcirculation, blood flow becomes impeded, and most importantly, the tissue cells become ischemic. The shock state becomes irreversible. Acidosis, increased capillary permeability, vasomotor failure (dilation), cardiac failure, and hepatic failure are some of the causes of a patient's demise.

Classes of Hemorrhagic Shock

Shock due to hemorrhage is classified into four classes based on the percent of blood volume lost. Table 12 lists the physiologic responses to the four degrees of volume loss.[4]

Table 12

PHYSIOLOGIC RESPONSES TO HEMORRHAGE (Based on 70 kg male)						
Class % Blood Loss	Pulse	Blood Pressure	Pulse Pressure	LOC	Respiratory Rate	Urinary Output
Class One (I) Up to 15% (up to 750 ml)	<100	Normal	Normal or increased	Slightly anxious	14 to 20	>30ml/hr
Class Two (II) 15 to 30% (750-1,500 ml)	>100	Normal	Decreased	Mildly anxious	20 to 30	20 to 30 ml/hr
Class Three (III) 30 to 40% (1,500-2,000 ml)	>120	Decreased	Decreased	Anxious, confused	30 to 40	5 to 15 ml/hr
Class Four (IV) >40% (>2,000 ml)	>140	Decreased	Decreased	Confused, lethargic	>35	Minimal

NURSING CARE OF THE PATIENT IN HYPOVOLEMIC SHOCK

Assessment

A patient who arrives in the emergency department in profound shock due to trauma will require simultaneous assessment and intervention.

History

Refer to Chapter 3, Initial Assessment, for a description of general information that should be collected regarding every trauma victim. Only pertinent questions specific to patients in shock are listed below.

- Does the patient have any obvious bleeding sites?

- What is the estimate of external blood loss?

Physical Assessment

Refer to Chapter 3, Initial Assessment, for a description of the assessment of the patient's airway and effectiveness of breathing and circulation.

INSPECTION

- Determine level of consciousness (LOC)

  A patient's LOC may progressively deteriorate. Restlessness, anxiety, or confusion may occur <u>early</u> in shock as cerebral perfusion is diminished. After 30 to 40% of the blood volume is lost, the patient may be unresponsive to verbal and/or painful stimuli. A loss of greater than 40% of the total blood volume generally leads to unconsciousness. The early signs of cerebral ischemia are difficult to interpret if alcohol and/or drug use are suspected. Consider any alteration in LOC a result of cerebral ischemia until proven otherwise.

- Assess breathing effectiveness and rate of respirations

- Identify obvious sources of external bleeding

- Assess skin color

  Patient may be ashen or pale especially around the mouth; mucous membranes may be pale.

- Observe external jugular veins and peripheral veins for distention or flattening

- Inspect the chest, abdomen, and extremities for signs of obvious bleeding, fractures, or major soft tissue injury

AUSCULTATION

- Obtain blood pressure

  Due to vasoconstriction and low cardiac output, auscultated blood pressures may be difficult to obtain. A Doppler Ultrasonic Flow Meter may assist with blood pressure measurement.

- Calculate pulse pressure

Trends in blood pressure are extremely important. As total peripheral resistance rises in early shock, diastolic pressures rise as well. Early shock is characterized by a normal or falling systolic pressure and a rising diastolic pressure. Consequently, pulse pressure (the difference between systolic and diastolic pressures) narrows as cardiac output falls and blood vessels constrict. A narrowing pulse pressure is an ominous sign.

- Auscultate breath sounds

  Bleeding into the thoracic cavity may lead to diminished or even absent breath sounds.

- Auscultate heart sounds

  Heart sounds may sound distant or muffled if blood collects in the pericardial sac.

- Auscultate bowel sounds

  The absence of bowel sounds may indicate intra-abdominal bleeding. However, even though bowel sounds are present, bleeding may still be present. Absent or hypoactive bowel sounds are common in patients in profound shock.

PERCUSSION

Percuss chest and abdomen

Dullness of the chest or abdomen may indicate the presence of blood. Early identification of sources of internal blood loss is essential.

PALPATION

- Palpate carotid pulse

  Early in shock, tachycardia may indicate a strong positive chronotropic (rate) effect of circulating catecholamines. A positive inotropic effect (force of contraction) may be evidenced by a bounding carotid pulse.

- Palpate peripheral pulses

  Weak and thready pulses are caused by a decreased stroke volume as a result of hypovolemia.

- Palpate skin temperature and degree of diaphoresis

Diagnostic Procedures

Refer to Chapter 3, Initial Assessment, for frequently-ordered radiographic and laboratory studies. Additional studies for patients in shock are listed below.

RADIOGRAPHIC STUDIES

- Chest radiograph to determine the presence of a hemothorax or pneumothorax and to assess the size of the mediastinum. Widening of the mediastinum may indicate injury to the aorta or other mediastinal vessels.

- Pelvis radiograph to locate fractures, which may result in significant blood loss due to disruption of pelvic veins.

- Femur radiograph, if fracture is suspected

LABORATORY STUDIES

- Serum blood sample for typing

  Baseline levels of the patient's hemoglobin, hematocrit, serum osmolarity, electrolytes, BUN, creatinine, and serum lactate should be obtained.

- Urinalysis including specific gravity

- Arterial pH, PaO_2 and $PaCO_2$

  Decreasing pH reveals a worsening of the cellular oxygen debt as metabolic acidosis develops due to anaerobic metabolism and lactic acid production. An elevated $PaCO_2$ (normal = 35 to 45 mmHg, 4.7 to 6.0 KPa) indicates respiratory acidosis and impaired ventilation of the alveoli. A low PaO_2 (normal = 100 mmHg, 13.3 KPa) indicates hypoxia.

Nursing Diagnoses and Outcome Identification

In addition to the nursing diagnoses outlined in Chapter 3, Initial Assessment, the following nursing diagnoses are potential problems for the patient in shock. Once a patient has been assessed, diagnoses can be defined as either actual or risk. An actual nursing diagnosis is one derived from a decision based on the patient's presenting signs and symptoms. A risk nursing diagnosis is a judgment the nurse makes based on a particular patient's risk and potential for developing certain problems.

POSSIBLE NURSING DIAGNOSES AND EXPECTED OUTCOMES

Nursing Diagnosis	Expected Outcome

Gas exchange, impaired related to:
• Ineffective breathing pattern: deterioration of ventilatory efforts
• Ineffective airway clearance
• Aspiration
• Impaired tissue perfusion, secondary to acute blood loss
	The patient will experience adequate gas exchange as evidenced by:
	• ABG values within normal limits:
	  ■ PaO_2 80 - 100 mmHg (10.0 - 13.3 KPa)
	  ■ SaO_2 >95%
	  ■ $PaCO_2$ 35 - 45 mmHg (4.7 - 6.0 KPa)
	  ■ pH between 7.35 - 7.45
	• Skin normal color, warm, and dry
	• Improved level of consciousness
	• Regular rate, depth, and pattern of breathing
	• Symmetric, bilateral chest expansion
	• Clear and equal bilateral breath sounds

Fluid volume deficit related to: • Hemorrhage • Fluid shifts • Alteration in capillary permeability • Alteration in vascular tone • Myocardial compromise	The patient will have an effective circulating volume as evidenced by: • Stable vital signs appropriate for developmental age • Urinary output of 1 ml/kg/hr • Strong, palpable peripheral pulses • Improved level of consciousness • Skin normal color, warm, and dry • Maintains HCT = 30 ml/dl or Hgb = 12 - 14 g/dl or greater • CVP reading of 5 - 10 cm H_2O • External hemorrhage is controlled
Cardiac output, decreased related to: • Decreased venous return secondary to acute blood loss or massive peripheral vasodilation	The patient will maintain adequate circulatory function as evidenced by: • Strong, palpable peripheral pulses • Apical pulse rate of 60 - 100 beats/minute • Normal heart tones • ECG with normal sinus rhythm, absence of dysrhythmias • Absence of jugular vein distension, deviated trachea • Skin normal color, warm, dry • Improved level of consciousness • CVP reading 5 - 10 cm H_2O • Urinary output of 1 ml/kg/hr
Hypothermia related to: • Rapid infusion of intravenous fluids • Decreased tissue perfusion • Exposure	The patient will maintain a normal core body temperature as evidenced by: • Core temperature measurement of 36° - 37.5°C (98° - 99.5°F) • Absence of shivering, cool skin, pallor • Skin normal color, warm, and dry

90

Planning and Implementation

Refer to Chapter 3, Initial Assessment, for a description of the specific nursing interventions for patients with compromises to airway, breathing, and/or circulation.

- Administer oxygen via a nonrebreather mask at a flow rate sufficient to keep the reservoir bag inflated; usually requires 12 to 15 L/minute.

  Oxygen is essential for the patient in shock. Oxygen via a nonrebreather mask can deliver up to 90% O_2 with a snug fit of the mask around the nose and mouth. For the patient who requires bag-to-mask or bag-to-tube ventilation, oxygen must be delivered via a device with an appropriate oxygen reservoir.

- Control any uncontrolled external bleeding

  Rapid control of bleeding is essential to prevent the progression of shock. Control major external bleeding by direct pressure.

- Prepare for surgery if control of internal bleeding is indicated

  Prepare the patient for immediate transportation to surgery after appropriate interventions for stabilization have been instituted.

- Initiate intravenous replacement of fluids

  Prior to the administration of blood or colloid solutions, initiate an isotonic, electrolyte-based, crystalloid solution via two large-bore, 14- or 16-gauge intravenous catheters.[4-5] Lactated Ringer's solution is a "near-physiologic" solution that is similar to the electrolyte content of plasma.[6] Normal saline (0.9%) is considered the second fluid of choice for a hypovolemic patient.[4] Normal saline is not considered as physiologic as lactated Ringer's solution because it contains more sodium and chloride than the body's own extracellular fluid.

  An initial bolus of 1 to 2 liters of lactated Ringer's solution may be given to adult patients as rapidly as possible.[4] The use of large-bore, short catheters, short intravenous tubing, and a rapid infusor device will contribute to rapid infusion. It is important to observe the patient's response to the bolus by measuring blood pressure and heart rate as well as listening to breath sounds.

- Initiate blood replacement

  Patients who do not adequately respond to a crystalloid fluid bolus are potential candidates for blood volume replacement.

  - Type-specific and crossmatched blood

    Type-specific and crossmatched blood is the ideal but may take too long to procure.

  - Type-specific blood

    Type-specific blood is usually available within minutes from blood banks.

  - Type O-negative packed cells

    O-negative is considered the universal donor since there are no aggluntinogens (antigens) on the red blood cells of O-negative blood to possibly react with any agglutinins (antibodies) in the recipient's plasma. Rh negative blood has no type D antigen. O-negative blood is an option to consider.

  - O-positive blood

    If O-negative blood is scarce, type O-positive blood is sometimes used for male patients since the risk of their plasma having anti-D antibodies is remote (85% of white population and 95% of black population is Rh positive). Avoid O-positive blood in premenopausal women whose blood type is unknown.

  - When packed cells are given, consider replacement of clotting factors for patients receiving large volumes, e.g., 10 units in a 70 kg person. Therefore, fresh frozen plasma and platelets are administered.

  - Administer blood through a filtering device designed to trap any clots. Use macropore (160 microns) not micropore filters.

  - Infuse blood through an intravenous line using normal saline.

  - Warm fluids to 39°C (102.2°F) to prevent hypothermia.[4]

- Consider autotransfusion for a patient with a hemothorax

- Continue or consider application of a pneumatic antishock garment (PASG)

  - The controversial PASG may already have been applied by prehospital personnel. Indications are hypotension from hypovolemia due to abdominal or pelvic trauma and for splinting of suspected pelvic fractures. Transport time is an important determining factor for PASG application in the field. The PASG is recommended for short-term use only[7] and, in fact, some experts recommend that it never be used.[8,9]

  - Pulmonary edema, suspected ruptured diaphragm, and compromised left ventricular function are contraindications.[4] Under certain circumstances, do not inflate the abdominal section, i.e., pregnancy or abdominal evisceration.

  - The PASG causes an increase in tissue pressure with a subsequent increase in total peripheral resistance in those vessels it surrounds. It also attempts to improve blood flow to the brain, heart, and lungs, and increases afterload in an effort to restore blood pressure.[7]

  - Any compromise of respiratory or cardiac function during the inflation of the PASG should be considered a reason to abandon its use.

  - Once the blood pressure is stabilized by the replacement of volume, the PASG may be carefully removed by segmental deflation. Initially, the abdominal compartment is gradually deflated. The blood pressure must be monitored simultaneously. A drop of 5 mmHg is considered significant. Deflation is then halted until the blood pressure is again stabilized through the administration of intravenous fluid. Once the abdominal compartment is fully deflated, then one leg compartment is deflated. If the blood pressure is maintained or returns to the predeflation measure, the other leg can be deflated.

- Position patient with legs elevated

  The modified Trendelenburg position may be advantageous if spinal cord or head injuries are not suspected. In this position, the patient remains supine with the legs elevated. The elevation assists venous return to the right atrium, but abdominal viscera remain in their normal position. As the patient's blood pressure is stabilized, the legs may be lowered gradually while monitoring the blood pressure for changes.

93

- Insert a gastric tube

  Gastric distension may lead to vomiting and/or aspiration. Distension may stimulate the vagus nerve, which could lead to bradycardia. Insertion of a gastric tube provides for evacuation of stomach contents, relieves gastric distention, and prevents vagal stimulation. After insertion of the tube, test the aspirated contents for the presence of blood.

- Insert an indwelling urinary catheter

  A urinary catheter provides for bladder drainage, allows for frequent monitoring of urinary output, and is necessary for any shock patient who is being prepared for surgery. Suspected injury to the urethra is a contraindication to catheterization through the urethra.

- Attach leads and monitor the patient's cardiac rate and rhythm

  Electrocardiographic (ECG) changes, other than sinus tachycardia, may not be apparent until very late in the course of hypovolemic shock. However, a patient with compromised coronary artery circulation may demonstrate ST changes in response to ischemia.

- Attach a pulse oximeter, if available, to monitor the patient's arterial oxygen saturation

  Pulse oximetry readings may be inaccurate if the patient has peripheral vasoconstriction.

Evaluation and Ongoing Assessment

Refer to Chapter 3, Initial Assessment, for a description of the ongoing evaluation of the patient's airway, effectiveness of breathing, and circulation. Additional evaluations include:

- Monitoring urinary output for response to fluid resuscitation and for overall renal function. The ability of the kidneys to concentrate urine is a reflection of the patient's overall perfusion status.

- Collaborating with other trauma team members as diagnostic studies and physical assessment identify the cause and source of hemorrhage

- Monitoring temperature to determine hypothermia. Hypothermia in the patient with hemorrhagic shock has serious sequelae including:

  - Decreased tissue extraction of oxygen from hemoglobin.

  - Impaired cardiac contractility and decreased cardiac output.

  - Coagulopathies due to disruption of cellular enzymatic function, platelet disturbances, and increased fibrinolysis.

The combination of hypothermia, coagulopathy, and metabolic acidosis predisposes the patient to severe consequences.

ADDITIONAL SHOCK SYNDROMES

Refer to "Nursing Care of the Patient in Hypovolemic Shock" for a description of the phases of the trauma nursing process.

Cardiogenic Shock

Cardiogenic shock due to trauma is very rare. Contusions to the myocardium may lead to decreased myocardial contractility and some degree of cardiogenic shock. Assess the trauma patient for signs of a myocardial infarction (a more common underlying reason for cardiogenic shock), which may have preceded or followed a traumatic event. Myocardial contusion will be discussed in detail in Chapter 6, Thoracic and Neck Trauma.

Obstructive Shock

The most common injuries that lead to obstructive shock are cardiac tamponade and a tension pneumothorax. Signs, symptoms, and interventions for these two injuries are discussed in Chapter 6, Thoracic and Neck Trauma.

Neurogenic Shock

Neurogenic shock is due to decreased sympathetic tone, which leads to dilation of both arterial and venous systems and cardiodeceleration. The etiology of neurogenic shock can either be trauma-related or due to reactions to spinal anesthesia, insulin shock, damage to the vasomotor center in the medulla, or certain drug overdoses. Neurogenic shock can be a consequence of cervical or high thoracic spinal cord injury.[11]

Signs and Symptoms

- Hypotension

  Due to peripheral vasodilation and poor distribution of blood volume resulting in a decrease in central circulation and an increase in the peripheral distribution, especially in the venous system.

- Warm and dry skin

  Due to peripheral vasodilation and the inability of the patient to sweat.

- Bradycardia

  Due to the loss of sympathetic stimulation of the heart rate resulting in parasympathetic (vagal) control of the heart rate.

- Loss of heat control

  The patient is susceptible to hypothermia due to loss of hypothalamic influence on the control of the autonomic nervous system.

Interventions

- Monitor intravenous volume replacement. Since the patient is normovolemic, fluid overload must be avoided. The cause of hypotension may be related to hypovolemia from other injuries or neurogenic shock. Therefore, determining the patient's pulse rate is key to the differentiation between the two shock syndromes.

- Peripheral vasoconstrictors are contraindicated in a hypovolemic patient but may be considered in patients who present in neurogenic shock with no other injuries causing hypovolemia.

Neurogenic shock is discussed in Chapter 8, Spinal Cord and Vertebral Column Injuries.

SUMMARY

Shock is a syndrome resulting from inadequate perfusion of tissues leading to a decrease in the supply of oxygen and nutrients required to maintain the metabolic needs of the body. The four types of shock are hypovolemic, cardiogenic, obstructive, and distributive. Hypovolemic shock, the most common shock in trauma patients, results from an inadequate intravascular blood volume. The organs and certain structures of the body respond to shock in a compensatory fashion. If compensatory mechanisms fail and/or treatment is not initiated, organ, tissue, and cellular ischemia ensue. Adherence to the six phases of the trauma nursing process allows for an organized approach to the assessment and management of compromises to airway, breathing, and circulation.

REFERENCES

1. Guyton AC. *Textbook of Medical Physiology*. 8th ed. Philadelphia, Pa: WB Saunders Co; 1991.

2. Porth CM. *Pathophysiology Concepts of Altered States*. 4th ed. Philadelphia, Pa: JB Lippincott Co; 1994.

3. Weil MH, Rackow EC. Cardiovascular system failure and shock. In: Schwartz GR, Cayten CG, Mangelsen MA, Mayer TA, Hanke BK, eds. *Principles and Practice of Emergency Medicine*. 3rd ed. Philadelphia, Pa: Lea & Febiger; 1992:73-88.

4. American College of Surgeons Committee on Trauma. Shock. In: *Advanced Trauma Life Support® Course for Physicians (Instructor Manual)*. 5th ed. Chicago, Ill: Author; 1993:77-94.

5. Fantini GA, Shires GT. Management of shock. In: Moore EE, Mattox KL, Feliciano DV, eds. *Trauma*. 2nd ed. Norwalk, Conn: Appleton & Lange; 1991:147-164.

6. Metheny NM. Why worry about IV fluids? *Am J Nurs*. 1990:50-57.

7. McSwain NE. Pneumatic antishock garment: does it work? *Prehospital and Disaster Med*. 1989;4:42-44.

8. Mattox KL, Bickell W, Pepe PE, Burch J, Feliciano DV. Prospective MAST study in 911 patients. *J Trauma*. 1989;29:1104-1112.

9. Mattox KL. Blind faith, poor judgment and patient jeopardy. *Prehospital and Disaster Med*. 1989;4:39-41.

10. Cribari C, Mattox KL. Abdominal vascular complications. In: Mattox KL, ed. *Complications of Trauma*. New York, NY: Churchill Livingstone; 1994:503-520.

11. Mangiardi JR, Moser FG, Spitzer D, Bouzarth WF. Spinal injuries. In: Schwartz GR, Cayten CG, Mangelsen MA, Mayer TA, Hanke BK, eds. *Principles and Practice of Emergency Medicine*. 3rd ed. Philadelphia, Pa: Lea & Febiger; 1992:955-993.

CHAPTER FIVE

BRAIN AND CRANIOFACIAL TRAUMA

LECTURE BEGINS ON PAGE 106.

Preface

Prior to reading this chapter, it is strongly suggested that the learner read the following section entitled "Anatomy and Physiology." Specific anatomy and physiologic concepts are presented to enhance the learner's ability to correlate such concepts with specific injuries. This material related to anatomy and physiology will not be covered during lectures, nor will it be evaluated by testing. However, knowledge of normal anatomy and physiology serves as the foundation for understanding the anatomic derangements and pathophysiologic compromises that may ensue as a result of trauma.

ANATOMY

Scalp

The scalp consists of five layers of tissue. They are the skin, subcutaneous tissue, galea aponeurotica, areolar tissue, and periosteum. These layers provide a protective covering and may absorb some of the energy transferred during an injury event. The scalp is also highly vascular and, if lacerated or incised, may bleed profusely.

Skull

The bony skull, formed by the cranium and the face, provides protection to the contents of the cranial vault (see Figure 6). The temporal bone of the skull is thin and, therefore, more susceptible to fracture. If this bone is fractured and displaced, it can lead to intracranial bleeding as the jagged bone ends may lacerate the middle meningeal artery, which courses through a groove in the temporal bone. The surface of the base of the skull is rough and irregular.[1] When energy forces are applied to the head, the brain can move across this rough base producing contusions, lacerations, and shearing injuries.

The bony structures of the face help to protect the brain and underlying structures from injury. The immovable maxilla is located in the midface area. The mandible or lower jaw is one of the strongest bones of the body. The facial muscles covering the bones are responsible for facial movements. Mandibular muscles assist with the opening and closing of the jaw and mastication. Sinus cavities are located in the frontal and maxillary bones.

Figure 6
Views of Skull

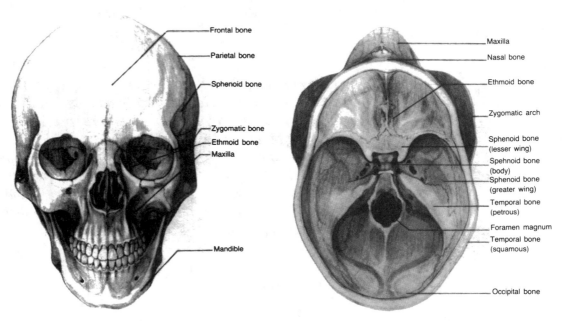

Anterior view of the skull   Superior view of the skull

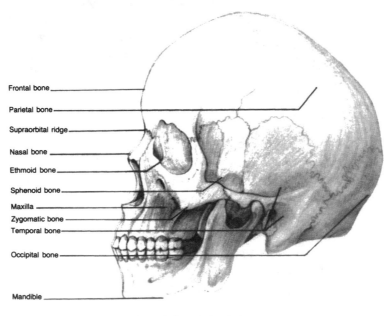

Lateral view of the skull

Intracranial Contents

Meninges

The meninges are three layers of connective tissue forming a protective covering for the brain and spinal cord (see Figure 7). These three layers are the dura mater, arachnoid membrane, and pia mater. The outermost layer, the dura mater, is close to the inner surface of the cranial bones. There are potential spaces both above (the epidural space) and below (the subdural space) the dural layer. The middle meningeal artery is located within the epidural space. Small bridging veins traverse the subdural space. The subarachnoid space is between the arachnoid membrane and the pia. Cerebrospinal fluid (CSF) is produced in the ventricles of the brain and circulates around the brain in the subarachnoid space and through the central canal of the spinal cord. The function of CSF is to cushion the brain and spinal cord.

Figure 7
Cerebral Meninges

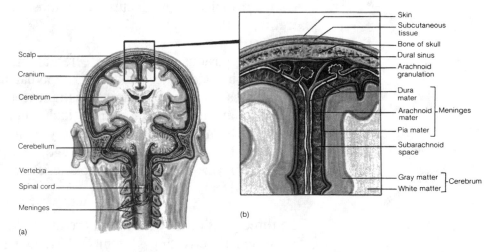

(Reprinted with permission from John W. Hole, Jr. *Human Anatomy and Physiology,* 6th ed. Copyright © 1993 Wm. C. Brown Communications, Inc., Dubuque, Iowa. Reprinted with permission of Times Mirror Higher Education Group, Inc., Dubuque, Iowa. All Rights Reserved.)

Cranial Compartments

The bones of the base of the skull form three hollow depressions termed fossae. They are the anterior, middle, and posterior fossae. Part of the dura mater extends from the occipital bone to near the center of the cranium forming the tentorium cerebelli. The tentorium divides the cranial cavity into supratentorial and infratentorial compartments. The supratentorial compartment contains the cerebral hemispheres in the anterior and middle fossae. The infratentorial compartment contains the medulla, pons, and cerebellum in the posterior fossa. The midbrain, the upper portion of the brainstem, and the oculomotor nerve (cranial nerve III) pass through an elongated gap in the tentorium.[1-5]

Brain (see Figure 8)

The two cerebral hemispheres are divided into frontal, parietal, temporal, and occipital lobes. These lobes are responsible for behavior, personality, and voluntary motor functions (frontal); sensory function (parietal); speech, auditory, and memory functions (temporal); and vision (occipital). Intellectual functions are processed within the cerebral cortex.

The diencephalon connects the cerebral hemispheres with the midbrain. It includes the thalamus, hypothalamus, subthalamus, and epithalamus. The hypothalamus has numerous key roles in hormonal regulation and metabolic functions including: temperature regulation; release of hormones from the pituitary gland and the adrenal cortex; emotional behaviors such as fear, rage, and pleasure; and activation of the sympathetic and parasympathetic functions of the autonomic nervous system.

The three parts of the brain stem are the midbrain, pons, and medulla. The reticular activating system (RAS), which originates in the midbrain and pons, is part of the system responsible for consciousness or the "awake state." Stimulation of the RAS, along with intact cerebral hemispheres, leads to consciousness. Conversely, a decrease in RAS stimulation results in a decreased level of consciousness. The vital cardiorespiratory centers that regulate respirations, blood pressure, and heart rate are located in the medulla and pons.

The cerebellum is composed of three lobes; two lateral hemispheres connected by a smaller third lobe. The cerebellum is in the posterior fossa and is responsible for activity coordination, movement, and balance.[1]

Figure 8
Brain Structures

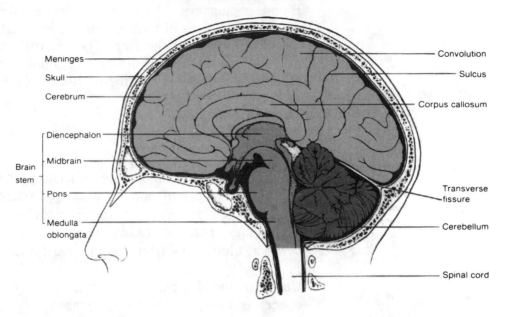

Cranial Nerves

There are 12 pairs of cranial nerves, of which nine (III - X, XII) have their origin (area of the brain where the nerve either exits or enters) in the brain stem. The olfactory nerve is actually a group of nerves within a fiber tract which connects the nasal mucosa to the olfactory bulb. The pair of optic nerves originate in the retina and are considered a fiber tract once they leave the optic chiasm. Millions of optic fibers travel to the occipital and temporal lobes of the cerebrum. Cranial nerve XI has both a cranial and spinal component. The spinal component is derived from the first five or six cervical spinal nerves.

Of particular importance in craniofacial trauma are the: olfactory nerve (I), which is involved with the sense of smell; optic (II) with vision; oculomotor (III), trochlear (IV), and abducens (VI) with eye movements; trigeminal (V) with movement and sensation of the face; facial (VII) with movements of the face and taste sensation of the anterior two thirds of the tongue; and glossopharyngeal (IX) with sensation to the tongue and pharynx and motor function related to the pharynx, i.e., swallowing and gag reflex. Any of these cranial nerve functions can be altered by injury.

Blood Supply

Blood is supplied to the brain through the carotid and vertebral arteries. Branches of the internal and external carotid arteries provide the blood supply to the face. The external maxillary artery branches off the external carotid artery and supplies blood to the nasal area. Hemorrhage from any of these arteries can be life-threatening.[5,6]

PHYSIOLOGY

Because the brain cannot store either oxygen or glucose, it requires a continuous supply of both. It uses approximately 20% of the body's total oxygen supply and metabolizes glucose at a rate of 60 mg/minute. These nutrients are delivered to the brain via a steady cerebral blood flow from the internal carotid and vertebral arteries.

Cerebral blood flow is affected by oxygen and carbon dioxide concentrations in the blood. Decreased oxygen concentration causes an increase in both cerebral blood flow and volume. Increased levels of carbon dioxide, a potent vasodilator, result in subsequent dilation of cerebral vessels, increased blood flow, and increased volume. Decreased carbon dioxide levels cause vasoconstriction, decreased blood flow, and decreased volume.[2-4,7,8]

The brain occupies approximately 80% of the cranial vault, blood approximately 10%, and cerebrospinal fluid approximately 10%. These volumes are relatively fixed and together create a normal intracranial pressure (ICP) within the skull of 10 to 15 mmHg. Through compensatory mechanisms, small changes in the individual volumes can occur without adversely changing the constant total volume or affecting ICP. According to the Monro-Kellie hypothesis, as one volume expands, compensatory mechanisms cause one or both of the other two volumes to decrease.[3] This compensatory mechanism is limited as the skull is a rigid and unyielding structure. Once this limitation is reached, there may be a significant increase in ICP. Elevations in ICP may result in a decrease in cerebral blood flow and a subsequent decrease in cerebral perfusion.

Adequate cerebral blood flow is dependent on the cerebral perfusion pressure (CPP), which is the difference between the mean arterial pressure (MAP) and the intracranial pressure (ICP). This relationship is expressed as follows:

$$CPP = MAP \text{ minus } ICP$$

CPP = Cerebral Perfusion Pressure
MAP = Mean Arterial Pressure
ICP = Intracranial Pressure

A close relationship exists between cerebral blood flow and the cerebral perfusion pressure (CPP). Cerebral perfusion pressure is a reflection of the adequacy of *perfusion* to the brain. Cerebral blood flow is regulated through sensitive autoregulatory mechanisms located in the cerebral arterioles or resistance vessels. These mechanisms cause the arterioles to vasoconstrict and vasodilate with changes in arterial pressure and in response to the cellular needs of the brain tissue. Cerebral autoregulation maintains a constant cerebral blood flow and functions well as long as the systemic mean arterial pressure is within the range of 60 to 180 mmHg.[9]

If the CPP falls below 50 to 60 mmHg due to an elevated ICP above the mean arterial pressure, cerebral and brainstem ischemia results from compression of the cerebral arteries. This ischemia of the central nervous system initiates a central nervous system ischemic response termed the Cushing response. The Cushing response stimulates an increase in systolic blood pressure and a reflex bradycardia. The result is an increase in cerebral perfusion pressure and cerebral blood flow due to an increase in arterial blood pressure.[2-4,8]

BRAIN AND CRANIOFACIAL TRAUMA

OBJECTIVES

Upon completion of this chapter/lecture, the learner should be able to:

1. Identify the common mechanisms of injury associated with brain and craniofacial injuries.
2. Analyze the pathophysiologic changes as a basis for signs and symptoms.
3. Discuss the nursing assessment of patients with brain and craniofacial injuries.
4. Based on the assessment data, identify appropriate nursing diagnoses and expected outcomes.
5. Plan appropriate interventions for patients with brain and craniofacial injuries.
6. Evaluate the effectiveness of nursing interventions for patients with brain and craniofacial injuries.

INTRODUCTION

Epidemiology

Brain injury is the leading cause of death related to trauma. There are more than 70,000 moderate to severe head injuries each year in the United States.[10] Head injury is responsible for nearly one half of all deaths from motor vehicle crashes.[11] Because the primary mechanism associated with brain and craniofacial injury is a motor vehicle crash, the majority of the population are at risk for injury during their life spans. However, there are certain groups of individuals who practice behaviors that place them at risk for sustaining brain or craniofacial injuries. These behaviors include:

- Acute or chronic alcohol abuse

- Use of mind-altering drugs

- Incorrect or nonuse of motor vehicle safety restraint systems[12]

- Nonuse of safety helmets when riding motorcycles or bicycles[13,14]

- Participating in team sports without protective equipment[15]

Mechanisms of Injury and Biomechanics

Motor vehicle crashes are the most common mechanism of injury associated with brain and craniofacial trauma. Falls, intentional assaults, use of firearms, and injuries occurring in recreational and sports activities also contribute to the incidence of brain and craniofacial trauma. The legislated use of safety restraints and, in some states, motorcycle helmets, has contributed to a decline in the severity of facial injuries.[13,14] Sports that involve high-speed objects are especially associated with facial trauma.[15]

The acceleration and deceleration forces responsible for trauma to the head frequently result in damage to the intracranial contents. When the head strikes a solid object, the sudden deceleration force may result in bony deformity and injury to cranial contents. A pressure wave is generated at the point of impact, travels across the cranial contents, and eventually dissipates. This initial impact and pressure wave may tear tissue within the cranial vault and result in injury on the side opposite the point of impact. The injury that may result on the same side of the impact is a coup injury, and if there is injury on the opposite side, it is a contrecoup injury.[2,7]

Types of Injuries

Injuries to the brain and craniofacial area may cause damage to the rigid cranial skull, the brain, facial bones, soft tissues, vascular structures, and/or cranial nerves. Blunt brain and craniofacial injuries are associated with acceleration, deceleration forces, or both. When forces are applied, shearing, tensile, and compressive stresses may lead to hemorrhage, hematomas, and/or contusions. As the force is applied, the brain may also be injured as it moves across the rough base of the cranial vault.

The sinus cavities of the frontal and maxillary bones are frequently injured with blunt facial trauma. The cavities and bony structures can collapse at the moment of injury and dissipate energy.

Penetrating brain and craniofacial injuries are associated with a high mortality rate. Missile type wounds may occur from rifles, handguns, semiautomatic weapons, or exploding objects, e.g., fireworks. Through-and-through penetrating wounds to the brain continue to carry a high mortality rate.[16]

Usual Concurrent Injuries

Patients who have sustained either brain and/or craniofacial injuries are at high risk for concomitant injury to the cervical spine. Therefore, **ALL** patients with a brain or craniofacial injury are assumed to have cervical spine injury until proven otherwise.[3,16,17] Of all patients who sustain major brain or craniofacial injury, 30% have at least one additional significant injury to another system.[3,6,17]

Injury to the airway can occur concurrently with facial injury. Injury to certain cranial nerves may alter the patient's appearance. Injuries to the face may be associated with severe hemorrhage from the branches of the internal and external carotid arteries and the external maxillary artery that supplies blood flow to the nasal area.

PATHOPHYSIOLOGY AS A BASIS FOR SIGNS AND SYMPTOMS

Injury to the brain leads to a primary injury, e.g., fractured skull, epidural hematoma, or intracerebral contusion. In addition to the primary injury, secondary brain injury may result from hypoxemia, cerebral edema, hypercarbia, hypotension, and a rise in intracranial pressure. Secondary injuries may diminish the effectiveness of autoregulatory and compensatory mechanisms of the brain.[3]

Airway Obstruction

Airway obstruction due to oral debris, accumulation of secretions, bleeding, facial edema, facial fractures, or occlusion by the tongue is a major cause of death in patients with brain or craniofacial trauma.

Increased Intracranial Pressure (ICP)

Adequate cerebral blood flow is dependent on the cerebral perfusion pressure (CPP), which is the difference between the mean arterial pressure (MAP) and the intracranial pressure (ICP). This relationship is expressed as follows:

$$CPP = MAP \text{ minus } ICP$$

CPP = Cerebral Perfusion Pressure
MAP = Mean Arterial Pressure
ICP = Intracranial Pressure

A close relationship exists between cerebral blood flow and the cerebral perfusion pressure (CPP). Cerebral perfusion pressure is a reflection of the adequacy of *perfusion* to the brain. Cerebral blood flow is a function of cerebral perfusion pressure (CPP) and the brain's ability to autoregulate cerebral blood vessels. Normally, autoregulation causes vasoconstriction or vasodilation, depending on the brain's changing metabolic needs.

Intracranial pressure is a reflection of three volumes: brain, cerebrospinal fluid, and blood. The normal ICP is approximately 10 to 15 mmHg. Injury to the brain may lead to a failure of the auto-regulatory mechanisms. This failure leads to cerebral vasodilation, increased blood volume in the brain, and cerebral engorgement. These mechanisms also contribute to the development of cerebral edema. The increase in volume of both the brain and blood causes a rise in ICP.

As the ICP rises, the CPP decreases, leading to cerebral ischemia and the potential for hypoxia and lethal secondary insults.[3] Cerebral ischemia can lead to an increased concentration of carbon dioxide and decreased concentration of oxygen in cerebral vessels. Carbon dioxide vasodilates cerebral blood vessels, leading to an increase in blood volume and contributing to the further increase in ICP. Increasing ICP produces different signs and symptoms, depending on the stage of increased pressure.

Early signs and symptoms:

- Headache

- Nausea and vomiting

- Amnesia for events before the injury and/or after the injury

- Altered level of consciousness

- Changes in speech, drowsiness, agitation, restlessness, and/or loss of judgment

Late signs:

- Dilated, nonreactive pupil due to pressure on the oculomotor nerve

- Unresponsiveness to verbal or painful stimuli

- Abnormal posturing patterns, e.g., flexion, extension, or flaccidity

- Increased systolic blood pressure resulting in a widening pulse pressure (hypotension is rarely caused by an isolated head injury)

- Decreased pulse rate

- Changes in respiratory rate and pattern

The last three signs are known as the Cushing response or reflex.[18]

Herniation Syndromes

As a result of increased ICP, portions of the brain can be displaced or herniate. Two types of supratentorial herniation are classified by the site of herniation (see Figure 9).

- Central or transtentorial herniation – A downward movement of the cerebral hemispheres with herniation of the diencephalon and midbrain through the elongated gap of the tentorium.

- Uncal herniation – Develops when the uncus (medial aspect of the temporal lobe) is displaced over the tentorium into the posterior fossa.

    - Leads to fixed, dilated pupil on the same side as the herniation due to compression of the oculomotor nerve.

    - Most common of the two types of herniation syndromes in the trauma patient.

Pressure on the pons and medulla result in blood pressure changes, cardiac deceleration, and asystole. If medullary/brain stem function has been altered due to severe brain injury, hypotension can occur as an event signifying imminent death.

Figure 9
Herniation Syndromes

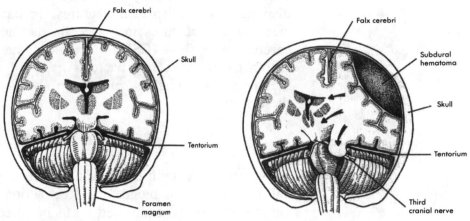

Normal relationship of intracranial structures

Uncal herniation syndrome

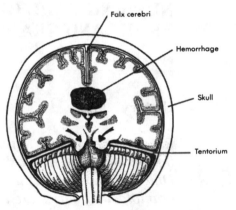

Central herniation syndrome

(Reprinted with permission from Pons PT. Head trauma. In: Rosen P, Barkin RM, Baker FJ, Braen GR, Dailey RH, Levy RL, eds. *Emergency Medicine: Concepts and Clinical Practice*. 3rd ed. St. Louis, Mo: Mosby-Year Book; 1992:340-341.)

Cerebrospinal Fluid Leakage

Disruption of the bony structures of the skull can result in either displaced or nondisplaced fractures. Fractures of the basilar skull or craniofacial structures may lacerate the dura, creating a passage for cerebrospinal fluid (CSF) either from the nose or ear. A potential entrance for invading bacteria is produced. Infections such as meningitis, encephalitis, or a brain abscess may be complications of these fractures.

Scalp and Facial Bleeding

Facial and scalp injuries bleed profusely due to their highly vascular nature and lack of blood vessel retraction. The bleeding is usually venous and can be controlled by using direct pressure. Disruption of the nasal bones can result in active bleeding from vessels and excessive epistaxis. These vessels can be lacerated through direct blunt forces or incised by fractured bones or other penetrating forces.[5,6,19]

NURSING CARE OF PATIENTS WITH BRAIN AND CRANIOFACIAL INJURY

Assessment

History

Refer to Chapter 3, Initial Assessment, for a description of general information that should be collected regarding every trauma victim. Only pertinent questions specific to patients with brain and craniofacial injuries are described below.

- What are the patient's complaints?

    - Headache, vomiting, or changes in memory are important early signs of increasing intracranial pressure.

    - Patients with facial injuries may complain of pain, facial sensory and/or motor disturbances, or dyspnea.

- Was there any loss of consciousness following the injury, and if so, for how long?

- Does the patient have any amnesia for the injury event?

- Have drugs or alcohol recently been used that may affect the level of consciousness?

- Does the patient have any previous neurological deficits or seizure history?

Physical Assessment

Refer to Chapter 3, Initial Assessment, for a description of the assessment of the patient's airway, and effectiveness of breathing, and circulation.

INSPECTION

- Assess the airway for obstruction, secretions, and foreign debris

  The airway can be compromised by:

  - Decreased level of consciousness and inability to keep the tongue from occluding the airway

  - Swelling or bleeding from oral or facial lacerations

  - Inability to open or close the jaw due to midface or mandibular fractures

- Observe respiratory rate and pattern

- Determine the level of consciousness using the Glasgow Coma Scale (GCS) (see Table 6)

  The initial GCS provides a baseline score and, through repeated assessments, determines whether the patient's neurological status is improving or deteriorating.

  - Eye opening response is measured by observing whether the patient opens eyes:

    - Spontaneously

    - In response to voice

    - In response to pain

    - Not at all

■ Verbal response is measured by the patient's response to questions. The response is characterized as:

  ◆ Oriented

  ◆ Confused but disoriented

  ◆ Inappropriate but comprehensible

  ◆ Incomprehensible sounds

  ◆ No verbal response

■ Motor response is measured by the patient's response to verbal or painful stimuli. Direct the patient to move an extremity. If the patient does not respond to verbal directions, painful stimuli should be applied, such as applying pressure to the patient's nailbeds or sternum. The response is characterized as:

  ◆ Localizes painful stimuli (pushing away of the stimuli)

  ◆ Withdrawal from stimuli

  ◆ Flexion

  ◆ Extension

  ◆ No movement or posturing

● Assess pupils for size, shape, equality, and reactivity to light

  ■ A unilaterally fixed and dilated pupil may indicate oculomotor nerve compression from increased intracranial pressure and/or herniation syndrome.

  ■ Bilateral fixed and pinpoint pupils may indicate pontine injury or lesion.

  ■ Use of alcohol or drugs can produce bilateral abnormal pupillary reactions leading to either pinpoint or dilated pupils.

● Observe for abnormal posturing patterns, e.g., flexion, extension, or flaccidity

114

- Inspect the craniofacial area for ecchymosis or contusions. Basilar skull fractures can be accompanied by bleeding into the three fossae, producing ecchymosis. The ecchymosis may not be present until several hours after injury.

  - Periorbital ecchymosis or raccoon's eyes indicates an anterior fossa fracture

  - Mastoid process ecchymosis or Battle's sign indicates a posterior fossa fracture

  - Blood behind the tympanic membrane may indicate a middle fossa fracture

- Inspect the nose and ears for drainage

  - If drainage is present and not mixed with blood, test fluid with chemical reagent strip. The presence of glucose indicates the drainage is CSF.

  - If drainage is present and mixed with blood (pink-tinged or red), test fluid by placing a drop of the fluid on linen or gauze. If a light outer ring forms around the dark inner ring (positive halo sign), the drainage contains CSF.

- Assess extraocular movements (EOMs) to test function of cranial nerves III, IV, and VI (see Figure 10)

  - The ability to perform EOMs indicates a functioning brainstem.

  - Limitation in range of ocular motion may indicate an orbital rim fracture with entrapment or paralysis of either nerve or muscle.

Figure 10
Eye Muscles and Function

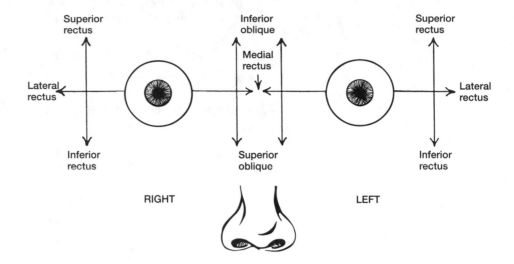

(Reprinted with permission from Waxman S, de Groot J, ed. In: Cranial nerves and pathways. *Correlative Neuroanatomy*. 22nd ed. Norwalk, Conn: Appleton & Lange; 1995:112.)

- Assess occlusion of the mandible and maxilla

    - Malocclusion or an inability to open and close the mouth is highly indicative of a maxillary or mandibular fracture.

PALPATION

- Palpate the craniofacial area for:

    - Point tenderness

    - Depressions or deformities

    - Hematomas

- Assess facial sensory function

    Craniofacial fractures can impinge on the infraorbital nerve causing numbness of the inferior eyelid, lateral nose, cheek, or upper lip on the affected side.

- Assess all four extremities:

    - Motor function and muscle strength

    - Sensory function

Diagnostic Procedures

Refer to Chapter 3, Initial Assessment, for frequently-ordered radiographic and laboratory studies. Additional studies for patients with brain and craniofacial trauma are listed below.

RADIOGRAPHIC STUDIES

- CT scan[3,4,20]

  - Patient movement may produce artifact and lead to an inaccurate CT reading.

  - Patients who are sedated or have received paralytic medications must be closely monitored during a CT procedure.[21]

  - May be indicated for complex facial fractures

- Skull series

  Not routinely ordered, especially if CT scan is available. If CT scan is unavailable, skull radiographs may be utilized to evaluate penetrating wounds to the head or suspected depressed skull fractures.

- Facial radiographs

- Magnetic Resonance Imaging (MRI)

Nursing Diagnoses and Outcome Identification

The following nursing diagnoses are potential problems for the patient with brain and craniofacial injuries. Once a patient has been assessed, diagnoses can be defined as either actual or risk. An actual nursing diagnosis is one derived from a decision based on the patient's presenting signs and symptoms. A risk nursing diagnosis is a judgment the nurse makes based on a particular patient's risk and potential for developing certain problems.

POSSIBLE NURSING DIAGNOSES AND EXPECTED OUTCOMES	
Nursing Diagnosis	**Expected Outcome**
Airway clearance, ineffective related to: • Pain • Decreased level of consciousness • Secretions and debris in airway • Soft tissue edema	The patient will maintain a patent airway as evidenced by: • Clear bilateral breath sounds • Regular rate, depth, and pattern of breathing • Effective cough reflex • Absence of pain with coughing • Appropriate use of splinting techniques with coughing

Aspiration, risk related to:
• Reduced level of consciousness secondary to injury, concomitant substance abuse
• Impaired cough and/or gag reflex
• Structural defect to head, face, or neck
• Facial and/or neck soft tissue edema
• Secretions and debris in airway
	The patient will not experience aspiration as evidenced by:
	• A patent airway
	• Clear and equal bilateral breath sounds
	• Regular rate, depth, and pattern of breathing
	• ABG values within normal limits:
	  ▪ PaO_2 80 - 100 mmHg (10.0 - 13.3 KPa)
	  ▪ SaO_2 >95%
	  ▪ $PaCO_2$ 35 - 45 mmHg (4.7 - 6.0 KPa)
	  ▪ pH between 7.35 - 7.45
	• Clear CXR without evidence of infiltrates
	• Ability to handle secretions independently

Gas exchange, impaired related to:
• Deterioration of ventilatory efforts secondary to acute brain injury
• Aspiration
• Shock
	The patient will experience adequate gas exchange as evidenced by:
	• ABG values within normal limits:
	  ▪ PaO_2 80 - 100 mmHg (10.0 - 13.3 KPa)
	  ▪ SaO_2 >95%
	  ▪ $PaCO_2$ 35 - 45 mmHg (4.7 - 6.0 KPa)
	  ▪ pH between 7.35 - 7.45
	• Skin normal color, warm, and dry
	• Improved level of consciousness
	• Regular rate, depth, and pattern of breathing

POSSIBLE NURSING DIAGNOSES AND EXPECTED OUTCOMES

Nursing Diagnosis	Expected Outcome

Tissue perfusion, altered cerebral related to:
• Cerebral edema, swelling, and expanding hematomas secondary to acute head injury
• Decreased cerebral perfusion secondary to hypoxemia and hypercarbia
	The patient will have optimal cerebral tissue perfusion as evidenced by:
	• GCS Score = 14 - 15 (spontaneous eye opening, obeys verbal commands, oriented to person, place, time, and purpose)
	• Vital signs within normal limits for developmental age: Absence of vital sign abnormalities, including hypertension, bradycardia, respiratory irregularities or increase in pulse pressure
	• Normal pupil size, shape, and reactivity to light
	• Absence of signs and symptoms of increased intracranial pressure: headache, vomiting, lethargy, restlessness, change in orientation or consciousness
	• ABG values within normal limits:
	  ■ PaO_2 80 - 100 mmHg (10.0 - 13.3 KPa)
	  ■ SaO_2 >95%
	  ■ $PaCo_2$ 35 - 45 mmHg (4.7 - 6.0 KPa)
	  ■ pH between 7.35 - 7.45
	• Ability for neck to maintain proper neutral alignment
	• Absence of, or quickly controlled, seizure activity

Injury, risk related to: • Increased intracranial pressure • Uncontrolled tonic/clonic movement • Altered sensorium secondary to head/facial injury • Visual field, motor, or perception deficits	The patient will be free from injury as evidenced by: • Patient will be seizure-free or seizures will be controlled rapidly once seizure activity evident • Absence of signs of injury such as bruises, broken teeth, or mucosal tears • Regains consciousness quickly following seizure activity • Airway patency is maintained • Identifies safety measures to prevent injury • Requests assistance when needed
Hyperthermia, risk related to: • Brain injury	The patient will maintain a normal core body temperature as evidenced by: • Core temperature measurement of 36° - 37.5°C (98° - 99.5°F) • Absence of shivering • Skin normal color, warm, and dry

POSSIBLE NURSING DIAGNOSES AND EXPECTED OUTCOMES	
Nursing Diagnosis	**Expected Outcome**
Infection, risk related to: • Contamination of wounds from accident or instrumentation • Prolonged immobility • Stress • Break in aseptic technique • Invasive procedures and devices	The patient will be free from infection as evidenced by: • Core temperature measurement of 36° - 37.5°C (98° - 99.5°F) • Absence of systematic signs of infection: fever, tachypnea, tachycardia • Wounds free from redness, swelling, purulent drainage, or odor • Urinary output 1 ml/kg/hr • WBC count within normal limits • Normal level of consciousness

Planning and Implementation

Refer to Chapter 3, Initial Assessment, for a description of the specific nursing interventions for patients with compromises to airway, breathing, and/or circulation.

Brain

- Open and clear the airway

  Minimize or avoid stimulation of the gag reflex, which can produce a transient increase in ICP or may cause vomiting and subsequent aspiration.

- Administer oxygen via a nonrebreather mask at a flow rate sufficient to keep the reservoir bag inflated; usually requires 12 to 15 L/minute.

- Assist with endotracheal intubation

  - Especially if the GCS is less than 8 or the level of consciousness acutely decreases.[22]

  - Administer neuromuscular blocking agents, as prescribed, to assist with intubation[21] (see Appendix 4).

  - Hyperventilate to maintain $PaCO_2$ between 26 and 30 mmHg (3.5 - 4.0 KPa) with 100% oxygen via a bag-valve device with an attached reservoir. Hypocarbia causes cerebral vasoconstriction, decreased cerebral blood flow, and decreased ICP. A $PaCO_2$ above 45 mmHg (6.0 KPa) may cause cerebral vasodilation and increases in blood

120

volume and ICP. Avoid hyperventilating to a $PaCO_2$ less than 26 mmHg (3.5 KPa), which results in cerebral vasoconstriction, causing further cerebral ischemia and secondary brain injury.[23]

- Apply direct pressure to bleeding sources except over depressed skull fractures

- Cannulate two veins with large-bore, 14- or 16-gauge catheters, and initiate infusions of lactated Ringer's solution; flow rate to be determined by patient's hemodynamic status.

  The goal of fluid support is to maintain hemodynamic stability without overhydration. Even brief periods of hypotension are to be avoided due to the resulting effect of decreased cerebral perfusion and subsequent secondary brain injury.[24,25] Research has investigated the use of hypertonic saline solution (3 to 5%) to maintain normovolemia and normotension without infusing large volumes of fluid.[25-27]

- Insert an orogastric or nasogastric tube. An orogastric tube should be inserted if a basilar skull fracture or severe midface fractures are suspected.[22]

- Position the patient as guided by institutional protocols. Elevation of the patient's head to decrease ICP is controversial. Some researchers believe an elevated head position reduces ICP, yet others have suggested it may also reduce CPP.[3]

  Position the head midline to facilitate venous drainage. Rotation of the head can compress the veins in the neck and result in both venous engorgement and decreased drainage from the brain.[28]

- Prepare for insertion of an ICP monitoring device and then monitor the ICP, as indicated

- Administer mannitol, as prescribed

  Mannitol, a hyperosmotic diuretic, decreases cerebral edema and ICP by pulling interstitial fluid into the intravascular space for eventual excretion by the kidneys. Although controversial, furosemide (Lasix), may be the diuretic utilized in some settings.

121

- Administer anticonvulsant medication, as prescribed

  Generally, anticonvulsant medication is administered only if the patient experiences seizure activity. Seizure activity is to be avoided as it increases both the cerebral metabolic rate and the ICP.

- Administer antipyretic medication, as prescribed, to treat hyperthermia. A hypothermia blanket may also be used.

  Hyperthermia may increase the cerebral metabolic rate and ICP. During the cooling process, avoid shivering as this activity further increases the cerebral metabolic rate and may precipitate a rise in ICP.

- Do not pack the ears or nose if a CSF leak is suspected

- Administer other medications, as prescribed

  These may include analgesics, sedatives, and naloxone (Narcan) if opiate use is suspected.

- Assist with wound repair for facial and scalp lacerations

- Administer antibiotics, as prescribed

  Patients with a basilar skull fracture may be given prophylactic antibiotics to prevent the development of meningitis.[3,6]

- Provide psychosocial support

- Prepare patient for operative intervention, hospital admission, or transfer, as indicated

Face

In addition to the above, interventions appropriate for patients with facial injuries are:

- Position the patient in a high-Fowler's position if no spinal injury is present

  Conscious patients instinctively seek their optimum position for airway maintenance. If at all possible, do not force a patient with severe facial trauma into a supine, flat position. High-Fowler's position may also decrease facial edema.

- Prepare for endotracheal intubation if necessary. Copious bleeding or secretions uncontrolled by suction may necessitate intubation to establish a patent airway. If intubation is unsuccessful, anticipate the need for a surgical airway.

- Apply ice compresses to the face to minimize edema

- Administer antibiotics, as prescribed

  Patients with open or penetrating wounds of the face, sinus, or oral areas may be given prophylactic antibiotics.

Evaluation and Ongoing Assessment

Refer to Chapter 3, Initial Assessment, for a description of the ongoing evaluation of the patient's airway, and effectiveness of breathing, and circulation. Additional evaluations include:

- Observing for increasing craniofacial edema

- Monitoring level of consciousness, using the GCS for trend analysis

- Monitoring pupillary changes

- Monitoring trends in blood pressure, pulse, respiratory rate, and patterns for signs of increasing ICP

- Monitoring motor and sensory function

- Evaluating response to fluid administration and/or diuretic therapy by frequently monitoring urinary output

SELECTED BRAIN AND CRANIOFACIAL INJURIES

Refer to "Nursing Care of Patients with Brain and Craniofacial Injuries" for a description of the phases of the trauma nursing process.

Concussion

"Classic cerebral concussion is a temporary, reversible neurologic deficiency associated with temporary (less than six hours) loss of consciousness."[24] However, mild concussion may occur without loss of consciousness, but with transient disruptions in other neurologic dysfunctions, as manifested by:

- Loss of memory

- Nausea and vomiting

- Confusion

- Dizziness

A concussion is a diffuse injury because there is no identifiable lesion. A concussion is a physiologic loss of the awake state due to transient disruption of the connection between the cerebral cortex and the brainstem center for wakefulness. Significant structural damage does not commonly occur, although patients may continue to experience memory problems.

Signs and Symptoms

- Brief loss of consciousness followed by drowsiness, restlessness, confusion, and/or possible periods of abnormal behavior

- Headache

- Nausea and vomiting

- Amnesia for events before the injury and/or after the injury

Interventions

Prepare for hospital admission if the loss of consciousness lasted for more than five minutes, or the patient's confusion does not clear.

Diffuse Axonal Injury (DAI)

The axon is the efferent nerve cell process that conducts the nerve impulse from one cell to the next. Acceleration and/or deceleration forces can produce shearing or tensile stresses causing damage to axons. DAI is manifested by diffuse, microscopic, hemorrhagic lesions. The brain stem and reticular activating system may be involved leading to prolonged coma. The overall mortality rate for DAI is 33%, but may be as high as 50% in severe cases.[22]

Signs and Symptoms

- Immediate unconsciousness. Coma may last from a few weeks to three months or longer.

- Hypertension with systolic blood pressure between 140 and 160 mmHg

- Hyperthermia with temperatures between 40 to 40.5C° (104 to 105°F). This may occur later during the hospital course.[3]

- Excessive sweating due to autonomic dysfunction

- Abnormal posturing (flexion, extension, or flaccidity)

Contusion

A contusion is a focal brain injury in which brain tissue is bruised and damaged in a local area. Contusions are often associated with a serious concussion and result in a depressed level of consciousness, confusion, or coma which may be prolonged. Contusions may occur at both the area of direct impact (coup) and/or on the opposite side (contrecoup) of impact. Patients may have multiple contusions. If the contused area and subsequent swelling are significant, a shift of the injured cerebral hemisphere to the opposite side can be visualized on CT scan. Delayed hemorrhage into the contused area may occur.

Signs and Symptoms

- Alteration in level of consciousness

- Unusual behavior may occur with frontal lobe contusions

- Abnormal posturing (flexion, extension, or flaccidity)

Epidural Hematoma

An epidural hematoma is a collection of blood between the skull and dura. It is frequently associated with fractures of the temporal or parietal skull that lacerate the middle meningeal artery. Since the bleeding is arterial, blood accumulates rapidly. The expanding hematoma can cause a rapid increase in ICP and lead to secondary brain injury. Epidural hematomas require immediate surgical intervention. Mortality rates associated with an epidural hematoma are related to the presence of coma prior to surgical intervention. The noncomatose patient with an epidural hematoma usually survives. However with coma, mortality rates can approach 20%.[22]

Signs and Symptoms

- Decreased level of consciousness that may follow one of two patterns:

    - Initial decreased level of consciousness, followed by a return of consciousness (lucid interval), and then followed by rapid unconsciousness. During the lucid phase, the patient is lethargic and frequently complains of a headache.

    - Persistent decreased level of consciousness.

- Hemiparesis or hemiplegia on the opposite side of the lesion, which may rapidly progress to abnormal posturing

- Unilateral fixed and dilated pupil on the same side as the hematoma

Subdural Hematoma

A subdural hematoma is a focal brain injury resulting from acceleration and/or deceleration forces. Subdural hematomas are usually venous in origin. A blow to the head can result in tearing of the bridging veins and bleeding into the subdural space. Additionally, injuries to tissue or vessels of the cerebral cortex may cause a subdural hematoma. These hematomas, unlike epidural hematomas, are not necessarily associated with a skull fracture. There is, in addition to the hematoma formation, an associated incidence of direct injury to underlying brain tissue. The formation of a subdural hematoma may be acute or chronic. Patients with acute subdural hematomas manifest symptoms within 48 hours of the injury event. Patients with chronic subdural hematomas manifest symptoms as long as two weeks after the injury event. Chronic subdural hematomas are frequently associated with minor injury in the elderly population and in chronic alcohol users due to fragility of bridging veins and coagulation defects. The mortality may be as high as 60%; with early surgical intervention, mortality has been reported as low as 30%.[22]

Signs and Symptoms

Onset varies depending on rapidity of hematoma formation and effect on neurologic function.

- Steady decline in level of consciousness

- Unilateral, fixed, dilated pupil on the same side as the hematoma

- Paresis on the opposite side of the hematoma

Intracerebral Hematoma

An intracerebral hematoma is a collection of blood greater than 5 ml within the brain tissue. This injury may be associated with acceleration and/or deceleration forces, which can produce either a blunt or penetrating injury. Increased local edema may lead to increased ICP.

Signs and Symptoms

Specific signs and symptoms are dependent on the location and size of the hematoma.

- Altered level of consciousness

- Progressive signs of increased ICP and herniation syndrome

Skull Fractures

Since significant force is required to fracture the skull, concurrent injury to the brain and cervical spine should always be considered. The three types of skull fractures are linear, depressed, and basilar. A linear skull fracture is a nondisplaced fracture of the cranium. It is of minor consequence unless the fracture site crosses an area where underlying vessels may be lacerated. A depressed skull fracture extends below the surface of the skull and can cause brain tissue compression and dural laceration. Basilar skull fractures are fractures of one or more of the five bones of the base of the skull. These fractures may accompany other injury to other intracranial structures, such as the brain, dura, or cranial nerves.

Signs and Symptoms: Depressed Skull Fracture

- Possible decreased level of consciousness

- Possible open fracture

- Palpable depression of skull over the fracture site

Interventions: Depressed Skull Fracture

Cover open fracture sites with a sterile dressing and do **NOT** apply pressure

Signs and Symptoms: Basilar Skull Fracture

- Headache

- Altered level of consciousness

- Periorbital ecchymosis (raccoon's eyes), mastoid ecchymosis (Battle's sign), or blood behind the tympanic membrane

- CSF rhinorrhea or CSF otorrhea

Interventions

- Do not pack or suction the nose or ears if a CSF leak is suspected

- Administer antibiotics, as prescribed

Mandibular Fracture

The mandible or lower jaw is a horseshoe-shaped bone attached to the cranium at the temporomandibular joints. The common fracture sites are the canine and third molar tooth area, the angle of the mandible, and the condyles.

Signs and Symptoms

- Malocclusion

- Inability to open the mouth (trismus)

- Pain especially on movement

- Facial asymmetry and a palpable step-off deformity

- Edema or hematoma formation at the fracture site

- Bloody and/or ruptured tympanic membrane[19]

- Anesthesia of the lower lip

Interventions

- Monitor for the development of airway obstruction

- Assist with repair of oral lacerations, as indicated

- Prepare patient for operative intervention, hospital admission, or transfer for definitive stabilization of the fracture, as indicated.

  The most common methods of operative treatment are intermaxillary wiring and the application of stabilizing arch bars. More complex fractures are treated by open reduction and interosseous wiring.

Maxillary Fracture

Maxillary fractures are commonly classified according to the LeFort classification system (see Figure 11).

LeFort I: A transverse maxillary fracture, which occurs above the level of the teeth resulting in a separation of the teeth from the rest of the maxilla.

Signs and Symptoms: LeFort I

- Slight swelling of the maxillary area

- Possible lip lacerations or fractured teeth

- Independent movement of the maxilla from the rest of the face

- Malocclusion

Figure 11
LeFort Maxillary Fractures

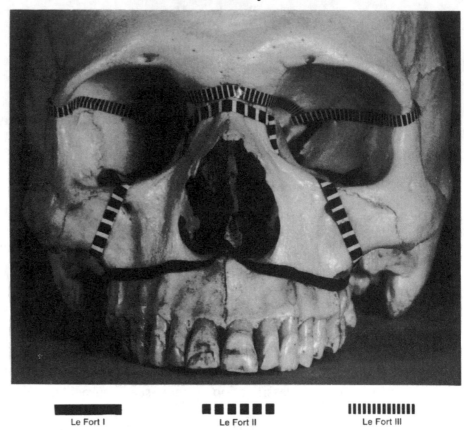

▬▬▬▬▬	■ ■ ■ ■ ■	▮▮▮▮▮▮▮▮▮▮
Le Fort I	Le Fort II	Le Fort III

(Reprinted with permission from Moore KL. The head. In: *Clinically Oriented Anatomy*. 3rd ed. Baltimore, Md: Williams & Wilkins; 1992:656.)

LeFort II: A pyramidal maxillary fracture involving the middle facial area. The apex of the fracture transverses the bridge of the nose. The two lateral fractures of the pyramid extend through the lacrimal bone of the face and ethmoid bone of the skull into the median portion of both orbits. The base of the fracture extends above the level of the upper teeth into the maxilla. A CSF leak is possible.

Signs and Symptoms: LeFort II

- Massive facial edema

- Obvious fracture of nasal bones

- Malocclusion

- CSF rhinorrhea

LeFort III: A complete craniofacial separation involving the maxilla, zygoma,[5] and bones of the cranial base. This fracture is frequently associated with leakage of CSF and/or a fractured mandible.

Signs and Symptoms: LeFort III

- Massive facial edema

- Mobility and depression of zygomatic bones

- Ecchymosis

- Anesthesia of the cheek

- Diplopia

- Open bite or malocclusion

- CSF rhinorrhea

Interventions

- Monitor for developing airway obstruction

- Administer antibiotics if a CSF leak is present, as prescribed

- Prepare patient for operative intervention, hospital admission, or transfer for definitive stabilization of the fracture, as indicated.

  Intermaxillary wiring, interosseous wiring, and suspension may be utilized to bring the teeth back into occlusion. LeFort III fractures require multiple methods of fixation due to the multiple number of bones involved.

Orbital Fracture

The orbit is composed of multiple bones including the frontal bone, zygoma, maxilla, sphenoid and ethmoid bones. On impact, there is an increase in intraorbital pressure, energy is dissipated through the area of least resistance, usually the medial wall or orbital floor. Entrapment of nerves and muscles may produce the signs associated with this injury. Visual disturbances may be due to hematoma formation, which may compress the globe, optic nerve, or retinal artery.

Signs and Symptoms

● Diplopia

● Loss of vision

● Altered EOMs (limited upward gaze)

● Enophthalmus

● Subconjunctival hemorrhage and/or ecchymosis of the eyelid

● Infraorbital pain or loss of sensation

● Orbital bony deformity

Interventions

● Monitor the patient's vision and EOMs

● Treat any concomitant eye injury

● Administer antibiotics, to prevent orbital cellulitis, as prescribed

SUMMARY

Head injury is the leading cause of trauma-related deaths. Appropriate and early intervention can prevent or minimize the development of irreversible brain injury. Secondary brain injury may result from cerebral hypoxemia, ischemia, cerebral edema, hypercarbia, hypotension, and increased intracranial pressure.

Maintaining adequate ventilation and cerebral blood flow are essential to preserve neurologic function. To maintain CPP, stabilize the patient's blood pressure and treat any increase in ICP through a collaborative team approach.

REFERENCES

1. Gray H. In: Goss C, ed. *Gray's Anatomy of the Human Body.* 30th ed. Philadelphia, Pa: Lea & Febiger; 1984.

2. Campbell VG. Neurophysiology. In: Clochesy J, Breu C, Cardin S, Rudy E, Whittaker A, eds. *Critical Care Nurse.* Philadelphia, Pa: WB Saunders Co; 1993:643-651.

3. Mitchell PH. Central nervous system I: Closed head injuries. In: Cardona VD, Hurn PD, Mason PJB, Scanlon AM, Veise-Berry SW, eds. *Trauma Nursing: From Resuscitation Through Rehabilitation.* 2nd ed. Philadelphia, Pa: WB Saunders Co; 1994:383-433.

4. Oman KS, Drury TE. Head trauma. In: Kitt S, Selfridge-Thomas J, Proehl JA, Kaiser J, eds. *Emergency Nursing: A Physiologic and Clinical Perspective.* 2nd ed. Philadelphia, Pa: WB Saunders Co; 1995:337-356.

5. Cantrill SV. Facial trauma. In: Rosen P, Barkin RM, Baker FJ, Braen GR, Dailey RH, Levy RC, eds. *Emergency Medicine: Concepts and Clinical Practice.* 3rd ed. St. Louis, Mo: Mosby-Year Book; 1992:355-370.

6. Bower, CT. Maxillofacial and soft tissue injuries. In: Cardona VD, Hurn PD, Mason PJB, Scanlon AM, Veise-Berry SW, eds. *Trauma Nursing: From Resuscitation through Rehabilitation.* 2nd ed. Philadelphia, Pa: WB Saunders Co; 1994:587-615.

7. Marshall SB, Marshall LF, Vos HR, Chestnut RM, eds. Consciousness, impaired consciousness and the neurological assessment. In: *Neuroscience Critical Care.* Philadelphia, Pa: WB Saunders Co; 1990:85-113.

8. Walleck C. Patients with head injury and brain dysfunction. In: Clochesy J, Breu C, Cardin S, Rudy E, Whittaker A, eds. *Critical Care Nurse.* Philadelphia, Pa: WB Saunders Co; 1993:677-707.

9. Guyton, AC. *Textbook of Medical Physiology.* 8th ed. Philadelphia, Pa: WB Saunders Co; 1991:10.

10. *Position Papers from the Third National Injury Control Conference.* Washington, DC: Dept Health and Human Services, Public Health Service, Centers for Disease Control, National Institute for Occupational Safety and Health, National Highway Traffic Safety Administration; 1992. US Government Printing Office 1922-634-666.

11. Sosin DM, Sacks JJ, Smith SM. Head injury – associated deaths in the United States from 1979 to 1986. *JAMA.* 1989;262:2251-2255.

12. Turnes C. Improperly positioned passenger-restraint systems as associated mechanisms of injury in motor vehicular collisions. *JEN.* 1991;17:373-379.

13. May C, Morabito D. Motorcycle helmet use, incidence of head injury, and cost of hospitalization. *JEN.* 1989;15:389-392.

14. Offner PJ, Rivara FP, Maier RV. The impact of motorcycle helmet use. *J Trauma.* 1992;32:636-642.

15. MacAfee K. Immediate care of facial trauma. *Physician Sportsmed.* 1992;20:79-91.

16. Gennarelli T. Triage of head-injured patients. In: Trunky D, Lewis F, eds. *Current Therapy of Trauma.* Philadelphia, Pa: BC Decker; 1991:157-162.

17. American College of Surgeons Committee on Trauma. Spine and spinal cord trauma. In: *Advanced Trauma Life Support ® Course for Physicians (Student Manual).* 5th ed. Chicago. Ill: Author; 1993:193-203.

18. Pons P. Head trauma. In: Rosen P, Barkin RM, Baker FJ, Braen GR, Dailey RH, Levy RC, eds. *Emergency Medicine: Concepts and Clinical Practice.* 3rd ed. St. Louis, Mo: Mosby-Year Book; 1992:338-354.

19. Emergency Nurses Association. Facial emergencies. In: *Emergency Nursing Core Curriculum.* 4th ed. Philadelphia, Pa: WB Saunders Co; 1994:211.

20. Reinus WR, Wippold FJ, Erickson KK. Practical selection criteria for noncontrast cranial computed tomography in patients with head trauma. *Ann Emerg Med.* 1993;22:1114-1118.

21. Redan J, Livingston D, Fortella B, Rush B. The value of intubating and paralyzing patients with suspected head injury in the emergency department. *J Trauma.* 1991;31:371-375.

22. American College of Surgeons Committee on Trauma. Head trauma. In: *Advanced Trauma Life Support® Course for Physicians (Student Manual).* 5th ed. Chicago, Ill: Author; 1993:159-183.

23. Kerr ME, Brucia J. Hyperventilation in the head-injured patient: an effective treatment modality? *Heart Lung.* 1993;22:516-521.

24. Gennarelli T, Kotapka M. Trauma to the head. In: Schwartz GR, Cayten CG, Mangelsen MA, Mayer TA, Hanke BK, eds. *Principles and Practice of Emergency Medicine.* 3rd ed. Philadelphia, Pa: Lea & Febiger; 1992:936-943.

25. Shackford SR. Fluid resuscitation in head injury. *J Intensive Care Med.* 1990;5:59-68.

26. Vassar MJ, Perry CA, Holcroft JW. Prehospital resuscitation of hypotensive trauma patients with 7.5% NaCl versus 7.5% NaCl with added dextran: a controlled trial. *J Trauma.* 1993;34:622-633.

27. Freshman SP, Battistella FD, Matteucci M, Wisner DH. Hypertonic saline versus mannitol: a comparison for treatment of acute head injuries. *J Trauma.* 1993;35:344-348.

28. Duffy KR, Becker DP. State-of-the-art management of severe closed head injury. *J Intensive Care Med.* 1988;3:291-302.

CHAPTER SIX

THORACIC AND NECK TRAUMA

LECTURE BEGINS ON PAGE 142.

Preface

Prior to reading this chapter, it is strongly suggested that the learner read the following section entitled "Anatomy and Physiology." Specific anatomy and physiologic concepts are presented to enhance the learner's ability to correlate such concepts with specific injuries. This material on anatomy and physiology will not be covered during lectures, nor will it be evaluated by testing. However, knowledge of normal anatomy and physiology serves as the foundation for understanding the anatomic derangements and pathophysiologic compromises that may ensue as a result of trauma.

ANATOMY AND PHYSIOLOGY

Respiratory System

The respiratory system's primary function is the transport of oxygen to cells and removal of carbon dioxide. This is achieved by the following processes: 1) pulmonary ventilation, the movement of air between the atmosphere and alveoli; 2) diffusion, the movement of oxygen and carbon dioxide between the alveoli and the blood; 3) transport of oxygen to the peripheral tissues, exchange of carbon dioxide at the cellular level, and return of carbon dioxide to the lungs; and 4) regulation of ventilation.[1]

The anatomy of the respiratory system is divided into those structures considered the upper airways, such as the nose, oropharynx, larynx and trachea. These structures filter, warm, and humidify inhaled air. The bronchi and bronchioles are lower airway structures and conduct atmospheric air to the alveoli where gas exchange takes place. The alveoli and pulmonary capillaries are responsible for gas exchange.[2]

The thoracic cavity extends from the top of the sternum to the diaphragm. Key structures within the thoracic cavity include the lungs and the space between the lungs termed the mediastinum. The mediastinum is bound anteriorly by the sternum, posteriorly by the 12 thoracic vertebrae, and inferiorly by the diaphragm. The contents of the mediastinal space include the heart, thoracic aorta, esophagus, trachea, inferior and superior vena cavae, vagus nerves, phrenic nerves, and other vascular structures. Correlation of anatomical structures and surface landmarks can be important in physical assessment of the chest.

Ventilation or breathing is accomplished by the alternate contraction and relaxation of the diaphragm and intercostal muscles. The diaphragm divides the abdominal and thoracic cavities. During inspiration, the diaphragm contracts and flattens, increasing the size of the thorax. During expiration, the diaphragm relaxes and the lungs recoil to decrease the chest size.[3] The diaphragm rises to the fourth intercostal space during expiration and extends to the 10th or 12th intercostal space during inspiration.

The lungs are expanded and contracted by increasing and decreasing the anterior-posterior diameter of the chest cavity by elevation and depression of the ribs.[1] The intercostal muscles also contribute to increasing the anterior to posterior diameter of the thoracic cavity by raising the rib cage. Other muscles, such as the sternocleidomastoids and the scaleni, raise the sternum and the first two ribs and are frequently termed accessory muscles. The muscles of expiration are the internal intercostals and abdominal recti.

The lungs are cone-shaped. The base of each lung rests against the diaphragm, and the apex of each lung extends to approximately 1½ inches above the clavicle. The pleura is a double-layered, thin, transparent membrane. The outer layer, the parietal pleura, lines the thoracic cavity, and the inner layer, the visceral pleura, surrounds each lung. A potential space, the pleural space, exists between the two layers, and is filled with 5 to 15 ml of lubricating fluid. The parietal and visceral pleura are in contact with each other to prevent any separation of the lungs from the chest cavity wall, yet slide smoothly over each other during breathing.

To keep the lungs fully expanded, the pressure within the pleural cavity must always remain slightly negative, –4 mmHg, in relation to atmospheric pressure. The lungs have an elastic tendency to recoil, while the thoracic cavity has an elastic tendency to expand. These opposing forces pull the two pleural membranes and generate the negative intrapleural pressure. The opposing forces create a slight negative pressure, much like a suction cup or vacuum. This suction or negative intrapleural pressure keeps the two pleural membranes in contact.[1,4] There is an increase in the negative intrapleural pressure during inspiration and a decrease during exhalation. The intrapleural pressure may become positive during expiration.[1]

Heart and Thoracic Great Vessels

The heart is situated in the mediastinum, with the most anterior chamber, the right ventricle, located beneath the sternum. The left ventricle is anterior to the thoracic spine. The heart is enclosed by the pericardium (pericardial sac). The double-layered pericardium is composed of a tough, outer, fibrous layer and a thinner, serous layer referred to as the epicardium. Between the two layers is approximately 30 to 50 ml of lubricating fluid that allows frictionless motion during systole and diastole.

Cardiac function and cardiac output are affected by:

- Preload, which refers to the volume in the left and right ventricles at the end of diastole[1]

- Afterload, which refers to the resistance or pressure in the arteries against which the ventricles must contract

- Myocardial contractility

- Heart rate

Factors affecting preload are blood volume, right atrial pressure, and intrathoracic pressure. Afterload is affected by the arterial pressure in the aorta and pulmonary arteries. Cardiac contractility can be affected by hypoxemia, ventricular diastolic volume, and stimulation of the sympathetic nervous system.

The thoracic aorta, the main vessel carrying oxygenated blood out of the left ventricle, is located in the mediastinum. It is divided into three portions: the ascending aorta, the aortic arch, and the descending thoracic aorta. The portion of the aorta immediately proximal to the heart is referred to as the ascending aorta. The aortic arch is attached to the pulmonary artery by the fetal remnant of the ductus arteriosus, termed the ligamentum arteriosum. The aortic isthmus is that portion of the aorta near the ligamentum where the left subclavian artery originates. This portion of the aorta is part of the descending aorta which is tethered in position and, therefore, has less ability to tolerate acceleration and/or deceleration forces.

Segmental arteries arise from the descending aorta. The segmental arteries branch into the intercostal and radicular arteries. The radicular arteries, which supply the anterior and posterior spinal arteries, are the primary vascular supply for the spinal cord[5] (see Figure 12).

Figure 12
Vascular Supply of the Spinal Cord

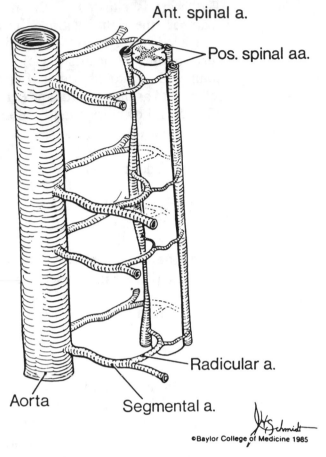

Ant. spinal a.

Pos. spinal aa.

Radicular a.

Aorta

Segmental a.

©Baylor College of Medicine 1985

(Reprinted with permission from Mattox KL. Approaches to trauma involving major vessels of the thorax. *Surg Clin North Am.* 1989;69:80.)

Neck

The neck contains a large concentration of anatomic structures relative to its size. The structures contained within the neck are the airway, common and internal carotid arteries, the internal and external jugular veins, the vertebral arteries, the vagus nerves, thoracic duct, trachea, pharynx, esophagus, spinal cord, cervical vertebral column, thyroid gland, parathyroid glands, lower cranial nerves, brachial plexus, muscle, and soft tissue.

The neck is commonly divided into three anatomic regions referred to as zones. The zones are based on bony and superficial landmarks. They are important in defining the potential structures injured, the diagnostic evaluation needed, and the management approach. Zone I extends from the level of the cricoid cartilage down to the clavicles.

The area above the cricoid cartilage to the angle of the mandible is described as Zone II. The angle of the mandible to the base of the skull is Zone III.[6,7]

The structures within the neck are enclosed by two fascial layers. The superficial fascia encompasses the platysma muscle and the deep cervical fascia, supports the muscles, vessels, and organs of the neck. The compartments formed by the fascia limit external bleeding, but bleeding within the closed spaces may compromise the airway with hematoma formation. The platysma muscle protects the underlying structures within the neck. If the platysma has been damaged, then underlying injury may be suspected.[8]

The vascular supply for the brain and brainstem arises from the vertebral arteries and the internal carotids. Abrupt interruption in the blood flow through these structures will result in cerebral hypoxia and neurological deficits.

The brachial plexus is a network of nerve fibers that incorporates the nerve roots of C-5 through T-1. These nerves subdivide to form the axillary, musculocutaneous, median, ulnar, and radial nerves. These nerves are responsible for arm and hand function.[9]

THORACIC AND NECK TRAUMA

OBJECTIVES

Upon completion of this chapter/lecture, the learner should be able to:

1. Identify the mechanisms of injury associated with thoracic and neck trauma.
2. Analyze the pathophysiologic changes as a basis for the signs and symptoms.
3. Discuss the nursing assessment of patients with thoracic and neck trauma.
4. Based on the assessment data, identify the appropriate nursing diagnoses and expected outcomes.
5. Plan appropriate interventions for patients with thoracic or neck trauma.
6. Evaluate the effectiveness of nursing interventions for patients with thoracic or neck injuries.

INTRODUCTION

Epidemiology

Patients with trauma to the chest and neck present some of the most life-threatening conditions in emergency care. Thoracic injuries are second only to brain and spinal cord injuries as the leading causes of traumatic death.[10]

Improvements in the overall provision of trauma care have contributed to a continued decline in mortality related to neck injuries. Most studies have reported a 2 to 6% mortality rate from neck injuries.[6] The increase in interpersonal violence has had an impact on the pattern of injuries to the chest and neck. Currently, there is an increasing number of chest and neck injuries due to gunshot wounds and stabbings.[10]

Mechanisms of Injury and Biomechanics

Mechanical energy is the most common energy source associated with chest and neck injuries. Acceleration and deceleration forces may be responsible for injuries to intrathoracic contents. The first and second ribs and the sternum tend to resist energy loads better than other bones of the body. Therefore, if these bones are fractured, suspect significant injury to underlying structures. Mechanical energy applied to the chest can lead to fractures as well as contusions of the myocardium and lung as energy is dissipated. Due to the relative fixation of the descending aorta distal to the ligamentum arteriosum, this structure is more susceptible to injury produced by deceleration forces. Forces that cause penetrating cardiac injury most often injure the right ventricle.

Motor vehicle crashes account for an estimated two-thirds of all chest trauma-related deaths (see Table 13). Additional mechanisms of injury commonly associated with thoracic injuries are falls, crush injuries, assaults, use of firearms, stabbings, and motor vehicle versus pedestrian incidents. Injuries to the neck are most commonly associated with motor vehicle crashes. Other mechanisms include strangle or choke holds, hangings, assaults, falls, and sudden neck hyperextension, such as with a "clothesline- type" of injury.[6]

Table 13

TYPE OF IMPACT AND ASSOCIATED THORACIC INJURIES	
Mechanism	**Associated Thoracic Injuries**
Frontal impact	• Anterior flail chest • Myocardial contusion • Pneumothorax • Transection of aorta (decelerating injury)
Side impact	• Lateral flail chest • Pneumothorax • Traumatic aortic rupture • Diaphragmatic rupture
Motor vehicle-pedestrian	Thoracic and abdominal injuries

(Adapted with permission from American College of Surgeons Committee on Trauma. Initial assessment and management. In: *Advanced Trauma Life Support® Course for Physicians (Student Manual)*. 5th ed. Chicago, Ill: Author; 1993:29.)

Types of Injuries

The most common type of injury associated with chest trauma is blunt, accounting for approximately 70% of all thoracic injuries.[11] Penetrating injuries to the chest are commonly the result of firearm injuries or stabbings.

Neck injuries also result in blunt and penetrating injuries. Penetrating injuries to the neck may appear benign based on the appearance of the wound but, due to the number and variety of vital structures in a small anatomic region, the potential for underlying organ injury is significant.[7] Slashing or cutting wounds are less likely to cause injury to underlying structures than penetrating wounds that puncture the platysma muscles of the neck.

Usual Concurrent Injuries

Injuries to the neck and chest are frequently associated with immediate life-threatening conditions. Life-threatening injuries of the neck may include upper airway trauma, vascular injuries, or cervical vertebral and spinal cord trauma. Chest and/or neck trauma may disrupt the airway, impair breathing, and/or result in serious alterations in circulation.

Isolated blunt thoracic injury is uncommon. Head, extremity, and abdominal injuries frequently occur concurrently. Penetrating trauma to the thorax, particularly gunshot or shotgun injuries, are frequently associated with abdominal trauma due to the anatomical proximity of the chest and abdomen. Patients with penetrating injuries to the lower thoracic region should be assumed to have both chest and abdominal injuries until proven otherwise.

Table 14 lists organs that may be injured when the sternum or ribs are fractured.

Table 14

| THORACIC SKELETAL FRACTURES ||
Injury	Associated Injury
Sternal fractures[12,13]	• Myocardial contusion
First and second rib fractures	• Great vessel injuries • Brachial plexus injuries • Head and spinal cord injuries
Rib fractures Flail chest	• Pulmonary contusions • Pneumothorax • Hemothorax
Fractures of lower ribs (seventh to twelfth)	• Liver and spleen injuries

PATHOPHYSIOLOGY AS A BASIS FOR SIGNS AND SYMPTOMS

Ineffective Ventilation

Ineffective ventilation can be a result of thoracic or neck trauma. The resulting pathophysiology is related to the loss of integrity of anatomical structures as well as compromises to the normal physiologic process of respiration.

Blunt or penetrating neck injuries can directly damage or destroy anatomical structures or indirectly occlude the airway through localized hematoma formation. Tears or lacerations in the tracheobronchial tree interrupt the integrity of the lower airway.[10] Patients with these injuries manifest dramatic symptoms early during resuscitation with massive air leaks into the subcutaneous tissue.

Ineffective ventilation may also result from rib fractures and/or sternal fractures which injure underlying organs. Pain resulting from these fractures may impair the patient's ability to adequately ventilate.

Penetrating injury of the chest wall and/or laceration of lung tissue affects the patient's ability to maintain negative intrapleural pressure. Air or blood leaking into the intrapleural space collapses the lung. The degree of the lung collapse is dependent on the severity of the underlying lung injury.

Interstitial and alveolar edema may occur, in addition to hemorrhage and laceration, when the lung is contused or punctured. The interstitial and alveolar edema results in impaired diffusion of gases across the alveolar membrane. Damaged alveoli and/or capillary injuries produce abnormalities in the ventilation to perfusion ratio.[1]

Ineffective Circulation

Injury to the heart and thoracic great vessels reduces the amount of circulating blood volume, leading to hemorrhage, hypovolemia, and shock. Direct trauma to the heart and/or myocardial contusion may lead to a reduction in cardiac output due to reduced myocardial contractility.

Air or blood that continues to accumulate in the thoracic cavity will increase the intrapleural pressure. If the pressure rises to an abnormally high level, the heart and great vessels will shift, causing compression of the vena cavae, obstruction of venous return, and collapse of the lung. Compression of the vena cavae with obstruction of venous return will result in a decreased cardiac output. The patient may present with respiratory distress, tachycardia, hypotension, tracheal deviation, unilateral absence of breath sounds, and neck vein distention due to increased intrathoracic pressure.

Rapid accumulation of even small amounts of blood in the pericardial sac (pericardial tamponade) will result in compression of the heart and inability of the heart to fill during diastole. This results in decreased cardiac output. The patient may exhibit hypotension, tachycardia, muffled heart tones, and neck vein distention.

Neurologic Deficits

Paraplegia associated with aortic injuries is related to ischemia or infarction of the spinal cord due to hematoma formation or occlusion of the blood flow from the aorta to the spinal arteries.[5,14] Injuries in the neck region may also cause spinal cord or brachial plexus injuries, impairing motor or sensory function. Neck injuries may also produce cerebral ischemia and/or infarction resulting in motor or sensory impairment.[8,15]

NURSING CARE OF PATIENTS WITH THORACIC AND NECK TRAUMA

Assessment

History

Refer to Chapter 3, Initial Assessment, for a description of general information that should be collected regarding every trauma victim. Only pertinent questions specific to patients with thoracic or neck injuries are described below.

- What was the mechanism of injury?

    - What was the type of motor vehicle collision?

        Head-on collision or impact with a stationary object, such as a tree or cement wall, will result in deceleration forces that may be associated with chest and neck injuries, such as a traumatic aortic rupture.

    - What was the damage to the exterior and interior of the vehicle?

        A bent steering wheel or steering column imprint on the patient's chest may be associated with sternal fractures, myocardial contusions, or a transected aorta. The amount of structural intrusion into the passenger compartment may be useful to identify patterns of injury, such as lateral rib fractures.

- What are the patient's complaints?

    - Dyspnea

    - Dysphagia (difficulty swallowing)

■ Dysphonia (hoarseness)

- What were the patient's vital signs prior to admission?

  Were vital signs or signs of life observed by prehospital care personnel or another reliable source? If cardiopulmonary resuscitation is being performed, when was it started? When did the patient lose signs of life? This information is important in determining the indications for an emergency department thoracotomy.

Physical Assessment

Refer to Chapter 3, Initial Assessment, for a description of the assessment of the patient's airway, and effectiveness of breathing, and circulation.

INSPECTION

- Observe the chest wall for injuries that may severely impair the adequacy of breathing, such as open sucking chest wounds. This requires the removal of debris or blood to avoid overlooking any wounds.

- Assess breathing effectiveness and rate of respirations

- Observe the chest wall for symmetrical movement

  The presence of a flail segment may produce paradoxical movement.

- Inspect the neck for signs of trauma, such as ecchymosis, swelling, or hematomas, that may result in airway obstruction. Listen for noisy air movement. Swelling of the face and/or neck may indicate a mediastinal, esophageal, or tracheobronchial injury.

- Inspect the jugular veins

  Distended neck veins may indicate increased intrathoracic pressure as a result of a tension pneumothorax or pericardial tamponade. Flat external jugular veins may reflect hypovolemia.

- Identify the zone of neck injury

- Inspect the upper abdominal region for evidence of blunt or penetrating injury

147

PERCUSSION

Percuss the chest

Dullness is associated with hemothorax, and hyperresonance suggests a pneumothorax.

PALPATION

- Palpate the chest wall, clavicles, and neck for:

  - Tenderness

  - Swelling or hematoma

  - Subcutaneous emphysema (esophageal, pleural, tracheal, or bronchial tear)

- Note the presence of bony crepitus (possible fractured ribs and/or sternum)

- Palpate central and peripheral pulses and compare quality between:

  - Right and left extremities

  - Upper and lower extremities

- Palpate the trachea

  Locate the suprasternal notch and palpate the trachea directly above it. A shifted trachea may indicate a tension pneumothorax or massive hemothorax.

- Palpate extremities for motor and sensory function

  Lower extremity paresis or paralysis may indicate aortic injury.[5,16] Hemiplegia may occur with vascular injury of the neck. A motor and/or sensory deficit in the upper extremities may indicate ulnar or radial nerve damage secondary to a brachial plexus injury.[8]

AUSCULTATION

- Auscultate and compare blood pressure in both upper and lower extremities

- Auscultate breath sounds

  Decreased or absent breath sounds may indicate the presence of a pneumothorax or hemothorax. Diminished sounds may result from splinting. Shallow respirations may be due to pain.

- Auscultate the chest for the presence of bowel sounds

  Bowel sounds present in mid to lower lung fields may occur with diaphragmatic rupture.

- Auscultate heart sounds

  Muffled heart sounds may be associated with pericardial tamponade.

- Auscultate the neck vessels for bruits (abnormal murmurs), which may indicate vascular injury

Diagnostic Procedures

Refer to Chapter 3, Initial Assessment, for frequently-ordered radiographic and laboratory studies. Additional studies for patients with thoracic and neck injuries are listed below.

RADIOGRAPHIC STUDIES

- Chest

  An upright chest radiograph may be necessary to evaluate the presence of a hemothorax, especially if blood accumulation is less than 300 ml.[17]

- Arteriography

  - Arteriography is used to evaluate suspected vascular injuries in the neck[19] and chest.

  - Aortography may be done if there is a mechanism of injury, or physical or radiographic signs that result in a high index of suspicion for aortic injury.[13,18]

- Esophagoscopy

- Bronchoscopy and laryngoscopy

- CT scan

    A thoracic CT evaluates pulmonary parenchymal injuries, pulmonary contusions,[20] and/or aortic injuries. Thoracic CT does not replace aortography in the evaluation of aortic injury.[5]

LABORATORY STUDIES

Cardiac enzymes

OTHER

- Electrocardiogram

    Premature ventricular contractions and atrioventricular blocks are most frequently observed following blunt chest injury.[21]

- Central venous pressure (CVP)

    Patients with cardiac tamponade or tension pneumothorax may have an elevated CVP. Patients with hypovolemia may have a decreased CVP. Normal CVP is 5 to 10 cm H_2O.

- Echocardiography

Nursing Diagnoses and Outcome Identification

The following nursing diagnoses are potential problems for the patient with thoracic and/or neck injury. Once a patient has been assessed, diagnoses can be defined as either actual or risk. An actual nursing diagnosis is one derived from a decision based on the patient's presenting signs and symptoms. A risk nursing diagnosis is a judgment the nurse makes based on a particular patient's risk and potential for developing certain problems.

POSSIBLE NURSING DIAGNOSES AND EXPECTED OUTCOMES	
Nursing Diagnosis	**Expected Outcome**
Airway clearance, ineffective related to: • Neck injury	The patient will maintain a patent airway as evidenced by: • Regular rate, depth, and pattern of breathing • Bilateral chest expansion • Effective cough/gag reflex • Absence of signs and symptoms of airway obstruction: stridor, dyspnea, hoarse voice • Clear sputum of normal amount without abnormal color or odor • Absence of signs and symptoms of retained secretions: fever, tachycardia, tachypnea

Breathing pattern, ineffective related to:
• Pain
• Musculoskeletal impairment
• Unstable chest wall segment
• Lung collapse
	The patient will have an effective breathing pattern as evidenced by:
	• Normal rate, depth, and pattern of breathing
	• Symmetrical chest wall expansion
	• Absence of stridor, dyspnea, or cyanosis
	• Clear and equal bilateral breath sounds
	• ABG values within normal limits:
	  ■ PaO_2 80 - 100 mmHg (10.0 - 13.3 KPa)
	  ■ SaO_2 >95%
	  ■ $PaCO_2$ 35 - 45 mmHg (4.7 - 6.0 KPa)
	  ■ pH between 7.35 - 7.45
	• Trachea midline

Gas exchange, impaired related to:
• Ineffective breathing pattern: loss of integrity of thoracic cage, impaired chest wall movement, loss of negative intrathoracic pressure
• Retained secretions
• Accumulation of blood in thoracic cavity
• Decrease in inspired air
• Pulmonary contusion
• Shock
	The patient will experience adequate gas exchange as evidenced by:
	• ABG values within normal limits:
	  ■ PaO_2 80 - 100 mmHg (10.0 - 13.3 KPa)
	  ■ SaO_2 >95%
	  ■ $PaCo_2$ 35 - 45 mmHg (4.7 - 6.0 KPa)
	  ■ pH between 7.35 - 7.45
	• Skin normal color, warm, and dry
	• Improved level of consciousness
	• Regular rate, depth, and pattern of breathing

POSSIBLE NURSING DIAGNOSES AND EXPECTED OUTCOMES	
Nursing Diagnosis	**Expected Outcome**
Fluid volume deficit related to: • Hemorrhage • Impaired cardiac filling and ejection • Mechanical compression of heart and great vessels	The patient will have an effective circulating volume as evidenced by: • Stable vital signs appropriate for developmental age • Urinary output 1 ml/kg/hr • Strong, palpable peripheral pulses • Improved level of consciousness • Skin normal color, warm, and dry • Maintains HCT = 30 ml/dl or Hgb = 12 - 14 g/dl or greater • CVP reading of 5 - 10 cm H_2O • Control of external hemorrhage
Cardiac output, decreased related to: • Hypovolemic shock secondary to acute blood loss • Compression of heart and great vessels • Impairment of cardiac filling and ejection	The patient will maintain adequate circulatory function as evidenced by: • Strong palpable peripheral pulses • Apical pulse rate of 60 - 100 • Normal heart tones • EKG with normal sinus rhythm • Absence of jugular vein distension, deviated trachea • Skin normal color, warm, and dry • Improved level of consciousness • CVP reading of 5 - 10 cm H_2O
Pain related to: • Trauma to rib cage • Pleural irritation • Invasive procedures	The patient will experience relief of pain as evidenced by: • Diminishing or absent level of pain through patient's self-report using an objective measurement tool • Absence of physiologic indicators of pain that include: tachycardia, tachypnea, pallor, diaphoretic skin, increasing blood pressure • Absence of nonverbal cues of pain: crying, grimacing, inability to assume position of comfort • Ability to cooperate with care as appropriate

Planning and Implementation

Refer to Chapter 3, Initial Assessment, for a description of the specific nursing interventions for patients with compromises to airway, breathing, and/or circulation.

- Ensure patent airway

  Prepare for endotracheal intubation or surgical airway with cervical spine stabilization, if the patient has severe neck or chest trauma.

- Administer oxygen via a nonrebreather mask at a flow rate sufficient to keep the reservoir bag inflated; usually requires 12 to 15 L/minute.

- Prepare for ventilatory support, as necessary. Administer 100% oxygen using either a bag-valve device with an attached reservoir system or a mechanical ventilator.

- Prepare for chest tube insertion

  A chest tube is inserted to decompress a pneumothorax or hemothorax. Chest tubes may be placed prophylactically in patients with blunt or penetrating chest trauma who require positive pressure ventilation.

- Cannulate two veins with large-bore, 14- or 16-gauge catheters, and initiate infusions of lactated Ringer's solution

- Assist with emergency department thoracotomy

  The indications for this procedure have been subject to considerable controversy. The use of emergency department thoracotomy for patients with no documented vital signs and/or with blunt injuries has been demonstrated to have questionable benefit. The best results are obtained in patients with a single penetrating injury of the anterior or precordial thoracic area, and in patients who had deteriorating vital signs. In such patients, especially those with stab wounds, a timely thoracotomy may lead to complete recovery.[22-25]

  This procedure is recommended only in situations where physicians are experienced in the technique and surgical resources are available for continuing surgical therapy.[18]

- Cover open wounds with a nonporous dressing at the end of expiration. Tape securely on three sides.

- Stabilize impaled objects

- Administer analgesics, as prescribed

- Provide psychosocial support

Evaluation and Ongoing Assessment

Refer to Chapter 3, Initial Assessment, for a description of the ongoing evaluation of the patient's airway, effectiveness of breathing, and circulation. Additional evaluations include:

- Monitoring airway patency, respiratory effort, and arterial blood gases

- Monitoring respiratory effort after covering a wound since this may lead to the development of a tension pneumothorax

- Monitoring CVP for changes

- Monitoring chest tube drainage to determine the amount and any change in drainage characteristics

SELECTED THORACIC AND NECK INJURIES

Refer to "Nursing Care of Patients with Thoracic and Neck Injuries" for a description of the phases of the trauma nursing process.

Rib and Sternal Fractures

Rib fractures are the most common type of blunt chest injury.[11,26] The injured area of lung underlying the fracture is usually of more clinical significance than the fracture. Fracture of the sternum, first, and/or second rib requires significant force and, therefore, may be associated with serious injuries of underlying structures. Left lower rib fractures may be associated with splenic injury, right lower rib fractures with hepatic injury, and sternal fractures with heart and/or great vessel injury.[26] Sternal fracture is associated with a blunt injury, e.g., impact with steering wheel. The most common fracture site is the junction of the manubrium and the body of the sternum.

Signs and Symptoms

- Dyspnea

- Localized pain on movement, palpation, or inspiration

- Patient assumes a position intended to splint chest wall to reduce pain

- Chest wall or sternal contusion or ecchymosis

154

- Bony crepitus or deformity

Interventions

- Administer analgesic medication, as prescribed. Pain control helps to prevent hypoventilation. Prepare to assist with intercostal nerve block, if prescribed.

- Monitor and treat cardiac dysrhythmias or dysfunction if significant myocardial contusion is suspected

- Prepare for hospitalization if:

  - Fracture of more than three ribs

  - Fracture of first or second rib

  - Displaced, comminuted rib fractures

  - The patient is elderly or has chronic pulmonary disease

Flail Chest

Flail chest is defined as a fracture of two or more sites on two or more adjacent ribs or when rib fractures produce a free-floating sternum. The unsupported chest wall or flail segment moves paradoxically or opposite from the rest of the chest wall during inspiration and expiration. Nearly 50% of flail segments are not clinically evident in the first several hours after injury because of muscle spasms that splint the flail segment.[26] A flail chest may be associated with the following:

- Ineffective ventilation

- Pulmonary contusion

- Lacerated lung parenchyma

Signs and Symptoms

- Dyspnea

- Chest wall pain

- Paradoxical chest wall movement – the flail segment moves in during inspiration and out during expiration.

155

Interventions

Interventions for patients with a flail chest in addition to those listed for rib and sternal fractures are:

- Anticipate the need for endotracheal intubation and mechanical ventilation

- Sandbags, strapping, or rib belts are not used since therapy is aimed at correcting abnormalities in gas exchange rather than providing chest wall stability.[26]

Pneumothorax

A pneumothorax (simple) results when an injury to the lung leads to accumulation of air in the pleural space with a subsequent loss of intrapleural pressure. Partial or total collapse of the lung may ensue.

An open pneumothorax is a pneumothorax resulting from a wound through the chest wall. Air enters the pleural space both through the wound and the trachea.

A tension pneumothorax is a life-threatening lung injury. Air enters the pleural space on inspiration, but the air cannot escape on expiration. Rising intrathoracic pressure collapses the lung on the side of the injury causing a mediastinal shift that compresses the heart, great vessels, trachea, and ultimately, the uninjured lung. Venous return is impeded, cardiac output falls, and hypotension results. A tension pneumothorax may occur as a result of an open or closed chest injury.

Signs and Symptoms

- Dyspnea, tachypnea

- Tachycardia

- Hyperresonance on injured side

- Decreased or absent breath sounds on the injured side

- Chest pain

- Open, sucking wound on inspiration (open pneumothorax)

Signs: Tension Pneumothorax

- Worsening of the above signs

- Hypotension

- Distended neck veins

- Tracheal deviation – shift toward uninjured side

Interventions

- Prepare for chest tube insertion

  If pneumothorax is small, the physician may decide to defer chest tube placement.

- Cover open wound with sterile, nonporous dressing, e.g., petroleum-impregnated dressing, and tape securely on three sides

  If signs or symptoms of a tension pneumothorax develop after application of the dressing, remove the dressing and re-evaluate the patient.

- IMMEDIATELY prepare for a needle thoracentesis if a tension pneumothorax is suspected. A 14-gauge needle is inserted into the second intercostal space in the midclavicular line or fifth intercostal space in the midaxillary line on the injured side. Prepare for subsequent chest tube insertion (see Figure 13).

Figure 13
Anatomical Landmarks for Needle Thoracentesis

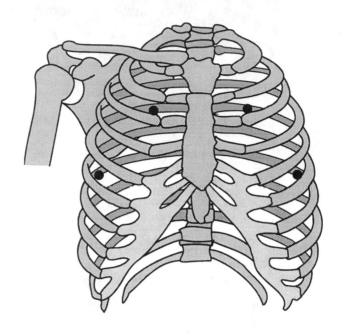

Hemothorax

A hemothorax is an accumulation of blood in the pleural space. A massive hemothorax is a rapid accumulation of 1,500 ml or more in the intrapleural space.[18] Massive, intrapleural hemorrhage may result in a mediastinal shift, decreased venous return, and hypotension.

Signs and Symptoms

- Dyspnea, tachypnea

- Chest pain

- Signs of shock

- Tracheal deviation

- Decreased breath sounds on injured side

- Dullness on the injured side

Interventions

- Prepare for chest tube insertion

- Prepare for transport to the operating room for emergency thoracotomy if there is an initial output of 1,500 ml or more of blood from the chest tube, or if there is continuing blood loss of greater than 200 ml/hour.[18]

- Prepare for autotransfusion, as indicated

  Consider autotransfusion if a large blood loss is anticipated or greater than 500 ml of blood is collected. Blood contaminated with abdominal contents is a relative contraindication to auto-transfusion.

Pulmonary Contusion

Pulmonary contusions may occur as a result of direct impact, deceleration, or high velocity bullet wounds.[27] Pulmonary contusions are seen on chest radiographs as consolidation and pulmonary infiltration. A pulmonary contusion may be demonstrated on a CT scan as a "pulmonary laceration surrounded by intra-alveolar hemorrhage without significant interstitial injury."[20] The degree of respiratory insufficiency is related to the size of the contusion, the severity of injury to the alveolar-capillary membrane, and the development of atelectasis.

Signs and Symptoms

- Dyspnea

- Ineffective cough

- Hemoptysis

- Hypoxia

- Chest pain

- Possible chest wall contusion or abrasions

Interventions

- Restrict fluid administration if no signs of hypovolemic shock are present, to prevent pulmonary complications

- Provide mechanical ventilatory assistance, as required

Ruptured Diaphragm

A ruptured diaphragm is a potentially life-threatening injury that may result from forces that penetrate the body, e.g., gunshot wounds, or from acceleration or deceleration forces, e.g., motor vehicle crashes. Since the right leaf is somewhat protected by the liver, the left leaf of the diaphragm is more likely to be injured. A rupture or tear of the diaphragm may allow herniation of abdominal contents, such as the stomach, small bowel, or spleen into the thorax. Herniation may result in respiratory compromise due to impairment of lung capacity and displacement of normal lung tissue. Mediastinal structures may shift to the opposite side of the injury.[28]

Penetrating injuries below the nipple line should be evaluated for the potential of diaphragmatic injury and concurrent abdominal injury. Stab wounds to the lateral chest walls and flanks can be associated with diaphragmatic lacerations due to the close proximity, steep slope, and large surface area of the diaphragm.

Signs and Symptoms

- Dyspnea

- Dysphagia

- Abdominal pain

- Sharp epigastric or chest pain radiating to the left shoulder

- Bowel sounds in lower to middle chest

- Decreased breath sounds on the injured side

Interventions

- Insert gastric tube

- Prepare for surgical intervention

Tracheobronchial Injury

Blunt ruptures or tears of the lower trachea or mainstem bronchus may be caused by such mechanisms of injury as striking the dashboard or steering wheel, karate-type blows, or "clothesline-type" injuries. Penetrating wounds are more common than blunt injuries.[29] Injuries causing large defects in the trachea or bronchial tree require bronchoscopy and/or bronchogram and immediate surgical intervention.

Signs and Symptoms

- Dyspnea, tachypnea

- Hemoptysis

- Potential airway obstruction

- Subcutaneous emphysema in neck, face, or suprasternal area

- Decreased or absent breath sounds

Interventions

- Suction airway to maintain patency, as needed

- If intubated, the end of the endotracheal tube must be positioned distal to injury

- Prepare for chest tube insertion

- Prepare for aggressive ventilatory support if a major bronchial air leak exists after chest tube insertion

  A tracheobronchial laceration can result in persistent bubbling in the chest drainage unit, and the involved lung will not re-expand despite suction.[30]

- Consult with physician before inserting an orogastric or nasogastric tube

- Monitor for possible tension pneumothorax

- Prepare for surgical intervention

Myocardial Contusion

Myocardial contusion should be suspected following any blow to the chest. It is most commonly associated with motor vehicle crashes, especially with direct impact of the chest with the steering wheel. The anterior wall of the right ventricle is the most frequent site of injury. On autopsy, myocardial contusions are clearly delineated areas, without the zones of ischemia seen with myocardial infarction.[21] Echocardiography and cardiac enzymes, especially CPK-MB, may be indicated.

Signs and Symptoms

- ECG abnormalities ranging from dysrhythmias (premature ventricular contractions and AV blocks are most common) to ST and T wave changes[21]

- Chest pain

- Chest wall ecchymosis

Interventions

- Monitor and treat cardiac dysrhythmias

Pericardial Tamponade

Pericardial tamponade is a collection of blood in the pericardial sac. This life-threatening cardiac injury occurs most often with penetrating injury, although a closed injury may also result in pericardial tamponade.[18] As blood accumulates in the noncompliant pericardial sac, it exerts pressure on the heart, inhibiting or compromising ventricular filling. A subsequent decrease in stroke volume leads to a decrease in cardiac output. Impairment in cardiac function is related to both the rate and amount of fluid accumulation.

Signs and Symptoms

- Dyspnea

- Penetrating chest wound

- Fracture of left third, fourth, or fifth ribs

- Cyanosis

- Beck's Triad:

    - Distended neck veins (may be absent if shock is present)

    - Hypotension

    - Muffled heart sounds

- Signs of shock

- Progressive decreased voltage of ECG complexes[10]

Interventions

- Prepare for pericardiocentesis, as indicated

  Pericardiocentesis is an emergency procedure to relieve a cardiac tamponade. The patient is placed with head and torso elevated at a 45° angle. A 16- or 18-gauge, 6-inch (15 cm) or longer, over-the-needle catheter is attached to a 60 ml syringe. The needle is inserted at a 45° angle, lateral to the left side of the xiphoid, 1 to 2 cm inferior to the left of the xiphochondral junction. Blood is aspirated during introduction of the needle until as much nonclotted pericardial blood is withdrawn as possible.[18, 31]

  Blood removed from the pericardial sac will generally not clot (because blood is defibrinated from agitation during systole), and the hematocrit will be lower than venous blood.[10] Blood clots may be present in the pericardial sac and require operative removal.

- Prepare for possible emergency department thoracotomy

- Prepare for operative intervention

Aortic Injuries

Injuries to the thoracic aorta may be the result of penetrating or blunt trauma. The descending thoracic aorta is susceptible to rupture from rapid deceleration forces, resulting in blunt trauma. The mechanism of injury is associated with a combination of shearing forces, compression of the aorta on the vertebral column, and an increase in pressure inside the vessel during the episode of the trauma.[17] The usual site of damage to the descending aorta is at the aortic isthmus distal to the ligamentum arteriosum and the take-off of the left subclavian artery where the aorta is relatively fixed. Ascending aortic injuries are immediately fatal in most cases.[14] Patients with descending aortic injury have a 85% mortality prior to arrival at a hospital. There is a 10 to 30% mortality in those patients who are admitted and who receive surgical intervention.[14,16]

Signs and Symptoms

- Hypotension

- Decreased level of consciousness

- Hypertension in upper extremities[5,16,32]

- Decreased quality (amplitude) of femoral pulses compared to upper extremity pulses

- Loud systolic murmur in parascapular region

- Chest pain

- Chest wall ecchymosis

- Widened mediastinum on chest radiograph

- Paraplegia

Interventions

- Prepare for operative intervention

Neck Injuries

The neck is commonly divided into three zones (see Figure 14).

- Zone I extends from the clavicle to the cricothyroid cartilage

- Zone II extends upward to the angle of the mandible

- Zone III extends from the angle of the mandible to the base of the skull

The clinical significance of these zones is related to:

- Identification of structures potentially injured

- Potential for deciding selective surgical management or observation with diagnostic testing

- Potential to control bleeding

The evaluation and treatment of blunt neck injuries includes an evaluation of the integrity of the cervical vertebrae and the spinal cord. Neck trauma may result in injuries to airway structures (trachea or larynx), blood vessels (subclavian, jugular, and carotid), esophagus, endocrine structures (thyroid and parathyroid gland), and thoracic duct. Additional diagnostic studies for neck injuries are arteriography, bronchoscopy, laryngoscopy, and rigid esophagoscopy.

Figure 14
Zones of the Neck

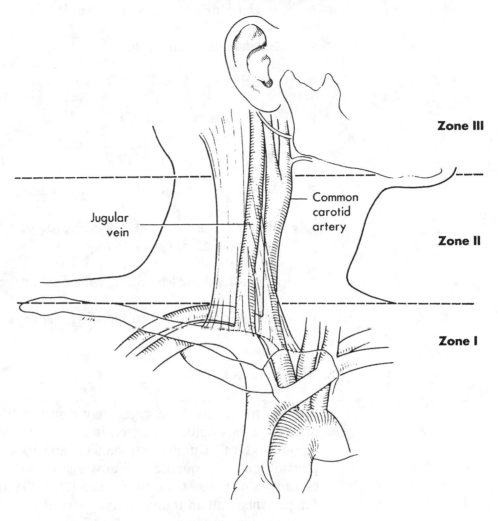

Jugular vein

Common carotid artery

Zone III

Zone II

Zone I

(Reprinted with permission from Yellin A, Weaver F. Evaluation and early management. In: Donovan AI. *Trauma Surgery Techniques in Thoracic, Abdominal, and Vascular Surgery*. St. Louis, Mo: Mosby-Year Book; 1994:31.)

Signs and Symptoms

- Penetrating wounds

- Pulsatile or expanding hematoma

- Loss of normal anatomic prominence of the laryngeal region

- Bruits

- Active external bleeding

- Neurological deficit, such as aphasia or hemiplegia

165

- Cranial nerve deficits

- Facial sensory or motor nerve deficits

- Subcutaneous emphysema

- Hoarseness

- Dysphagia or dysphonia

Interventions

- Monitor for progressive airway edema

  Prepare to assist in emergency procedures to maintain a patent airway, e.g., surgical airway.

- Control external bleeding with direct pressure

- Monitor for continued bleeding and expanding hematomas

SUMMARY

Trauma to the neck and chest may result in life-threatening injuries due to catastrophic compromises in breathing and circulation. Knowledge of anatomy, mechanism and pattern of injury, and the physiologic consequences of any disruption of the pulmonary and cardiovascular systems is the foundation of the trauma nursing process for patients with an injury to the chest or neck.

Early identification of all injuries requires a collaborative team approach to conduct the necessary diagnostic and therapeutic interventions. Determining the patient's need for operative management and/or transfer to a comprehensive trauma center is a major consideration for members of the trauma team.

REFERENCES

1. Guyton AC. *Textbook of Medical Physiology*. 8th ed. Philadelphia, Pa: WB Saunders Co; 1991.

2. Porth CM. *Pathophysiology: Concepts of Altered Health States*. 4th ed. Philadelphia, Pa: JB Lippincott Co; 1994.

3. Gray H. In: Goss C, ed. *Gray's Anatomy of the Human Body*. 30th ed. Philadelphia, Pa: Lea & Febiger; 1984.

4. Erickson RS. Mastering the ins and outs of chest drainage. *Nursing*. 1989;19:37-43.

5. Mattox KL. Approaches to trauma involving the major vessels of the thorax. *Surg Clin North Am*. 1989;69:77-91.

6. Thal ER. Injury to the neck. In: Moore EE, Mattox KL, Feliciano DV, eds. *Trauma*. 2nd ed. Norwalk, Conn: Appleton & Lange; 1991:306-317.

7. Garramone RR, Jacobs LM, Sahdev P. Diagnosis and management of penetrating neck trauma. *Contemporary Surgery*. 1990;36:11-20.

8. Asensio JA, Valenziano CP, Falcone RE, Grosh JD. Management of penetrating neck injuries: the controversy surrounding Zone II injuries. *Surg Clin North Am*. 1991;71:267-296.

9. Strange JM, Kelly PM. Musculoskeletal injuries. In: Cardona VD, Hurn PD, Mason PJB, Scanlon AM, Veise-Berry SW, eds. *Trauma Nursing: From Resuscitation through Rehabilitation*. 2nd ed. Philadelphia, Pa: WB Saunders Co; 1994:566-568.

10. Hurn PD, Harstock RL. Thoracic injuries. In: Cardona VD, Hurn PD, Mason PJB, Scanlon AM, Veise-Berry SW, eds. *Trauma Nursing: From Resuscitation through Rehabilitation*. 2nd ed. Phildelphia, Pa: WB Saunders Co; 1994:466-509.

11. LoCicero J, Mattox KL. Epidemiology of chest trauma. *Surg Clin North Am*. 1989;69:15-19.

12. Demling RH, Pomfret EA. Blunt chest trauma. *New Horizons*. 1993;1:402-420.

13. Hills WH, Delprado AM, Deane SA. Sternal fractures: associated injuries and management. *J Trauma.* 1993;35:55-60.

14. Bednarski JJ, Bayduch DA. Thoracic aorta rupture as the cause of paraplegia: a diagnostic dilemma. *J Trauma.* 1989;29:531-533. Case report.

15. Haas MJ. Penetrating neck injuries. *Crit Care Nurse.* 1988;8:42-49.

16. Mattox KL. Injury to the thoracic great vessels. In: Moore EE, Mattox KL, Feliciano DV, eds. *Trauma.* 2nd ed. Norwalk, Conn: Appleton & Lange; 1991:393-408.

17. Eddy AC, Carrico CJ, Rusch VW. Injury to the lung and pleura. In: Moore EE, Mattox KL, Feliciano DV, eds. *Trauma.* 2nd ed. Norwalk, Conn: Appleton & Lange; 1991:357-369.

18. American College of Surgeons Committee on Trauma. Thoracic trauma. In: *Advanced Trauma Life Support® Course for Physicians (Student Manual).* 5th ed. Chicago, Ill: Author; 1993:127-140.

19. Alexander JB, DelRossi AJ. Head and neck vascular injuries. *Topics in Emerg Med.* 1991;13:39-47.

20. Wagner RB, Jamieson PM. Pulmonary contusion: evaluation and classification by computed tomography. *Surg Clin North Am.* 1989;69:31-46.

21. Christensen MA, Sutton KR. Myocardial contusion: new concepts in diagnosis and management. *Am J Crit Care.* 1993;2:28-34.

22. Washington B, Wilson RF, Steiger Z, Bassett JS. Emergency thoracotomy: a four-year review. *Ann Surg.* 1985;40:188-191.

23. Hoyt DB, Shackford SR, Davis JW, Mackersie RC, Hollingsworth-Fridlund P. Thoracotomy during trauma resuscitations: an appraisal of board-certified general surgeons. *J Trauma.* 1989;29:1318-1321.

24. Esposito TJ, Jurkovich GJ, Rice CL, Maier RV, Copass MK, Ashbaugh DG. Reappraisal of emergency room thoracotomy in a changing environment. *J Trauma.* 1991;31:881-887.

25. Boyd M, Vanek VW, Bourguet CC. Emergency room resuscitative thoracotomy: when is it indicated? *J Trauma*. 1992;33:714-721.

26. Cogbill TH, Landercasper J. Injury to the chest wall. In: Moore EE, Mattox KL, Feliciano DV, eds. *Trauma*. 2nd ed. Norwalk, Conn: Appleton & Lange; 1991:327-341.

27. Besson A, Saegesser F. *Color Atlas of Chest Trauma: Volume I*. Oradell, NJ: Medical Economics Books;1983:329-341.

28. Root HD, Harman PK. Injury to the diaphragm. In: Moore EE, Mattox KL, Feliciano DV, eds. *Trauma*. 2nd ed. Norwalk, Conn: Appleton & Lange; 1991:427-437.

29. Pate JW. Tracheobronchial and esophageal injuries. *Surg Clin North Am*. 1989;69:111-123.

30. Mulder DS, Barkun JS. Injury to the trachea, bronchus, and esophagus. In: Moore EE, Mattox KL, Feliciano DV, eds. *Trauma*. 2nd ed. Norwalk, Conn: Appleton & Lange; 1991:343-355.

31. Harman PK, Trinkle JK. Injury to the heart. In: Moore EE, Mattox KL, Feliciano DV, eds. *Trauma*. 2nd ed. Norwalk, Conn: Appleton & Lange; 1991:373-391.

32. Wolfe WG, Duhaylongsod FG. Traumatic thoracic aortic rupture. In: Moylan JA, ed. *Principles of Trauma Surgery*. New York, NY: Gower Medical Publishing; 1992:6-2-6-12.

CHAPTER SEVEN

ABDOMINAL TRAUMA

LECTURE BEGINS ON PAGE 176.

Preface

Prior to reading this chapter, it is strongly suggested that the learner read the following section entitled "Anatomy and Physiology." Specific anatomy and physiologic concepts are presented to enhance the learner's ability to correlate such concepts with specific injuries. This material on anatomy and physiology will not be covered during lectures, nor will it be evaluated by testing. However, knowledge of normal anatomy and physiology serves as the foundation for understanding the anatomic derangements and pathophysiologic compromises that may ensue as a result of trauma.

ANATOMY AND PHYSIOLOGY

The abdominal cavity extends from the diaphragm to the pelvis and is bounded anteriorly by the abdominal wall and posteriorly by the vertebral column. The left side of the diaphragm is slightly lower than the right and may extend to the level of the fifth rib in the mammary line. The abdominal contents are located in the peritoneal cavity, retroperitoneal space, or pelvic cavity.

For the purposes of abdominal evaluation, the abdomen can be divided into four quadrants (see Figure 15).

Figure 15
Abdominal Viscera

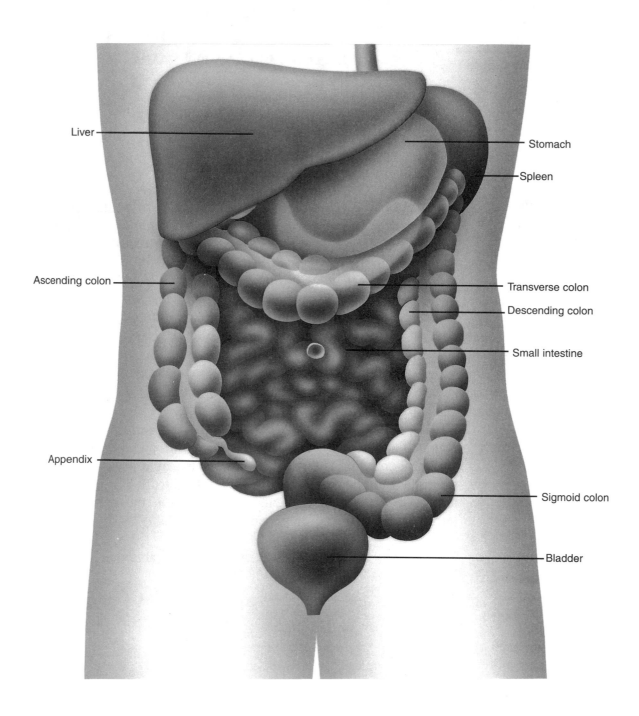

Liver

Ascending colon

Appendix

Stomach

Spleen

Transverse colon

Descending colon

Small intestine

Sigmoid colon

Bladder

The abdominal structures are covered by a serous, smooth membrane called the peritoneum. The parietal peritoneum lines the abdominal wall. The visceral layer surrounds organs of the abdomen. Because the peritoneum is a smooth, lubricated layer of tissue, the viscera can move within the abdomen without friction. Mesenteries are sheets of connective tissue covered by peritoneum, and they carry blood vessels. Certain organs, i.e., large and small bowel, are surrounded by peritoneum and are suspended from the abdominal wall by mesenteries. Other organs are only partially covered by the peritoneum. These organs are in the retroperitoneal space, e.g., kidneys, pancreas, aorta, vena cava and a portion of the duodenum. In men, the peritoneum is a closed sac. In women, the peritoneum is open where the distal ends of the fallopian tubes enter the peritoneal cavity.[1]

Solid Organs

Liver

The liver, spleen, kidneys, and pancreas are solid organs. The liver is an extremely vascular organ in the upper right quadrant and extends transversely across the midline. It has a solid consistency, but is friable enough to be lacerated, ruptured, or fragmented. The liver substance, hepatic parenchyma, forms lobules that are surrounded by a capsule. The diaphragmatic surface of the liver is smooth and convex, lying at the level of the sixth to 10th ribs on the right side, and at the seventh and eighth ribs on the left side. The circulation through the liver is via the hepatic artery and portal vein. Blood flow to the liver is approximately 30% of the total cardiac output.

Besides its role in metabolism, the liver has two other major functions. The first is as a secretory gland releasing bile. Bile salts help emulsify fat particles in food and absorb fatty acids. The second major function is to filter and store blood. The liver has a large vascular capacity and can store as much as 500 ml of blood at one time.

Spleen

The spleen is located in the upper left quadrant under the diaphragm and lateral to the stomach. The vascular, friable spleen has a diaphragmatic surface at the level of the ninth through 11th ribs. It is covered by peritoneum, which forms the external layer of the spleen's capsule. The spleen acts as a blood filter and reservoir for up to 200 ml of blood.

Kidneys

The kidneys are in the retroperitoneal space at the level of T-12 to L-3. The right kidney is slightly lower than the left because of the position of the liver. The kidneys are behind the stomach, spleen, colic flexure, and small bowel. Because they are not fixed to the abdominal wall, they move with inspiration and exhalation. The kidneys are surrounded by a capsule of fatty tissue and a layer of renal fascia. This fascia, along with the renal vessels, maintain the position of the kidneys. The ureters are a conduit for urine from the kidney to the bladder.

Pancreas

The pancreas is a gland that lies along the abdomen's posterior wall in the retroperitoneum. The head of the pancreas is close to the duodenum and the transverse colon, while the upper border is near the hepatic and splenic arteries. As an exocrine organ, it produces fluid containing enzymes, electrolytes, and bicarbonate to aid in digestion and nutrient absorption. Its endocrine function includes the secretion of insulin and glucagon, the hormones involved in carbohydrate metabolism.

Hollow Organs

Stomach

The stomach, small bowel, colon, and bladder are hollow organs. The stomach is in the upper left quadrant of the abdomen between the liver and spleen at the level of the seventh to ninth ribs. The stomach contains acidic gastric secretions.

Small Bowel

The small bowel is approximately seven meters long and is divided into three sections. In descending order from the stomach, the sections are the duodenum, jejunum, and ileum. The first portion of the duodenum, part of the second portion of the duodenum, the jejunum, and the ileum are in the peritoneal cavity. The rest of the duodenum is retroperitoneal. The small bowel is held in position by the adjacent viscera, the peritoneal membrane attachments to the posterior abdominal wall, and ligaments. Enzymes are secreted into the small bowel to aid in digestion and absorption.

Large Bowel

The large bowel is approximately 1½ meters long. The four sections of the large bowel are the cecum, colon, rectum, and anal canal. The colon is further divided into four sections. The first section, the ascending colon, travels past the right lobe of the liver. The second section, the transverse colon, crosses the abdomen from the upper right quadrant to the upper left quadrant. As it crosses the end of the spleen, it curves to become the descending colon located in the left quadrants. The last section, the sigmoid colon, is S-shaped and ends at the level of S-3. The rectum continues for approximately 13 cm where it dilates and forms the anal canal. The anal canal has both an internal and an external sphincter.

Bladder

The bladder is a membranous sac that stores urine. When it is empty, the bladder is located in the pelvic cavity. When full, it can expand into the abdomen. In women, the bladder is anterior to the uterus and behind the symphysis pubis. The urethra is a membranous canal that conducts urine from the bladder to the exterior of the body at the urinary meatus. The urethra in females is shorter than in males. The prostate is a gland in the male surrounding the neck of the bladder and part of the urethra.

ABDOMINAL TRAUMA

OBJECTIVES

Upon completion of this chapter/lecture, the learner should be able to:

1. Identify the mechanisms of injury associated with abdominal trauma.
2. Analyze the pathophysiologic changes as a basis for signs and symptoms.
3. Discuss the nursing assessment of patients with abdominal trauma.
4. Based on the assessment data, identify appropriate nursing diagnoses and expected outcomes.
5. Plan appropriate interventions for patients with abdominal trauma.
6. Evaluate the effectiveness of nursing interventions for patients with specific types of abdominal injuries.

INTRODUCTION

Epidemiology

Abdominal injuries are common in patients who sustain major trauma. Unrecognized abdominal injuries are frequently the cause of preventable death.[2] Abdominal injuries rank third as a cause of traumatic death preceded by head and chest injuries. Abdominal trauma results in a mortality rate of 13 to 15%. Patients with multiple abdominal organ injuries (with or without an injury to another body system) have significantly higher mortality rates than those with an isolated abdominal injury. Approximately one fifth of all traumatized patients requiring operative intervention have sustained trauma to the abdomen. The use of the lap belt and shoulder harness has significantly decreased the number and severity of injuries.[3]

Mechanisms of Injury and Biomechanics

The abdomen is vulnerable to injury since there is minimal bony protection for underlying organs. Because of the retroperitoneal location of certain organs and vascular structures, e.g., vena cava, aorta, pancreas, and duodenum, these structures are less frequently injured. The physical examination of the abdomen may not be successful in identifying intra-abdominal pathology; therefore, a description of the mechanism of injury is important.[4]

The most common mechanism of injury is a motor vehicle crash. Firearms, stabbings, and physical assaults are associated with penetrating abdominal trauma. Injuries to the abdomen can result from acceleration, deceleration, or a combination of both forces. The abdominal viscera may be compressed or directly impacted. Crushing forces may compress the duodenum or the pancreas against the vertebral column. During energy transfer, abdominal structures attached by either ligaments or blood vessels may be stressed at their attachment points. Forces applied to a solid organ can rupture a surrounding capsule and injure the parenchyma as well.

Safety restraint devices, particularly three-point safety belts, provide significant protection. However, if they are improperly positioned, they can cause deceleration injuries to the lower abdomen.[5] Lap belt use has been associated with injury to the hollow organs, particularly the small bowel and colon, lumbar spine, and abdominal wall.[6] Frontal impact crashes with a bent steering wheel and broken windshield are associated with spleen and liver injuries as well as head and chest trauma. Depending on the side of the impact, side impact crashes can result in injuries to the liver and spleen. Rear impact crashes can result in neck or abdominal injuries in unrestrained drivers who hit the steering column. Ejected motorcyclists may sustain pelvic fractures or intra-abdominal trauma from collisions with the handlebars or ground.

Types of Injuries

Blunt and penetrating abdominal injuries may be associated with extensive damage to the viscera resulting in massive blood loss. Blunt or penetrating abdominal injuries are related to the:

- Type of force applied

- Tissue density of structure injured, e.g., fluid-filled, gas-filled, solid, or encapsulated

The liver and spleen are the most commonly injured organs from blunt trauma.

The organs of the abdomen are vulnerable to penetrating injury not only through the anterior abdominal wall, but through the back, flank area, and lower chest.[4] Patients with penetrating abdominal injuries may present with single or multiple wounds. The liver, small bowel, and stomach are the most commonly injured organs from penetrating trauma.

Usual Concurrent Injuries

Due to their anatomical location, fractures of the lower rib cage are often associated with spleen or liver injuries. The patient with abdominal trauma, particularly esophageal and gastric injuries, may have associated chest trauma. Patients with pelvic fractures frequently have associated intra-abdominal trauma, e.g., bladder laceration. Patients with penetrating wounds at the nipple line anteriorly or at the inferior border of the scapula posteriorly are considered to be at risk for intra-abdominal injury.

PATHOPHYSIOLOGY AS A BASIS FOR SIGNS AND SYMPTOMS

Patient manifestations of abdominal trauma are frequently subtle. The abdomen may sequester large amounts of fluid without apparent distention. Signs and symptoms of blood loss, abdominal tenderness, specific pain patterns, and absent bowel sounds are associated with abdominal injury.

Blood Loss

Injuries to organs or abdominal blood vessels may lead to extensive hemorrhage. Some abdominal organs are semi-fixed by ligaments, such as the mesenteric attachments of the intestines. When these organs are stressed at their points of attachment, tears often occur at the point where the vessels enter the organ.

The spleen and the liver have a rich blood supply and store blood. Rapid loss of large blood volumes from their parenchyma or vascular structures can occur. Because they are encapsulated, compression of the abdomen may rapidly increase pressure within the capsule, resulting in rupture and hemorrhage. In addition, the consistency of the tissues makes hemostasis difficult.

Bleeding from organs in the anterior abdomen is usually confined to that cavity. Bleeding from structures in the retroperitoneum leads to hemorrhage in the retroperitoneum, which is more difficult to evaluate and diagnose (see Figure 16).

Figure 16
Retroperitoneal Structures

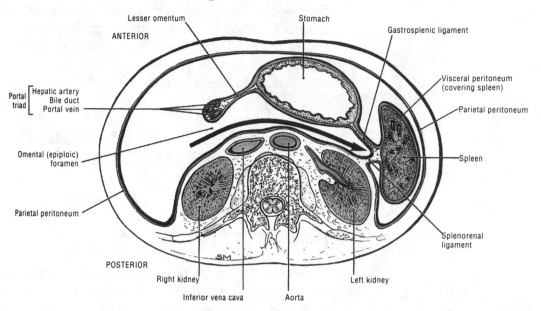

(Reprinted with permission from Moore KL. The abdomen. In: *Clinically Oriented Anatomy*. 3rd ed. Baltimore, Md: Williams & Wilkins; 1992:153.)

Pain

Pain, rigidity, guarding, or spasm of the abdominal musculature are classic signs of intra-abdominal pathology. Rebound tenderness and guarding of the abdominal muscles are caused by sudden movement of irritated peritoneal membranes against the abdominal wall. Irritation may be due to the presence of free blood or gastric contents in the peritoneal cavity. Manifestations of pancreatic and duodenal injury are related to hemorrhage in the area and the effect of active enzymes on their surrounding tissues. The resultant "chemical peritonitis" from the enzymes released into the retroperitoneum and the significant tissue swelling may not appear as signs and symptoms for several hours after injury.[4] The patient with pancreatic and duodenal injury may also complain of diffuse abdominal tenderness and pain radiating from the epigastric area to the back.

Pain can be referred to other areas of the body. An example is the referred shoulder pain known as Kehr's sign associated with splenic rupture. The blood that collects under the diaphragm causes irritation of the phrenic nerve which innervates the diaphragm. The pain is perceived along the course of the nerve and is commonly located in the left subscapular region. Pain referred to the testicles may be indicative of duodenal injury.[5]

179

Peristalsis

Following abdominal injury, bowel sounds are frequently hypo-dynamic. Blood in the abdominal cavity, direct bowel injury, or any number of conditions including stress may decrease peristaltic activity. However, hypoactive or absent bowel sounds combined with tenderness and guarding should be viewed with a high index of suspicion.

NURSING CARE OF THE PATIENT WITH ABDOMINAL TRAUMA

Assessment

History

Refer to Chapter 3, Initial Assessment, for a description of general information that should be collected regarding every trauma victim. Only pertinent questions specific to patients with abdominal injuries are described below.

- Was the patient wearing any restraints or protective devices? Inappropriately positioned lap belts may injure lower abdominal structures. The use of a lap belt without a shoulder belt is associated with hyperflexion injury to the lumbar spine.

- What is the location, intensity and quality of pain?

- Is nausea or vomiting present?

- Does the patient feel an urge to defecate or urinate?

Physical Assessment

Refer to Chapter 3, Initial Assessment, for a description of the assessment of the patient's airway, and effectiveness of breathing, and circulation.

INSPECTION

- Observe the contour of the abdomen, i.e., flat or distended

- Inspect the lower chest, abdomen, flanks, and back for seat belt abrasions or other soft tissue injuries

  - Ecchymosis over the upper left quadrant suggests soft tissue trauma or splenic injury

180

- Ecchymosis around the umbilicus suggests intraperitoneal bleeding, and ecchymosis of the flank suggests retroperitoneal bleeding.[4] Ecchymotic signs such as these take hours or days to develop and may not be noted on initial presentation.

- Inspect gunshot and stab wounds, and note size and location. Wounds should **NOT** be labeled as entrance and exit, but clearly identified and numbered.

- Inspect the pelvic area for soft tissue bruising

- Inspect the perineum for hematomas, bloody drainage from the urethral meatus, and vaginal or rectal bleeding

AUSCULTATION

- Auscultate all four quadrants of the abdomen for bowel sounds. Absence of bowel sounds in combination with abdominal distention and guarding are highly indicative of visceral injury.

- Auscultate the chest. If bowel sounds are heard in the chest, it is an indication of diaphragmatic rupture with herniation of the stomach or small bowel into the thoracic cavity.

PERCUSSION

Percuss the abdomen for hyperresonance or dullness. Hyperresonance indicates air while dullness indicates fluid accumulation.

PALPATION

- Begin palpating in an area where the patient has not complained of pain. Gently palpate each of the four quadrants separately for involuntary guarding, rigidity, spasm, and localized pain. Press on the abdomen and quickly release to determine the presence of rebound tenderness. Any positive findings of involuntary guarding, rigidity, pain, or spasm during palpation indicate peritoneal irritation. These signs may be absent if the patient has:

  - Competing pain from another injury

  - A retroperitoneal hematoma

  - A spinal cord injury

- ■ Ingested alcohol or narcotics

- ■ A decreased level of consciousness

- ● Palpate the pelvis for bony instability, asymmetry, or pain, which indicate possible dislocations or fractures

- ● Palpate the flanks for tenderness

- ● Palpate anal sphincter for presence or absence of tone

Diagnostic Procedures

Refer to Chapter 3, Initial Assessment, for frequently-ordered radiographic and laboratory studies. Additional studies for patients with abdominal trauma are listed below.

RADIOGRAPHIC STUDIES

- ● Computerized tomography (CT)

  A CT scan may be used to identify solid organ lacerations, hematomas, or small amounts of blood or air in the abdominal cavity.[7,8]

- ● Intravenous pyelogram (IVP)

  Extravasation of the contrast media into surrounding tissues indicates a disruption in the integrity of the kidney, ureters, or bladder.

- ● Flat plate, lateral, or upright abdominal films

  These studies are used to:

  - ■ Visualize foreign bodies and associated visceral damage

  - ■ Identify the path of penetrating objects

  - ■ Visualize free air in the abdomen indicating disruption of the gastrointestinal tract

- ● Cystogram/urethrogram

- ● Ultrasonography

LABORATORY STUDIES

- Serum amylase

- Analysis of urine, stool, and/or gastric contents for blood

- Pregnancy testing for women of childbearing age

OTHER STUDIES

Diagnostic peritoneal lavage (DPL)

- DPL is one method used to detect intra-abdominal bleeding (see Figure 17). A diagnostic peritoneal lavage is not useful for identifying retroperitoneal bleeding.[9] After decompressing the bladder with an indwelling catheter and the stomach with a gastric tube to avoid inadvertent puncture, a peritoneal catheter is inserted into the abdomen (usually below the umbilicus). The catheter is introduced via a puncture or a small incision. Withdrawal of gross blood from the catheter is considered a positive finding. If gross blood is not initially aspirated, a liter of warmed lactated Ringer's solution or normal saline is rapidly infused through the catheter. The lavage fluid is then allowed to drain out via gravity and analyzed for the presence of red or white blood cells, bile, amylase, food fiber, or feces. DPL has a 98% accuracy rate in correctly identifying intra-abdominal bleeding.[2] A positive DPL requires a surgical consult.

- The American College of Surgeons Committee on Trauma recommends that a DPL be performed early to evaluate the severely injured, hypotensive patient, especially if the abdominal examination is[2]:

  - Suggestive of injury

  - Unreliable, e.g., patient is unresponsive

- Diagnostic peritoneal lavage may be contraindicated in the following circumstances[2]:

  - When the decision has already been made to perform abdominal surgery

  - When the patient has had previous abdominal surgery increasing the potential for adhesions

- When the patient has known cirrhosis of the liver

- When the patient is extremely obese, making technical performance of the procedure difficult

- When the patient has a known medical history of coagulopathy

Figure 17
Diagnostic Peritoneal Lavage

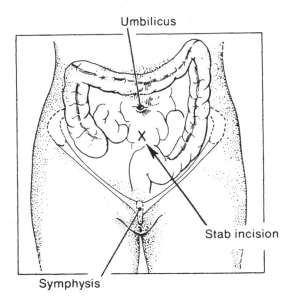

(Reprinted with permission from Moncure A. Peritoneal lavage. Illustrated techniques. In: *Emergency Medicine Scientific Foundations and Current Practice*. 3rd ed. Baltimore, Md: Williams & Wilkins; 1989:1030.)

Nursing Diagnoses and Outcome Identification

The following nursing diagnoses are potential problems for the patient with abdominal injuries. Once a patient has been assessed, diagnoses can be defined as either actual or risk. An actual nursing diagnosis is one derived from a decision based on the patient's presenting signs and symptoms. A risk nursing diagnosis is a judgment the nurse makes based on a particular patient's risk and potential for developing certain problems.

POSSIBLE NURSING DIAGNOSES AND EXPECTED OUTCOMES

Nursing Diagnosis	Expected Outcome
Fluid volume deficit related to: • Hemorrhage secondary to evisceration, disruption in integrity of intra-abdominal organs, drainage	The patient will have an effective circulating volume as evidenced by: • Stable vital signs appropriate for developmental age • Urinary output of 1 ml/kg/hr • Strong, palpable peripheral pulses • Improved level of consciousness • Skin normal color, warm, and dry • Maintains HCT = 30 ml/dl or Hgb = 12 - 14 g/dl or greater • CVP reading of 5 - 10 cm H_2O • External hemorrhage is controlled
Cardiac output, decreased related to: • Decreased venous return secondary to acute blood loss or massive peripheral vasodilation	The patient will maintain adequate circulatory function as evidenced by: • Strong, palpable peripheral pulses • Normal heart tones • ECG with normal sinus rhythm, absence of dysrthythmias • Absence of jugular vein distension, deviated trachea • Skin normal color, warm, and dry • Improved level of consciousness • CVP reading of 5 - 10 cm H_2O • Urinary output of 1 ml/kg/hr
Infection, risk related to: • Presence of invasive lines and procedures • Contamination of peritoneal cavity by blood, urine, feces, gastric contents, bile • Loss of immune support secondary to splenic injury	The patient will be free from infection as evidenced by: • Core temperature measurement of 36° - 37.5°C (98° - 99.5°F) • Absence of systemic signs of infection: fever, tachypnea, tachycardia • Wounds free from redness, swelling, purulent drainage or odor • Urinary output 1 ml/kg/hr • Negative blood cultures • WBC within normal limits • Normal level of consciousness • Abdomen is nontender, nondistended, with bowel sounds in all quadrants
Urinary elimination, altered related to: • Urethral or renal trauma	The patient will have normal patterns of urinary elimination as evidenced by: • Urine output of 1 ml/kg/hr • Absence of or decreasing hematuria • Adequate bladder emptying

185

POSSIBLE NURSING DIAGNOSES AND EXPECTED OUTCOMES	
Nursing Diagnosis	**Expected Outcome**
Pain related to: • Blunt or penetrating injury • Stimulation of nerve fibers, secondary to abdominal distension • Invasive procedures	The patient will experience relief of pain as evidenced by: • Diminishing or absent level of pain through patient's self-report, using an objective measurement tool • Absence of physiologic indicators of pain, including: tachycardia, tachypnea, pallor, diaphoretic skin, increasing blood pressure • Absence of nonverbal cues of pain: crying, grimacing, inability to assume position of comfort • Ability to cooperate with care as appropriate

Planning and Implementation

Refer to Chapter 3, Initial Assessment, for a description of the specific nursing interventions for patients with compromises to airway, breathing, and/or circulation.

- Cannulate two veins with large bore, 14- or 16-gauge catheters, and initiate infusions of lactated Ringer's solution

- Administer blood, as prescribed

- Insert indwelling urinary catheter

  Suspected injury to the urethra is a contraindication of catheterization though the urethra.

- Insert gastric tube and aspirate gastric contents, in order to:

  ■ Decompress the stomach and prevent aspiration

  ■ Prevent vagal stimulation and resultant bradycardia

  ■ Minimize gastric content leakage and subsequent contamination of the abdominal cavity

  ■ Test the gastric aspirate for the presence of blood

- Cover open abdominal wounds with a sterile dressing. If evisceration of abdominal contents has occurred, place a sterile, moist dressing over the injury.

186

- Stabilize impaled objects

- Continue or apply a pneumatic antishock garment (PASG) for patients with severe hypotension due to hemorrhage. Although use of the garment is controversial, if used it may reduce intra-abdominal hemorrhage.[10]

- Administer antibiotics, as prescribed. Leakage of gastric and bowel contents will result in peritonitis and possibly sepsis.

- Administer analgesics, as prescribed

- Prepare the patient for operative intervention, hospital admission, or transfer, as indicated

- Provide psychosocial support

Evaluation and Ongoing Assessment

Refer to Chapter 3, Initial Assessment, for a description of the ongoing evaluation of the patient's airway, and effectiveness of breathing, and circulation. Additional evaluations include:

- Monitoring cardiovascular status for changes suggestive of hypovolemic shock

- Reassessing the abdomen frequently and thoroughly to detect subtle changes

SELECTED ABDOMINAL INJURIES

Refer to "Nursing Care of Patients with Abdominal Trauma" for a description of the phases of the trauma nursing process.

Hepatic Injuries

Due to its size and location, the liver is frequently injured when force is applied to the abdomen. The severity of hepatic injuries ranges from a controlled subcapsular hematoma and lacerations of the parenchyma to a severe vascular injury of the hepatic veins, retrohepatic cava, and/or hepatic avulsion (see Figure 18 and Appendix 7). The friability of liver tissue, the extensive blood supply, and the blood storage capacity cause hepatic injury to result in profuse hemorrhage. These types of injuries require surgical control of bleeding.

Figure 18
Types of Hepatic Injuries

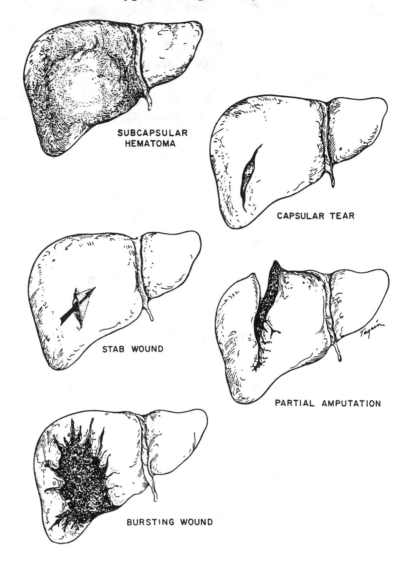

(Reprinted with permission from Malt RA. In: Burke JF, Boyd RJ, McCabe CJ, eds. *Trauma Management: Early Management of Visceral Nervous System, and Musculoskeletal Injuries.* Chicago, Ill; Year Book Medical Publishers, Inc; 1988:119.)

Signs and Symptoms

- Upper right quadrant pain

- Abdominal wall muscle rigidity, spasm, or involuntary guarding

- Rebound tenderness

- Hypoactive or absent bowel sounds

- Signs of hemorrhage and/or hypovolemic shock

Diagnostic Procedures

- Peritoneal lavage may reveal the presence of red blood cells and, occasionally, bile

- CT scan may show densities consistent with hematomas or bleeding

- Liver function studies

Splenic Injuries

Injury to the spleen is usually associated with mechanisms of injury resulting in blunt trauma. Fractures of the left 10th to 12th ribs are associated with underlying damage to the spleen. Injuries to the spleen range from laceration of the capsule or a non-expanding hematoma to ruptured subcapsular hematomas or parenchymal laceration. The most serious splenic injury is a severely fractured spleen or vascular tear, producing splenic ischemia and massive blood loss (see Appendix 7).

Signs and Symptoms

- Signs of hemorrhage and/or hypovolemic shock

- Pain in the left shoulder (Kehr's sign)

- Tenderness in the upper left quadrant

- Abdominal wall muscle rigidity, spasm, or involuntary guarding

Diagnostic Procedures

- Peritoneal lavage may reveal the presence of red blood cells

- CT scan may show densities consistent with hematomas or bleeding

Hollow Organ Injury

Forces causing injuries to hollow organs may result in either blunt or penetrating injuries. The small bowel is the hollow organ most frequently injured. Deceleration may lead to shearing, which causes avulsion or tearing of the small bowel. The areas of the small bowel most commonly affected are the areas relatively fixed or looped.

Signs and Symptoms

- Peritoneal irritation manifested by abdominal wall muscle rigidity, spasm, involuntary guarding, rebound tenderness, and/or pain

- Evisceration of the small bowel or stomach

- DPL may show presence of bile, feces or food fibers

Renal Injuries

The most common injury to the kidney is a blunt contusion (see Figure 19). Suspect renal injury if there are fractures of the posterior ribs or lumbar vertebrae. Renal parenchyma can be damaged by shearing and compression forces causing lacerations or contusion. The deeper the laceration, the more serious the bleeding. Rupture of the kidney is usually not associated with hypovolemia unless a laceration of a renal artery has occurred. Deceleration forces may cause vascular damage to the renal artery. Since there is little collateral circulation in the area of the renal artery, any ischemia is serious and may lead to acute tubular necrosis.

Signs and Symptoms

- Ecchymosis over the flank

- Flank or abdominal tenderness elicited during palpation

- Gross or microscopic hematuria – the absence of hematuria does not rule out renal injury

Diagnostic Procedures

Arteriography

Figure 19
Classification of Renal Trauma

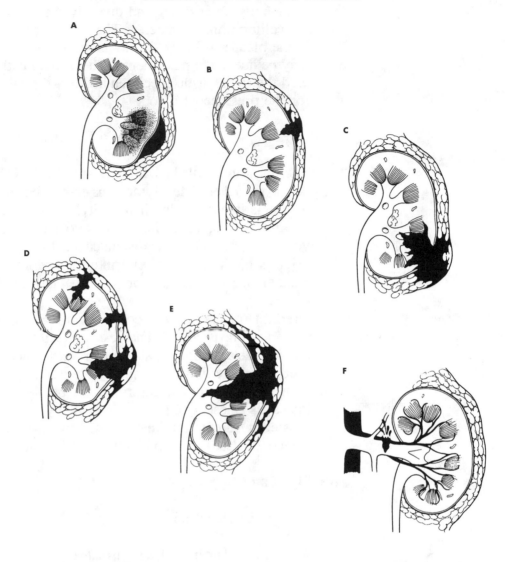

Figure Legend: A: minor injury – renal contusion with or without a subcapsular hematoma; B: minor laceration that does not include the collecting system; C-D-E: major lacerations resulting in some degree of urinary extravasation; F: shattered kidney, renal pedicle injury with injury to renal vein, artery, or branches.

(Reprinted with permission from Skinner E. Genitourinary trauma. *Trauma Surgery Techniques in Thoracic, Abdominal and Vascular Surgery*. St. Louis, Mo: Mosby-Year Book; 1994:166.)

Interventions

Frequently observe for and quantify the degree of hematuria with an indwelling urinary catheter. The initial urine obtained may have been in the bladder prior to the traumatic event. If hematuria is noted, this may be due to the placement of the urinary catheter. Measure and discard the initial urine specimen and test the subsequent urine specimen for the presence of blood.

Bladder and Urethral Injuries

The majority of bladder injuries are blunt. Normally, the bladder lies below the level of the symphysis pubis, but when full, it rises above the pubis into the abdominal cavity. If the bladder is not full when the rupture occurs, urine may leak into the surrounding pelvic tissues, vulva, or scrotum. If a distended bladder ruptures or is perforated, urine is likely to extravasate into the abdomen. Most ruptures of the bladder occur in association with pelvic fractures.

Urethral trauma is more common in males than females because the male urethra is longer and less protected. Suspicion of an anterior pelvic fracture should raise the index of suspicion of a concomitant urethral injury. Urethral injury in females is almost always associated with pelvic fractures. Injury to the penile portion of the urethra in males is most commonly caused by straddle trauma. Prostatic (posterior) urethral injury is usually caused by pelvic fractures and frequently leads to incontinence and impotence.[11]

Signs and Symptoms

- Suprapubic pain

- Urge, but inability to urinate

- Hematuria, may be microscopic

- Blood at the urethral meatus

- Blood in scrotum

- Rebound tenderness

- Abdominal wall muscle rigidity, spasm, or involuntary guarding

- Displacement of prostate gland

Diagnostic Procedures

- Analysis of urine

- IVP

- CT

- Arteriography

- Cystogram/urethrogram

Interventions

Drain urine via an indwelling urinary catheter to minimize urine leakage into the abdomen or supporting tissues. If a urethral injury is suspected, consider catheterizing the bladder through a suprapubic approach.

SUMMARY

Abdominal trauma is frequently associated with injuries to other body regions, including the chest. Due to the high vascularity of the solid organs and the presence of major vessels, abdominal trauma has the potential to produce hemorrhage and hypovolemic shock. Patients with abdominal injuries may not present with obvious signs and symptoms. Frequent assessments and ongoing evaluation are essential components of the trauma nursing process to detect changes in the patient's condition. Unrecognized abdominal trauma is a frequent cause of preventable death.[2]

The trauma nurse is part of a team who recognize the nature of multi-system trauma and the need for an organized, methodical approach to the assessment, diagnosis, and interventions for the management of the patient. The nurse, who is familiar with the anatomy of the abdomen, mechanisms and patterns of injury, and the pathophysiologic consequences of injury as a basis for signs and symptoms, contributes significantly to the collaborative efforts of the trauma team.

193

REFERENCES

1. Moore KL. The abdomen. In: *Clinically Oriented Anatomy*. 3rd ed. Baltimore, Md: Williams & Wilkins; 1992:127-242.

2. American College of Surgeons Committee on Trauma. Abdominal trauma. In: *Advanced Trauma Life Support® Course for Physicians (Student Manual)*. 5th ed. Chicago, Ill: Author; 1993:141-154.

3. Trunkey D, Hill AC, Schecter WP. Abdominal trauma and indications for celiotomy. In: Moore EE, Mattox KL, Feliciano DV, eds. *Trauma*. Norwalk, Conn: Appleton & Lange; 1991:409-426.

4. Marx, JA. Abdominal trauma. In: Rosen P, Barkin RM, Baker FJ, Braen GR, Dailey RH, Levy RC, eds. *Emergency Medicine: Concepts and Clinical Practice*. 3rd ed. St. Louis, Mo: Mosby-Year Book; 1992:471-496.

5. Mason PJB. Abdominal trauma. In: Cardona VD, Hurn PD, Mason PJB, Scanlon AM, Veise-Berry SW, eds. *Trauma Nursing: From Resuscitation Through Rehabilitation*. 2nd ed. Philadelphia, Pa: WB Saunders Co; 1994:512-547.

6. Hayes C, Conway W, Walsh J. Seat belt injuries: radiologic findings and clinical correlation. *Radiographics*. 1991;11:23.

7. Gay SB, Sistrom CL. Computed tomographic evaluation of blunt abdominal trauma. *Radiol Clin of North Am*. 1992;30:367-368/877.

8. Wolfman NT, Bechtold RE, Scharling ES, Meredith JW. Blunt upper abdominal trauma: evaluation by CT. *Am J Roentgenology*. 1992;158:493-501.

9. Trunkey D. Diagnostic laboratory investigation and diagnostic and interventional radiology. In: Champion HR, Robb J, Trunkey D, eds. *Robb & Smith's Operative Surgery: Trauma Surgery*. 4th ed. London, England: Butterworth; 1989:91.

10. American College of Surgeons, Committee on Trauma. Shock. In: *Advanced Trauma Life Support® Course for Physicians (Student Manual)*. 5th ed. Chicago, Ill: Author; 1993:75-94.

11. Zoller GW. Genitourinary trauma. In: Rosen P, Barkin RM, Baker FJ, Braen GR, Dailey RH, Levy RC, eds. *Emergency Medicine: Concepts and Clinical Practice*. 3rd ed. St. Louis, Mo: Mosby-Year Book; 1992:497-519.

CHAPTER EIGHT

SPINAL CORD AND
VERTEBRAL COLUMN TRAUMA

LECTURE BEGINS ON PAGE 205.

Preface

Prior to reading this chapter, it is strongly suggested that the learner read the following section entitled "Anatomy and Physiology." Specific anatomy and physiologic concepts are presented to enhance the learner's ability to correlate such concepts with specific injuries. This material on anatomy and physiology will not be covered during lectures, nor will it be evaluated by testing. However, knowledge of normal anatomy and physiology serves as the foundation for understanding the anatomic derangements and pathophysiologic compromises that may ensue as a result of trauma.

ANATOMY AND PHYSIOLOGY

Vertebral Column

The vertebral column is a series of stacked bones that support the head and trunk and provide the bony encasement for the spinal cord. The vertebral column is composed of 33 vertebrae divided into regions. The first seven vertebrae are the cervical vertebrae. There are 12 thoracic vertebrae, five lumbar vertebrae, five sacral vertebrae (fused into one), and four coccygeal vertebrae (fused into one) (see Figure 20). The typical vertebra is composed of a body (anterior or ventral) and a vertebral arch, which forms the enclosure, the vertebral foramen, for passage of the spinal cord. The spinal cord fills about 35% of the vertebral foramen at the origin of the spinal cord at C-1. In the remainder of the cervical and thoracolumbar regions, the spinal cord fills 50% of the foramen.[1] The arch is made of two pedicles, two laminae, four articular processes (facets), two transverse processes, and one spinous process. The spinous process can be felt by an examiner when palpating the back (see Figure 21).

Figure 20
Vertebral Column

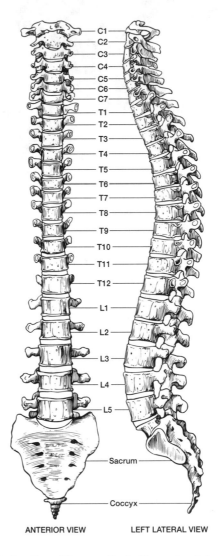

ANTERIOR VIEW   LEFT LATERAL VIEW

(Reprinted with permission from Waxman S, de Groot J, ed. In: The spinal cord in situ. *Correlative Neuroanatomy*. 22nd ed. Norwalk, Conn: Appleton & Lange; 1995:74.)

Cervical Vertebrae

The cervical vertebrae are the smallest and most flexible. The first cervical vertebra, the atlas, supports the weight of the head and articulates with the occipital condyles of the skull. The atlas is different from the other vertebrae since it has no spinous process or vertebral body. In addition, the foramen opening for the spinal cord is larger than the rest of the vertebrae. The axis, C-2, has a perpendicular projection called the odontoid process or dens. The atlas articulates with the axis on the odontoid process.

196

Figure 21
Structure of Vertebrae

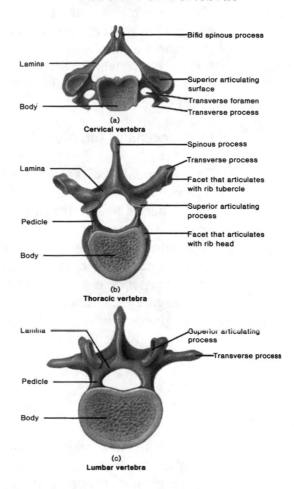

Thoracic Vertebrae

The thoracic vertebrae, T-1 through T-12, articulate with the ribs. The attachment to the ribs limits flexion and extension, but permits more rotation than the lumbar region and less than the cervical region. The vertebrae in this region are strong, and additional support is provided by the ribs. Extreme forces are required to produce fractures and dislocations in this region of the vertebral column. Therefore, vertebral fractures in the thoracic region can be frequently accompanied by spinal cord injury.

Lumbar, Sacral, and Coccygeal Vertebrae

The five lumbar vertebrae (L-1 to L-5) are the largest and strongest in the vertebral column. This area of the spine has some freedom of movement and rotation, but not as much as the cervical region. The five sacral vertebrae (S-1 to S-5) are fused to form the sacrum in the adult, and the final four coccygeal vertebrae are fused to form the coccyx.[2]

Ligaments and Intravertebral Discs

The vertebral bodies are connected by a series of ligaments which provide support and stability for the vertebral column. The anterior and posterior longitudinal ligaments are major ligaments that run the length of the vertebral column and hold the discs and vertebral bodies in position. The ligaments prevent the vertebral column from experiencing excessive flexion and extension. The spinous and transverse processes serve as attachment points for muscles and other ligaments (see Figure 22). Located between the vertebral bodies are fibro-cartilaginous discs, which act as shock absorbers during weight bearing and articulating surfaces for the subsequent vertebral bodies. The more flexible cervical and lumbar regions contain thicker intervertebral discs.[2]

Spinal Cord

The spinal cord is an elongated mass of nerve tissue. The spinal cord occupies the vertebral foramen of the vertebral column and extends from the superior border of C-1 to the superior border of L-2. In the lower thoracic area, the cord tapers and terminates into a cone-shaped structure called the conus medullaris. Spinal nerve roots continue to exit below the conus medullaris and are collectively referred to as the cauda equina.

The spinal cord, when viewed in a cross section, has an H-shaped core. The core is made up of gray matter, which consists of nerve cell bodies. The gray matter is surrounded by white matter. The white matter is composed of longitudinal nerve projections composed of ascending and descending tracts. The descending pathways are motor tracts, and the ascending pathways are sensory tracts. The descending pathways are termed the corticospinal tracts. The ascending pathways are termed the spinothalamic and posterior tracts.

Figure 22
Section of Vertebral Column

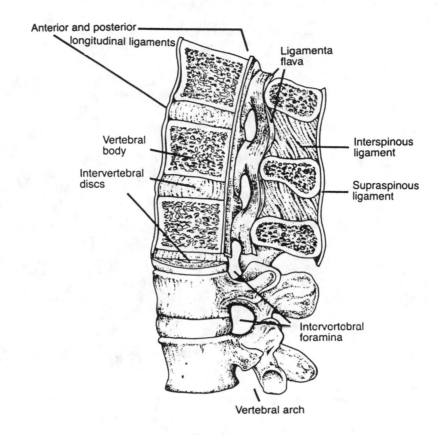

Anterior and posterior longitudinal ligaments

Ligamenta flava

Vertebral body

Interspinous ligament

Intervertebral discs

Supraspinous ligament

Intervertebral foramina

Vertebral arch

(Reprinted with permission from Romero-Sierra C. In: *Neuroanatomy: A Conceptual Approach*. New York, NY: Churchill Livingstone; 1986.)

Motor

Voluntary motor movement originates from cells in the frontal lobe of the cerebral cortex (upper motor neurons). Upper motor neurons cross to the opposite side in the medulla of the brainstem and then descend in the corticospinal (pyramidal) tract. Upper motor neurons synapse with cell bodies of lower motor neurons on the anterior horn of the gray matter in the spinal cord. The lower motor neurons innervate skeletal muscle. The cervical nerve fibers of the corticospinal tract, which innervate the upper extremities, are located in the central portion of the anterior horn or gray column of the spinal cord (see Figure 23). The sacral fibers of the corticospinal tract, which innervate the lower extremities, are located in the peripheral portion of the anterior horn or gray column of the spinal cord.[1,3]

Figure 23
Cross Section of Spinal Cord

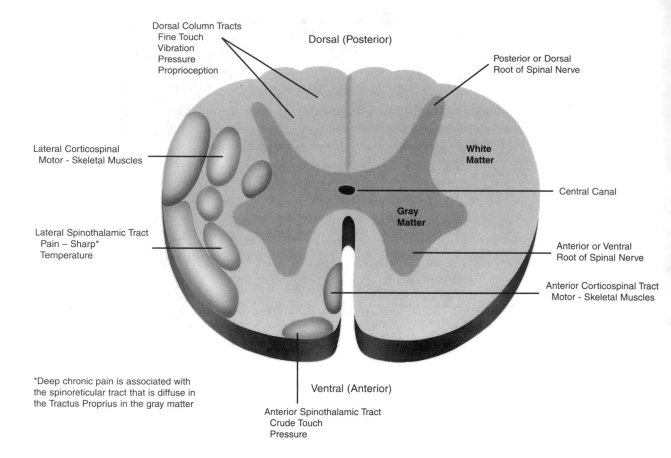

Dorsal Column Tracts
Fine Touch
Vibration
Pressure
Proprioception

Dorsal (Posterior)

Posterior or Dorsal
Root of Spinal Nerve

Lateral Corticospinal
Motor - Skeletal Muscles

White Matter

Central Canal

Gray Matter

Lateral Spinothalamic Tract
Pain – Sharp*
Temperature

Anterior or Ventral
Root of Spinal Nerve

Anterior Corticospinal Tract
Motor - Skeletal Muscles

*Deep chronic pain is associated with
the spinoreticular tract that is diffuse in
the Tractus Proprius in the gray matter

Ventral (Anterior)

Anterior Spinothalamic Tract
Crude Touch
Pressure

Sensory

Sensory input can be integrated into spinal reflexes or relayed to higher centers in the brain for interpretation. Sensation is classified as superficial, deep, and/or combined. Superficial sensation is related to touch, pain, and temperature. Deep sensation is muscle or joint position sense (proprioception), vibration sensation, and deep muscle pain.[3] The afferent (ascending) impulses transmit sensory information from specific segments of skin referred to as dermatomes (see Figure 24). Afferent impulses enter the spinal cord via the posterior (dorsal) roots and ascend in a tract of the spinal cord, depending on the type of sensation. Proprioception and vibration fibers ascend via the posterior column and cross in the medulla. Pain and temperature fibers cross immediately on entering the spinal cord, or within one to two spinal segments, before ascending in the spinothalamic tract. Touch sensation fibers cross immediately upon entering the spinal cord and then ascend in the spinothalamic tract[1,3] (see Table 15).

200

Figure 24
Dermatomes

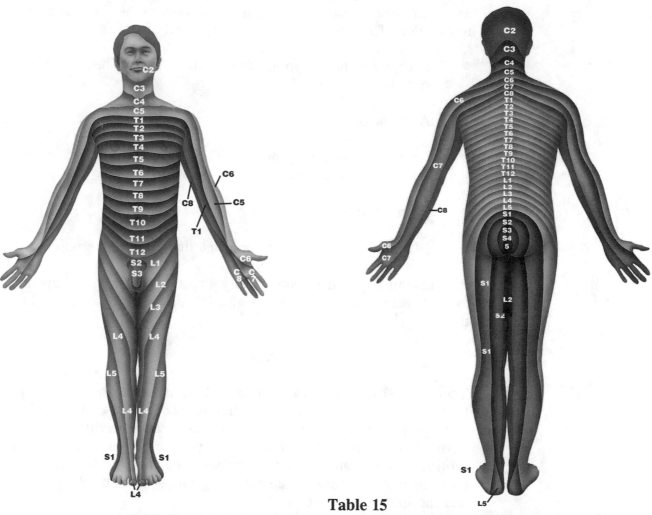

Table 15

MOTOR AND SENSORY SPINAL NERVE TRACTS				
Nerve Tracts	**Origin**	**Cross Over**	**Function**	**Location in Spinal Cord**
DESCENDING TRACTS • Corticospinal (Pyramidal)	Cerebral cortex	Medulla	• Voluntary motor	Anterolateral
ASCENDING TRACTS • Spinothalamic	Sensory receptors located throughout body	Level they enter spinal cord	• Pain • Temperature • Crude touch • Crude pressure	Anterolateral
• Posterior tracts (Dorsal)	Sensory receptors located throughout body	Medulla	• Proprioception • Vibration • Fine touch • Fine pressure	Posterior (Dorsal)

The Reflex Arc

The reflex arc is a stimulus-response mechanism that does not require ascending or descending spinal cord pathways to the cerebral cortex to function. The essential structures of the reflex are[3]:

- Receptor (sense organ, cutaneous end-organ, or neuromuscular spindle)

- Afferent (sensory) neuron

- Intercalated neuron (neuron within the spinal cord that relays impulse to the efferent neuron)

- Efferent (motor) neuron

- Effector (muscle, tendon, or gland that produces response)

An anatomically and physiologically intact reflex arc will function even if there is disruption of spinal cord function above the level of the reflex.[1]

Spinal Nerves

There are 31 pairs of spinal nerves, which include eight cervical, 12 thoracic, five lumbar, five sacral, and one coccygeal (see Figure 25). Each pair of spinal nerves exit the spinal cord bilaterally, and each have a posterior (dorsal) root and anterior (ventral) root. The posterior (dorsal) root transmits sensory impulses. The anterior (ventral) roots transmit motor impulses from cells originating in the cerebral cortex and the spinal cord to the body.

The thoracic nerves innervate the thorax, abdomen, buttocks (skin), and portions of the upper arm. The intercostal muscles are innervated by spinal nerves T-2 through T-8. The lumbar nerves innervate the groin region and lower extremities. The sacral nerves S-3 to S-5 supply the perianal muscles, which control voluntary contraction of the external bladder sphincter and the external anal sphincter.

Figure 25
Spinal Nerves and Plexuses

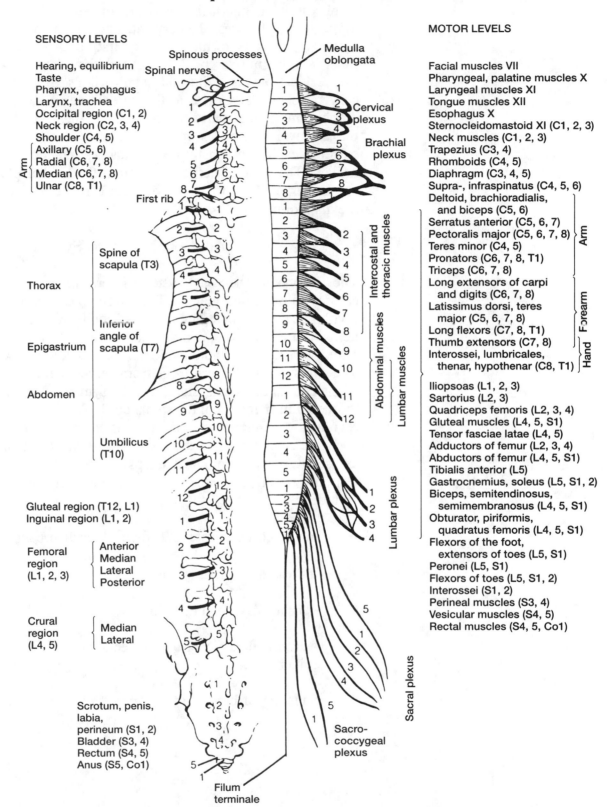

SENSORY LEVELS

Hearing, equilibrium
Taste
Pharynx, esophagus
Larynx, trachea
Occipital region (C1, 2)
Neck region (C2, 3, 4)
Shoulder (C4, 5)

Arm
Axillary (C5, 6)
Radial (C6, 7, 8)
Median (C6, 7, 8)
Ulnar (C8, T1)

Spinous processes
Spinal nerves
First rib

Spine of scapula (T3)

Thorax

Inferior angle of scapula (T7)

Epigastrium

Abdomen

Umbilicus (T10)

Gluteal region (T12, L1)
Inguinal region (L1, 2)

Femoral region (L1, 2, 3)
Anterior
Median
Lateral
Posterior

Crural region (L4, 5)
Median
Lateral

Scrotum, penis, labia, perineum (S1, 2)
Bladder (S3, 4)
Rectum (S4, 5)
Anus (S5, Co1)

Filum terminale

Medulla oblongata
Cervical plexus
Brachial plexus
Intercostal and thoracic muscles
Abdominal muscles
Lumbar muscles
Lumbar plexus
Sacral plexus
Sacro-coccygeal plexus

MOTOR LEVELS

Facial muscles VII
Pharyngeal, palatine muscles X
Laryngeal muscles XI
Tongue muscles XII
Esophagus X
Sternocleidomastoid XI (C1, 2, 3)
Neck muscles (C1, 2, 3)
Trapezius (C3, 4)
Rhomboids (C4, 5)
Diaphragm (C3, 4, 5)
Supra-, infraspinatus (C4, 5, 6)

Arm
Deltoid, brachioradialis, and biceps (C5, 6)
Serratus anterior (C5, 6, 7)
Pectoralis major (C5, 6, 7, 8)
Teres minor (C4, 5)
Pronators (C6, 7, 8, T1)
Triceps (C6, 7, 8)

Forearm
Long extensors of carpi and digits (C6, 7, 8)
Latissimus dorsi, teres major (C5, 6, 7, 8)
Long flexors (C7, 8, T1)
Thumb extensors (C7, 8)

Hand
Interossei, lumbricales, thenar, hypothenar (C8, T1)

Iliopsoas (L1, 2, 3)
Sartorius (L2, 3)
Quadriceps femoris (L2, 3, 4)
Gluteal muscles (L4, 5, S1)
Tensor fasciae latae (L4, 5)
Adductors of femur (L2, 3, 4)
Abductors of femur (L4, 5, S1)
Tibialis anterior (L5)
Gastrocnemius, soleus (L5, S1, 2)
Biceps, semitendinosus, semimembranosus (L4, 5, S1)
Obturator, piriformis, quadratus femoris (L4, 5, S1)
Flexors of the foot, extensors of toes (L5, S1)
Peronei (L5, S1)
Flexors of toes (L5, S1, 2)
Interossei (S1, 2)
Perineal muscles (S3, 4)
Vesicular muscles (S4, 5)
Rectal muscles (S4, 5, Co1)

(Reprinted with permission from Waxman S, de Groot J, ed. Appendix C. In: *Correlative Neuroanatomy*. 22nd ed. Norwalk, Conn: Appleton & Lange; 1995:358.)

203

Plexuses

A plexus is an interlacing network of nerve fibers. There are four major nerve plexuses: the cervical, brachial, lumbar, and sacral. The cervical plexus is formed by the first four cervical nerves, which innervate the muscles of the neck and shoulders. In addition, C-4 of the cervical plexus, with additional origins from the third and fifth cervical nerve, gives rise to the phrenic nerve, which innervates the diaphragm. Spinal nerves C-5 to C-8, and T-1, form the brachial plexus, which supplies motor control and sensation to the upper extremities. The brachial plexus branches include the ulnar and radial nerves. The femoral nerve arises from the lumbar plexus, formed by spinal nerves T-12 to L-4. The sciatic nerve arises from the sacral plexus, formed by L-4 to L-5, and S-1 to S-3.[4]

Autonomic Nervous System

The autonomic nervous system fibers innervate smooth muscle, cardiac muscle, and glands. The autonomic nervous system controls involuntary vital functions such as blood pressure, heart rate, body temperature, appetite, fluid balance, gastrointestinal motility, and sexual function. The autonomic nervous system has two subdivisions. The parasympathetic originates from nerves in the craniosacral regions of the central nervous system, and the sympathetic originates from the thoracolumbar region of the spinal cord. The parasympathetic division regulates the function of smooth muscle, cardiac muscle, and glands under normal body conditions. Sympathetic system activity is increased during physiological and psychological stress. The generalized response resulting from stimulation of the sympathetic nervous system includes[4,5]:

- Increased heart rate and force of cardiac contraction

- Increased respiratory rate

- Peripheral vasoconstriction

- Adrenal gland release of catecholamines, norepinephrine, and epinephrine

- Shunting of blood to the core circulation

SPINAL CORD AND VERTEBRAL COLUMN TRAUMA

OBJECTIVES

Upon completion of this chapter/lecture, the learner should be able to:

1. Identify the mechanisms of injury associated with spinal cord and/or vertebral column trauma.
2. Analyze the pathophysiologic changes as a basis for signs and symptoms.
3. Discuss the nursing assessment of the patient with spinal cord and/or vertebral column trauma.
4. Based on the assessment data, identify appropriate nursing diagnoses and expected outcomes.
5. Plan appropriate interventions for spinal cord and/or vertebral column trauma patients.
6. Evaluate the effectiveness of nursing interventions for patients with spinal cord and/or vertebral column injuries.

INTRODUCTION

Epidemiology

Each year approximately 10,000 Americans sustain spinal cord injuries. Eighty percent of spinal cord injured victims are males. The majority of men injured are between 16 and 30 years of age (60%). Motor vehicle crashes account for the largest number of spinal cord and vertebral column injuries among young men, and frequently involve alcohol use. Falls are the second most common cause. Greater than 50% of the spinal cord injuries in people older than 60 years of age are associated with falls.[6] Gunshot or stab wounds, sports-related injuries, assaults, and diving injuries are responsible for the remaining spinal cord and vertebral column injuries.[5]

Mechanisms of Injury and Biomechanics

The type of vehicular crash is associated with certain movements of the vertebral column. The highest incidence of fatal and nonfatal injuries are a result of side impact collisions. Rear-end collisions usually result in hyperextension injuries to the vertebral column and/or spinal cord. Head-on collisions result in hyperflexion injuries. Persons ejected from vehicles are at an extremely high risk for serious neck injury.[7] Victims of motorcycle crashes are frequently ejected over the handlebars and may sustain spinal cord and/or vertebral column injury.[8]

The use of safety restraint systems minimizes the possibility of ejection. Incorrectly applied seat belts may be associated with injuries. Serious injury to the anterior neck may be associated with the use of diagonal torso belts. The use of a lap belt may contribute to fracture or dislocation of a lumbar vertebra.

Rapid acceleration or deceleration forces may cause the spine to move beyond its usual range of motion, resulting in hyperextension, hyperflexion, or flexion/rotation injuries. Axial loading results from vertical compressive forces applied to the vertebral column.

Hyperextension injuries are caused by the backward thrust of the head beyond the tolerance of the cervical vertebral column. Resultant damage to the anterior ligaments can vary from minor, as is demonstrated by whiplash, to the severely unstable injury involving ligamentous tears and bony dislocations (see Figure 26).[9]

Hyperflexion injuries may occur when a motor vehicle occupant's cervical spine is forcefully flexed forward and the head strikes an immovable object, such as the windshield. Flexion injuries are the most common cause of spinal cord injury.[9]

Figure 26
Neck Movement During a Rear-End Crash

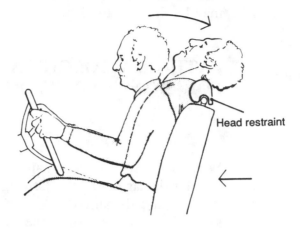

(Reprinted with permission from Moore KL. The back. In: *Clinically Oriented Anatomy*. 3rd ed. Baltimore, Md: Williams & Wilkins; 1992:347.)

Rotational injuries are frequently seen in motor vehicle crashes. Injury results from loss of posterior ligament integrity, and anterior fracture and/or dislocation of the vertebral body.[10] Flexion/rotation injuries may result in rupture of the posterior ligament, and/or anterior fracture or dislocation of the vertebral body.[11]

Axial loading results from direct forces transmitted along the length of the vertebral column. An example is the diver who strikes his or her head on the bottom of a swimming pool.[9] These compressive forces may cause deformity of the vertebral column and secondary edema of the spinal cord, resulting in neurological deficits.

Types of Injuries

Most injuries to the spinal cord and/or vertebral column are blunt injuries from acceleration and/or deceleration forces on the spinal cord and/or vertebral column. Most penetrating injuries result from gunshots that often disrupt the integrity of the vertebral column. Stab wounds do not often cause instability of the vertebral column. However, the wounding object may lacerate the spinal cord and/or nerve roots.

Usual Concurrent Injuries

Usual concurrent injuries include closed head injuries, long bone fractures, thoracic, and abdominal injuries. Rib fractures or chest injury may be associated with thoracic vertebral injury. Pelvic fractures are frequently associated with injuries of the lumbar spine. A fall from a height, resulting in calcaneus fractures, is an additional pattern of injury associated with compression fractures of the lumbar vertebrae.[1] Due to the patient's inability to feel pain, potentially serious injuries elsewhere in the body, such as abdominal injuries, may be difficult to identify.[12]

PATHOPHYSIOLOGY AS A BASIS FOR SIGNS AND SYMPTOMS

Neurologic Deficits

When excessive force is applied to the spinal cord, hemorrhage, cellular damage, structural changes, and/or biochemical responses to injury cause damage to the cord. The spinal cord is rarely actually severed or transected. The spinal cord is usually bruised or compressed initially, resulting in hemorrhage into the tissue and edema. Vasomotor activity is lost and blood flow to the injured area is diminished with resultant secondary ischemia.[1] Since the spinal cord occupies a small space of the cervical foramen, there is more space for swelling and edema to occur, prolonging the vascular occlusion and causing the development of ischemia.

Secondary damage to the spinal cord can occur from:

- Hypovolemic shock

- Shock, resulting in bradycardia, peripheral vasodilation, and hypotension[8,13]

- Injury due to inadequate spinal immobilization

- Endogenous biochemical responses causing edema and cellular necrosis[10]

- Hypoxia

Since spinal cord neurons do not regenerate, severe injury with cellular death results in permanent loss of function. Injury to the spinal cord may result in loss of all motor and sensory functions below the level of the lesion. Loss of function may be temporary if cellular death has not occurred.

Spinal Cord Pathology

Spinal cord pathology may be due to concussion, contusion, transection, or disruption of the blood supply to the cord.

- Concussion is a temporary loss of function lasting 24 to 48 hours. This injury may be observed in patients with pre-existing degenerative disease, with resultant narrowing of the vertebral foramen. The pathological changes are not identifiable.[5,8]

- Contusion is bruising of the cord with edema and possible necrosis of tissue from cord compression. The amount of neurological deficit is dependent on the physiologic changes and the presence of necrosis.

- A transection is the complete or incomplete severing of the cord. Although a complete transection of the spinal cord is rare, a complete physiologic transection may be seen. A laceration of the cord produces permanent residual deficits.

- Interruption in the vascular supply to the spinal cord may result in cord ischemia or necrosis. Temporary deficits may be caused by episodes of ischemia, while prolonged ischemia will result in necrosis of the spinal cord with permanent neurological deficits.[5]

Inadequate Ventilation

Injuries to the upper cervical region of the spinal cord are most critical as this region supports respiratory function. The most likely cause of death in a spinal cord injury above C-4 is respiratory arrest due to loss of phrenic nerve function and resultant paralysis of the diaphragm. Damage to the cord above the region of T-2 to T-8 may result in a loss of function of the intercostal muscles and disruption of the mechanics of ventilation.

Shock

Spinal Shock

Spinal shock usually occurs shortly after the spinal cord is suddenly injured or damaged. Spinal shock results in the temporary loss of motor, sensory, and reflex functions below the level of the lesion. The onset is usually immediate, but can occur several days after the initial injury. The intensity and duration of spinal shock varies with the level of the lesion. Spinal shock may last days or weeks. The patient presents with flaccid paralysis and bowel and bladder dysfunction. The conversion to spastic paralysis and return of reflexes indicates the resolution of spinal shock.[14]

Neurogenic Shock

Neurogenic shock, a form of distributive shock, is associated with spinal cord injuries at the level of T-6 or above. Impairment of the descending sympathetic pathways in the spinal cord results in loss of vasomotor tone and sympathetic innervation to the heart.[12] The sympathetic fibers of the autonomic nervous system are located from T-1 through L-2, and communicate with vasomotor centers in the brain. When these pathways are interrupted, loss of sympathetic activity leads to vasodilation, a maldistribution of blood volume, and cardiac deceleration. The patient presents with hypotension and bradycardia. The massive vasodilation results in a decreased preload, decreased cardiac filling, decreased stroke volume, and hypotension. The patient experiences hypotension despite a normal volume.[14]

NURSING CARE OF PATIENTS WITH SPINAL CORD AND VERTEBRAL COLUMN TRAUMA

Assessment

History

Refer to Chapter 3, Initial Assessment, for a description of general information that should be collected regarding every trauma victim. Only pertinent questions specific to patients with spinal cord or vertebral column injuries are described below.

- Does the patient complain of neck or back pain?

- Was there spontaneous movement or altered sensation of the extremities?

  Changes may indicate expansion of a hematoma or additional edema formation.

Physical Assessment

INSPECTION

- Assess breathing effectiveness and rate of respirations

  Spinal cord injury at the level of C-3 to C-5 interferes with diaphragmatic function. Although C-6 lesions spare the diaphragm, edema formation and hemorrhage may affect respiratory effort.[5] Lesions at T-2 to T-8 may spare the diaphragm but result in loss of intercostal muscle function. The higher the lesion, the greater the loss of intercostal muscle function.

- Assess motor and sensory functions

  Ask patient to wiggle his or her toes and fingers; gently lift an arm and a leg.

- Logroll patient and examine vertebral column for deformity or open wounds

- Observe for priapism (continuous erection of the penis), due to parasympathetic nervous system stimulation and loss of sympathetic nervous system control.[4]

PALPATION

- Palpate pulse rate and quality

  Pulse is slow and full in neurogenic shock, as opposed to rapid and weak in hypovolemic shock.

- Palpate skin temperature

  Skin is warm and dry in neurogenic shock as opposed to cool and moist in hypovolemic shock. The patient may assume the temperature of the environment (poikilothermy).[5]

- Assess all four extremities for motor function and muscle strength

  An inability to perform gross extremity movement indicates a lesion above the level:

  Extend and flex arms: C-5 to C-7
  Extend and flex legs: L-2 to L-4
  Flexion of foot, extension of toes: L-4 to L-5
  Tighten anus: S-3 to S-5

- Assess sensory function

  - The use of a touch stimulus to determine levels of sensory function should begin at the area of no feeling and proceed toward the area of feeling. This will aid in localizing the level of injury (see Figure 24).

C-5	Top of shoulder
T-4	Nipple line
T-10	Umbilicus
L-4	Great toe

- ■ Proprioception is the ability of the patient to sense the position of a particular body part. Move the patient's great toe up, down, or leave it neutral. Ask the patient to describe the various positions.

- ● Gently palpate vertebral column for pain, tenderness, or step deformities between vertebrae

- ● Palpate anal sphincter for presence or absence of tone

  Contraction of the anal sphincter is either voluntary or reflex.

- ● Assess for sacral sparing

  The presence of perianal sensation, anal sphincter tone, and great toe flexor activity represents an incomplete spinal cord injury.[1]

PERCUSSION

Assist with examination of deep tendon reflexes and Babinski reflex. In the presence of spinal shock, the patient will present with areflexia. A Babinski's reflex is a pathologic reflex, due to dysfunction of upper motor neurons of the corticospinal tract. A positive Babinski's reflex is extension of the great toe and fanning of the other toes when the sole of the relaxed foot is stroked.[15]

Diagnostic Procedures

Refer to Chapter 3, Initial Assessment, for frequently-ordered radiographic and laboratory studies. Additional studies for patients with spinal cord and/or vertebral trauma are listed below.

RADIOGRAPHIC STUDIES

- ● Vertebral column radiographs

  - ■ Obtain an initial cross-table lateral of the cervical spine. Additional views can determine the exact site and nature of the bony injury.[7,16] These views may include anterior/posterior, odontoid, and obliques. Cervical spine films should visualize all seven cervical vertebrae and T-1.

- Radiographic studies of the thoracic and lumbar spine, as indicated. Thorough radiographic evaluation is indicated if the patient has an altered mental status.

- CT scan

  If C-7 to T-1 cannot be visualized on x-ray, consider CT.[16]

- MRI

Nursing Diagnoses and Outcome Identification

The following nursing diagnoses are potential problems for the patient with spinal cord and/or vertebral column injuries. Once a patient has been assessed, diagnoses can be defined as either actual or risk. An actual nursing diagnosis is one derived from a decision based on the patient's presenting signs and symptoms. A risk nursing diagnosis is a judgment that the nurse makes based on a particular patient's risk and potential for developing certain problems.

POSSIBLE NURSING DIAGNOSES AND EXPECTED OUTCOMES	
Nursing Diagnosis	**Expected Outcome**

Airway clearance, ineffective related to:
 • Decreased strength of cough secondary to paralysis of chest and abdominal muscles
	The patient will maintain a patent airway as evidenced by:
	 • ABG values within normal limits:
	   ▪ PaO_2 80 - 100 mmHg (10.0 - 13.3 KPa)
	   ▪ SaO_2 >95%
	   ▪ $PaCO_2$ 35 - 45 mmHg (4.7 - 6.0 KPa)
	   ▪ pH between 7.35 - 7.45
	 • Clear, bilateral breath sounds
	 • Clear sputum of normal amount without color or odor
	 • Absence of signs and symptoms of retained secretions: fever, tachycardia, tachypnea
	 • Effective cough when assisted

POSSIBLE NURSING DIAGNOSES AND EXPECTED OUTCOMES

Nursing Diagnosis	Expected Outcome

Aspiration, risk related to:
• Reduced level of consciousness
• Impaired cough and gag reflex secondary to spinal cord injury
• Spinal immobilization devices
• Gastric distension secondary to paralytic ileus
	The patient will not experience aspiration as evidenced by:
	• A patent airway
	• Clear and equal bilateral breath sounds
	• Regular rate, depth, and pattern of breathing
	• ABG values within normal limits:
	  ■ PaO_2 80 - 100 mmHg (10.0 - 13.3 KPa)
	  ■ SaO_2 >95%
	  ■ $PaCO_2$ 35 - 45 mmHg (4.7 - 6.0 KPa)
	  ■ pH between 7.35 - 7.45
	• Clear CXR without evidence of infiltrates
	• Ability to handle secretions independently

Gas exchange, impaired related to:
• Lost innervation of respiratory muscles secondary to spinal cord injury
• Shock
	The patient will experience adequate gas exchange as evidenced by:
	• Patent airway
	• Vital signs within normal limits for developmental age
	• Clear and equal bilateral breath sounds
	• Regular rate, depth, and pattern of breathing
	• ABG values within normal limits:
	  ■ PaO_2 80 - 100 mmHg (10.0 - 13.3 KPa)
	  ■ SaO_2 >95%
	  ■ $PaCO_2$ 35 - 45 mmHg (4.7 - 6.0 KPa)
	  ■ pH between 7.35 - 7.45
	• Skin normal color, warm, and dry
	• Normal level of consciousness

Fluid volume deficit related to: • Spinal shock • Alteration in vascular tone secondary to spinal cord injury	The patient will have an effective circulating volume as evidenced by: • Stable vital signs appropriate for developmental age • Urinary output of 1 ml/kg/hr • Strong, palpable peripheral pulses • Improved level of consciousness • Skin normal color, warm, and dry
Thermoregulation, ineffective related to: • Loss of hypothalamic control secondary to spinal cord injury	The patient will maintain a normal core body temperature as evidenced by: • Core temperature measurement of 36° - 37.5°C (98° - 99.5°F) • Absence of shivering, cool skin, pallor • Skin normal color, warm, and dry

POSSIBLE NURSING DIAGNOSES AND EXPECTED OUTCOMES	
Nursing Diagnosis	**Expected Outcome**
Injury, risk related to: • Instability of vertebral column fracture • Altered level of consciousness • Lack of knowledge regarding spinal precautions	The patient will be free from increase in injury as evidenced by: • No iatrogenic extension of the injury • Movement of neck is minimized due to proper alignment and immobilization of the spinal column • Verbalizes and demonstrates understanding of need for no movement of neck • Absence of increase in extent of original injury
Impaired skin integrity, risk related to: • Pressure, shear, friction forces on skin and tissue • Mechanical irritants: fixation devices • Impaired mobility • Urinary and bowel incontinence • Sensory and motor deficits	The patient will demonstrate absence or resolution of impaired skin integrity as evidenced by: • Absence of signs of irritation: redness, ulceration, blanching, itching • Signs of progressive healing of dermal layer • Understanding and willingness to participate in frequent movement to relieve pressure • Verbalizes understanding of immobilization devices
Infection, risk related to: • Contact with contagious agents (community and nosocomial acquired) • Contamination of wounds • Prolonged immobility • Stress • Break in aseptic technique • Iatrogenic introduction of organisms during invasive procedures	The patient will be free from infection as evidenced by: • Core temperature measurement of 36° - 37.5°C (98° - 99.5°F) • Absence of systemic signs of infection: fever, tachypnea, tachycardia • Wounds free from redness, swelling, purulent drainage or odor • Urinary output 1 ml/kg/hr • Negative blood cultures • WBC count within normal limits • Normal level of consciousness

Planning and Implementation

Refer to Chapter 3, Initial Assessment, for a description of the specific nursing interventions for patients with compromises to airway, breathing, and/or circulation.

• Immobilize vertebral column

Spinal immobilization includes stabilization (as defined in Chapter 3) and the application of a backboard and straps.

- Suction airway, as needed

  Use caution since vigorous suctioning can lead to bradycardia. Bradycardia may be due to stimulation of the vagus nerve in combination with a loss of sympathetic function.[17]

- Administer steroids, as prescribed

  Large-dose steroid (methylprednisolone) administration has been reported to minimize the effects of certain biochemical responses to spinal cord injury. The primary benefit appears to be limitation of cord edema, ischemia, and the prevention of cellular death.[18] The recommended regime for administration is a 30 mg/kg loading dose over 15 minutes. Wait 45 minutes; then initiate a 5.4 mg/kg/hour intravenous infusion over the next 23 hours. For maximum effect, the initial dose must be administered within the first eight hours of injury.[19,20]

- Insert a gastric tube

- Provide psychosocial support

- Keep the patient warm

  Increase room temperature and/or cover patient with a warm blanket to prevent loss of body heat.

- Initiate skin care early

  Identify and document high-risk areas of abrasions or loss of skin integrity. Remove or pad the backboard as soon as possible. Keep clean, dry linen beneath the patient and protect all bony prominences from pressure with padding.

- Assist with application of skeletal tongs

  Skeletal tongs and traction are frequently applied in the emergency department to obtain and maintain spinal alignment, and reduce patient discomfort due to muscle spasm. The spring-loaded Gardner-Wells tongs are the most commonly used and are easily applied. Two other types of tongs are Vinke and Crutchfield. Once tongs are applied, assure that traction weights are hanging freely at all times.[4]

- Consider transferring the patient with a spinal cord injury, either suspected or confirmed, to a specialized facility. Consult the receiving facility regarding stabilization techniques during transfer.

Evaluation and Ongoing Assessment

Refer to Chapter 3, Initial Assessment, for a description of the ongoing evaluation of the patient's airway, and effectiveness of breathing and circulation. Additional evaluations include:

- Monitoring breathing effectiveness

  Patients with disruption of innervation to the intercostal muscles develop respiratory fatigue.

- Monitoring changes in sensory and/or motor function

- Monitoring temperature to avoid hypothermia

SELECTED VERTEBRAL COLUMN AND SPINAL CORD INJURIES

Refer to "Nursing Care of Patients with Spinal Cord and/or Vertebral Column Trauma" for a description of the phases of the trauma nursing process.

Vertebral Column Fractures and Dislocations

Vertebral fractures most often occur in the vertebral body, or in combination with another part. Due to the mobility of the cervical and lumbar regions, they are more frequently injured. Greater force is required to fracture the thoracic vertebrae since they are supported by the ribs. Vertebral fractures are classified into major categories (see Table 16).

- Simple fractures

- Compression or wedge fractures

- Comminuted or burst fractures

- Teardrop fractures

Injuries to the anterior and posterior ligaments may produce unilateral or bilateral facet dislocation, resulting in malalignment (dislocation) of the vertebrae. If the vertebrae are not completely dislocated, it is termed a subluxation. Dislocations and subluxations may occur simultaneously with a fracture.

217

Table 16

VERTEBRAL COLUMN FRACTURES		
Fracture/ Dislocation	**Mechanism of Injury**	**Description**
Simple	• Acceleration or deceleration forces	• Linear fracture of the spinous or transverse process, facets, or pedicles • Compression of spinal cord is rare • Vertebral column remains aligned
Compression (Wedge)	• Compression of vertebral body • Anterior or lateral flexion • Hyperflexion	• Fracture of vertebral body • Compression of the spinal cord may or may not be present
Burst	• Axial loading	• Comminuted fracture of vertebral body • May result in spinal cord compression
Teardrop	• Hyperflexion	• Small fracture of anterior edge of vertebra • Fragment may impinge on cord • May have associated posterior dislocation

Atlas and Axis Fractures

The region of C-1 and C-2, due to their articulation, have a wide range of motion.[4] Table 17 describes four fractures or dislocations of this region.

Table 17

C-1 AND C-2 FRACTURES AND DISLOCATIONS		
Fracture/ Dislocation	**Mechanism of Injury**	**Description**
(C-1) Atlanto-occipital dislocation	• Hyperextension and extreme force	• Dislocation of atlas from the occipital bone • Usually fatal
(C-1) Atlas fracture (Jefferson fracture)	• Axial loading forces transmitted from occiput to C-1	• Varies; may be a burst fracture, comminuted, arch fracture, or transverse process fracture • Compression of spinal cord is rare
(C-2) Hangman's fracture	• Axial loading • Lateral bending forces	• Fracture(s) of C-2 may be associated with dislocation of one or both facets • May or may not be displaced
(C-2) Odontoid fracture	• Hyperextension • Hyperflexion	• Disruption of the odontoid process projection of C-2

Vertebral Fracture Stability

Vertebral fractures are frequently classified as stable or unstable. Spinal stability is defined as[21]:

• No potential for progressive impingement or injury to the spinal cord

• No potential for displacement of injured bony area during the healing process

• No displacement or angulation from normal physiologic loading after healing has occurred

Stability of the vertebral column depends on the integrity of ligamentous and bony structures. The loss of ligamentous integrity results in an unstable spinal injury. During resuscitation, assume an unstable injury exists and maintain spinal immobilization.

Spinal Cord Injury

The initial evaluation and treatment of a spinal cord injury includes distinguishing between complete and incomplete lesions.

Incomplete Spinal Cord Lesions

A patient with an incomplete lesion may have preservation of some motor or sensory function below the level of the injury. Sacral sparing with any incomplete lesion represents some structural integrity of the ascending and descending tracts. Perianal sensation, anal sphincter tone, and great toe flexor function represent sacral sparing. In the presence of spinal shock in the patient with an incomplete lesion, sacral sparing may be absent. As spinal shock resolves, sacral sparing becomes evident. Patients with these syndromes demonstrate different signs and symptoms (see Table 18). Certain incomplete lesions are termed incomplete cord syndromes, such as: Central Cord Syndrome, Anterior Cord Syndrome, Posterior Cord Syndrome, and Brown-Sequard Syndrome. Analysis of upper to lower extremity motor and sensory function is important to discern the exact cord syndrome.

Table 18

INCOMPLETE CORD SYNDROMES			
Syndrome	Spinal Tract Involved[1]	Etiology[4]	Symptoms[1,4]
Central Cord		• Hyperextension injuries • Swelling in the center of the cord • Bony abnormality may be absent • Most common	• Loss of motor and sensory function below the level of the lesion with greater loss in arms than in legs
Anterior Cord	• Spinothalamic • Corticospinal (pyramidal)	• Acute anterior cord compression • Disruption of blood flow to anterior cord • Common	• Loss of motor function • Loss of pain, temperature, crude touch, and crude pressure • Intact proprioception, fine touch, fine pressure, and vibration
Posterior Cord	• Posterior tract (dorsal)	• Acute posterior cord compression • Rare	• Loss of proprioception, vibration, fine touch, and fine pressure • Intact motor function, pain, temperature, crude touch, and crude pressure

INCOMPLETE CORD SYNDROMES			
Syndrome	**Spinal Tract Involved[1]**	**Etiology[4]**	**Symptoms[1,4]**
Brown-Sequard	• Posterior tract (dorsal) on same side • Spinothalmic on opposite side • Corticospinal (pyramidal) on same side	• Transverse hemisection of cord • Usually due to penetrating injury • Uncommon	• Loss of motor function, proprioception, and vibration sense on side of injury • Loss of pain and temperature opposite the side of injury

Complete Spinal Cord Lesion

Patients with a complete spinal cord syndrome lose all motor and sensory function below the level of the lesion. Spinal shock is frequently the initial response resulting in loss of motor, sensory, and reflex function below the level of the injury.[1] The patient may also develop neurogenic shock resulting in loss of autonomic function.

SIGNS AND SYMPTOMS

- Loss of motor function below the level of the injury; initially flaccid paralysis

- Bilateral external rotation of the legs at the hips

- Loss of sensory function below the level of the injury

  Loss of pain, touch, temperature, deep pain, vibration, and proprioception.

- Loss of autonomic nervous system function (neurogenic shock)

- Hypotension due to loss of autonomic function, resulting in venous pooling in the extremities.

- Bradycardia and loss of thermoregulation is related to the loss of autonomic function. The patient may become poikilothermic, which means the patient assumes the environmental temperature. This is primarily due to the absence of vasoconstriction, but is also related to the inability of the patient to shiver or sweat to regulate body temperature.[5]

- Loss of voluntary bowel and bladder function, due to loss of autonomic function

- Loss of reflexes, if in spinal shock

INTERVENTIONS

- Administer fluids judiciously if neurogenic shock is suspected

- Administer vasopressors, as prescribed, if neurogenic shock is suspected

  In the absence of hypovolemia, vasopressor agents may be considered to increase the blood pressure and prevent secondary cord ischemia from hypotension.

SUMMARY

Blunt and penetrating injuries to the bony vertebral column may result in fractures, subluxations, or dislocations. Injury to the spinal cord may result in incomplete or complete spinal cord injuries. Anatomic transection of the cord is rare. However, physiologic cord damage may be demonstrated by motor, sensory, and sympathetic nervous system deficits.

Knowledge of the pattern of injury, including the type of forces applied to the vertebral column, and the resulting flexion, extension, and/or rotation, is important in the assessment phase of the trauma nursing process. Assess the patient's breathing effectiveness for inadequate ventilation from interruption of the nerves to the diaphragm and/or intercostal nerves. The patient in spinal shock (temporary loss of motor, sensory, and reflex function) or neurogenic shock (loss of vasomotor tone with maldistribution of blood volume in the venous system) needs collaborative team intervention to assure adequate ventilation and circulation.

REFERENCES

1. Keenen TL, Benson DR. Initial evaluation of the spine-injured patient. In: Browner BD, Jupiter JB, Levine AM, Trafton BG, eds. *Skeletal Trauma: Fractures, Dislocations, Ligamentous Injuries*. Philadelphia, Pa: WB Saunders Co; 1992;1:585-603.

2. de Groot J, ed. *Correlative Neuroanatomy*. 21st ed. Norwalk, Conn: Appleton & Lange; 1991.

3. Chusid JG. *Correlative Neuroanatomy and Functional Neurology*. 17th ed. Los Altos, Calif: Lange Medical Publications; 1979:65-71,195,211.

4. Hickey JV. *The Clinical Practice of Neurological and Neurosurgical Nursing*. 3rd ed. Philadelphia, Pa: JB Lippincott Co; 1991.

5. Walleck CA. Central nervous system II: Spinal cord injury. In: Cardona VD, Hurn PD, Mason PJB, Scanlon AM, Veise Berry SW, eds. *Trauma Nursing: From Resuscitation Through Rehabilitation*. 2nd ed. Philadelphia, Pa: WB Saunders Co; 1994:435-465.

6. *Position Papers from the Third National Injury Control Conference*. Washington, DC: Dept Health and Human Services, Public Health Service, Centers for Disease Control, National Institute for Occupational Safety and Health, National Highway Traffic Safety Administration; 1992. US Government Printing Office 1922-634-666.

7. O'Malley KF, DeLong WG. Cervical spine considerations in head and neck trauma. *Top Emerg Med*. 1991;13:8-16.

8. Marion D, Clifton G. Injury to the vertebrae and spinal cord. In: Moore EE, Mattox KL, Feliciano DV, eds. *Trauma*. 2nd ed. Norwalk, Conn: Appleton & Lange; 1991:263-272.

9. Jaworski MA, Wirtz KM. Spinal cord injuries. In: Kitt S, Selfridge-Thomas J, Proehl JA, Kaiser J, eds. *Emergency Nursing: A Physiologic and Clinical Perspective*. 2nd ed. Philadelphia, Pa: WB Saunders Co; 1995:357-376.

10. Coen SD. Spinal cord injury: preventing secondary injury. *AACN Clin Issues*. 1992;3:44-54.

11. Holdsworth F. Fractures, dislocations, and fracture-dislocations of the spine. *J Bone Joint Surg Am.* 1970;52A:1534-1551.

12. American College of Surgeons Committee on Trauma. Spine and spinal cord trauma. In: *Advanced Trauma Life Support® Course for Physicians (Student Manual).* 5th ed. Chicago, Ill: Author; 1993:191-203.

13. Ivatury RR, Simon RJ, Rohman M. Cardiac complications. In: Mattox KL, ed. *Complications of Trauma.* New York, NY: Churchill Livingstone; 1994:418.

14. Walleck CA. Neurological considerations in the critical care phase. *Crit Care Nurs Clin of North Am.* 1990;2:357-361.

15. Miller BF, Keane CB. *Encyclopedia and Dictionary of Medicine, Nursing, and Allied Health.* 4th ed. Philadelphia, Pa: WB Saunders Co; 1987:132-133.

16. Tyson GW, Rimer RW, Winn HR, Butler AB, Jane JA. Acute care of the spinal cord injured patient. *Crit Care Q.* 1987;2:45-60.

17. Nolan S. Current trends in the management of acute spinal cord injury. *Crit Care Nurs Q.* 1994;1:64-78.

18. Hall ED. The neuroprotective pharmacology of methylprednisolone. *J Neurosurg.* 1992;76:13-21.

19. Braken MB, Shepard MJ, Collins WF, et al. A randomized, controlled trial of methylprednisolone or naloxone in the treatment of acute spinal cord injury. *N Engl J Med.* 1990;322:1405-1411.

20. Braken MB, Shepard MJ, Collins WF, et al. Methylprednisolone or naloxone treatment after acute spinal cord injury: 1-year follow-up data. *J Neurosurg.* 1992;76:23-31.

21. Bucholz RW. Lower cervical spine injuries. In: Browner BD, Jupiter JB, Levine AM, Trafton BG, eds. *Skeletal Trauma: Fractures, Dislocations, Ligamentous Injuries.* Philadelphia, Pa: WB Saunders Co; 1992;1:699-721.

CHAPTER NINE

MUSCULOSKELETAL TRAUMA

LECTURE BEGINS ON PAGE 230.

Preface

Prior to reading this chapter, it is strongly suggested that the learner read the following section entitled "Anatomy and Physiology." Specific anatomical and physiologic concepts are presented to enhance the learner's ability to correlate such concepts with specific injuries. This material on anatomy and physiology will not be covered during lectures, nor will it be evaluated by testing. However, knowledge of normal anatomy and physiology serves as the foundation for understanding the anatomic derangements and pathophysiologic compromises that may ensue as a result of trauma.

ANATOMY AND PHYSIOLOGY

The musculoskeletal system and associated neurovascular structures are comprised of bones, joints, tendons, ligaments, muscles, vessels, and nerves. This system provides support, strength, movement, and protection to the human body. Additionally, bones store needed calcium for body fluids.

Types of Bone

Bone is composed of 65% mineral and 35% organic material, of which the majority is collagen. The two types of bone are compact and spongy (cancellous). Compact bone is dense and more rigid than spongy bone; it forms the shaft of long bones and the exterior surface of some bones, e.g., short bones. Spongy bone is located in the interior of the bone and is constructed in a lattice-like pattern. Spongy bone contains red marrow, which is involved in the production of red blood cells. By adulthood most red marrow is converted to yellow marrow that contains adipose cells. However, the vertebrae, ribs, sternum, and ileum maintain their red bone marrow.

Classification of Bones

There are 206 bones classified into four different categories: long, short, flat, and irregular. Long bones include the femur, tibia, fibula, humerus, radius, and ulna. Short bones, such as the tarsals, are spongy bone with a compact bone surface. Flat bones provide protection and include the skull, scapula, ribs, and sternum. Flat bones are made of a layer of spongy bone and two layers of compact bone. The vertebrae and facial bones are examples of irregular bones (see Figure 27).

Figure 27
Anterior View of Human Skeleton

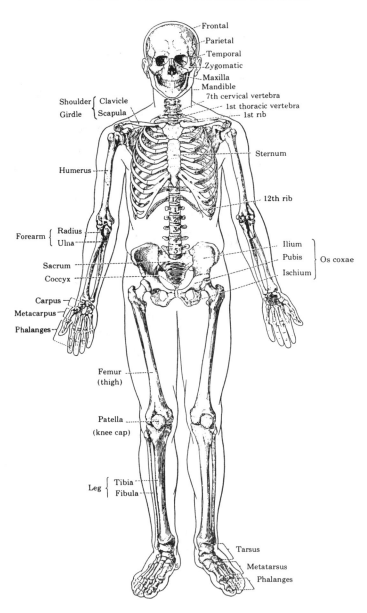

(Reprinted with permission from *Dorland's Illustrated Medical Dictionary*. 28th ed. Philadelphia, Pa: WB Saunders Co; 1994:Plate 44.)

Structure of Bone

The structural components of a long bone are (see Figure 28):

- Epiphyses – one located at each end of the bone.

- Epiphyseal plate – where longitudinal bone growth occurs (growth ceases between 18 and 25 years of age).

- Diaphysis – the compact bone that forms the shaft surrounding a medullary cavity.

- Medullary cavity – canal located within the shaft. The medullary cavity contains yellow marrow consisting mostly of fat cells.

- Articular cartilage – a thin layer of cartilage that covers the epiphyses.

- Periosteum – vascular layer that covers the bone except at articular surfaces. Tendons and ligaments are continuous with the periosteum.[1]

Joints

The body has three structural types of joints: fibrous (synarthroses), cartilaginous (amphiarthroses), and synovial (diarthroses). Fibrous joints allow for little or no movement and are found between the bones of the cranium, teeth and jaw, and maxillary bones. Cartilaginous joints allow for slight movement and are found between the vertebrae and between the pubic symphysis bones. The most common and most complex type of joints are synovial joints, which are freely movable. Examples include the knee, wrist, hip, and shoulder.

Supporting Structures

Tendons are thick, white fibrous material that attach muscles to bones. The white color is due to collagen fibers, which give tendons their tensile strength. Tendons allow for movement of the extremity by extension or flexion of the muscle groups. As the muscle group moves, the tendon pulls the distal bone in the desired direction. Tendons are not elastic and contain a minimal blood supply.

Ligaments are bands of fibrous connective tissue that attach bones to bones. They have elastic fibers to provide the stretch necessary to move bones. These structures help stabilize joints and assist in movement.

Skeletal (striated) muscles are voluntary muscles whose fibers fuse with tendon fibers and insert into bones. Muscles are covered by fascia, a fibrous membrane that supports and separates muscles.

Figure 28
Diagram of Longitudinal Section of a Long Bone

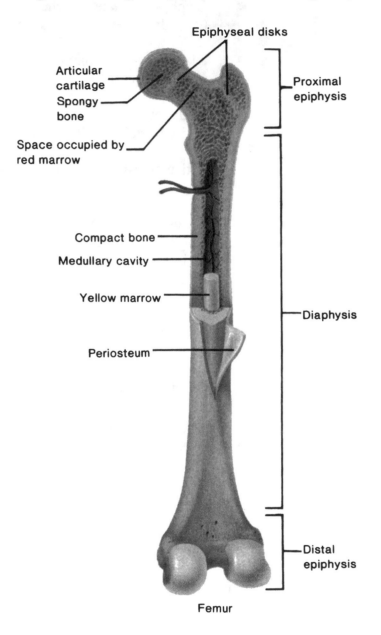

Epiphyseal disks

Articular cartilage

Spongy bone

Space occupied by red marrow

Proximal epiphysis

Compact bone

Medullary cavity

Yellow marrow

Periosteum

Diaphysis

Distal epiphysis

Femur

Blood and Nerve Supply

Small blood vessels permeate the bone and periosteum. Large vessels enter and exit through the articular ends and supply the open spaces of the spongy bone. The medullary canal is usually supplied by a medullary artery that enters through the middle of the diaphysis. Large and small vessels transverse the length of long bones often curving around the bone and through surrounding muscle and soft tissue.[2]

Nerves are distributed throughout the periosteum and usually accompany arteries. Nerves transmit impulses from the brain to the skeletal muscles along descending pathways to initiate fine and gross extremity movement.

Skin

The two layers of the skin are the epidermis and dermis. The outermost epidermis is nonvascular and consists of epithelium, which is 10% water. The innermost dermis contains connective tissue, elastic fibers, numerous blood vessels, lymph vessels, and motor and sensory nerves.[3]

Pelvis

The pelvis is a ring formed by the sacrum and two innominate bones (see Figure 29). Each innominate bone is formed by the fusion of the ilium, ischium, and pubis. The innominate bones are connected posteriorly to the sacrum at the sacroiliac joints and are joined anteriorly at the symphysis pubis. The stability of the pelvis is maintained by ligaments. A significant number of blood vessels are located in the pelvic cavity and along the inner wall of the pelvis. Those veins in the pelvis form a large venous plexus. The pelvis is a weight-bearing structure and provides protection to the lower abdominal viscera.[3,4]

Figure 29
The Pelvis

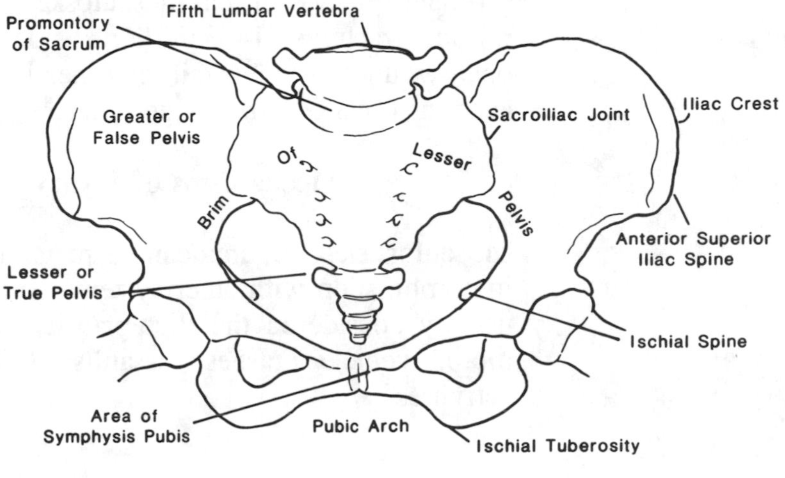

229

MUSCULOSKELETAL TRAUMA

OBJECTIVES

Upon completion of this chapter/lecture, the learner should be able to:

1. Identify the mechanisms of injury associated with musculo-skeletal trauma.
2. Analyze the pathophysiologic changes as a basis for signs and symptoms.
3. Discuss the nursing assessment of the patient with musculo-skeletal trauma.
4. Based on the assessment data, identify appropriate nursing diagnoses and expected outcomes.
5. Plan appropriate interventions for patients with musculoskeletal trauma.
6. Evaluate the effectiveness of nursing interventions for patients with specific types of musculoskeletal trauma.

INTRODUCTION

Epidemiology

Nearly half of all hospital admissions due to trauma are patients with some type of extremity injury, usually the lower limb.[5] The elderly are at a particularly high risk of being hospitalized for an extremity injury. The highest rate of pelvic fractures is in the female population over 85 years of age.[6] Of those injuries sustained by passengers involved in nonfatal motor vehicle crashes, 46% sustain pelvic fractures and 41% sustain femur fractures. Drivers sustain femur fractures (65%), pelvic fractures (46%), and ankle fractures (39%).[7]

The American Association of Orthopedic Surgeons reported an annual estimate of 32.7 million musculoskeletal injuries, which includes 6.1 million fractures, 14.6 million dislocations and sprains, 9.4 million open wounds, and 2.1 million other injuries. Musculoskeletal injuries account for 8,000 deaths per year.[8]

Mechanisms of Injury and Biomechanics

Musculoskeletal trauma can be sustained as a single system injury or in combination with other systems. Injuries to the extremities are not usually considered the first priority. Mechanisms of injury include motor vehicle crashes, assaults, falls, sports, leisure, or home activities.

Falls are a frequent mechanism of injury, especially for the elderly. Elderly patients who fall often sustain pelvic or lower extremity injuries. These injuries, even if not life-threatening, can seriously alter the elderly person's lifestyle and reduce his or her functional independence. Underlying bone disease, such as osteoporosis or cancer metastases, may predispose the patient to an extremity injury.

Differentiating between unintentional and intentional injury can be difficult. Abuse should be considered as a possible cause of the injury. Suspicion of abuse should be raised if the type or degree of injury does not correspond to the history.

Musculoskeletal injuries can result from the application of both acceleration and deceleration forces. Injuries to the bone result from tension, compression, bending, and torsion type forces.[9] When there is enough force to fracture the shaft of a bone, this force may be transmitted to the joints, e.g., fractures of the shaft of the radius and ulna may be associated with fractures to the wrist, elbow, and shoulder.[10]

Calcaneus fractures may occur when an individual falls or jumps landing on their feet. The force of the impact is transmitted upward, compressing the vertebral bodies. The person then tends to fall forward and extends the arms to cushion the fall, resulting in wrist fractures. Thus, patients with fractured calcaneus bones may have concurrent thoracolumbar vertebral fractures and/or bilateral wrist fractures.[10,11]

When the patella comes in contact with the dashboard during a motor vehicle crash, the impact often results in a femur fracture, posterior hip fracture/dislocation, and/or popliteal artery damage.[10,11]

Types of Injuries

Musculoskeletal injuries may be blunt or penetrating. They may involve bone, soft tissue, muscles, nerves, and/or blood vessels. Injuries include fractures and/or dislocations of the bone or joint, sprains, strains, ligamentous tears, tendon lacerations, and neurovascular compromises.

Bony extremity injuries may be associated with concurrent injury to nerves, arteries, veins, or soft tissue. Suspect neurovascular injury with any injury to the bones of an extremity. Severe pelvic fractures can be associated with injuries to pelvic organs and large blood loss. Genitourinary injuries, especially to the bladder or the urethra in males, can result from pelvic fractures.[4,10] Depending on the mechanism of injury, bony injury of the extremities may be associated with vertebral column injuries.

PATHOPHYSIOLOGY AS A BASIS FOR SIGNS AND SYMPTOMS

Blood Loss

Musculoskeletal trauma can be associated with large blood loss either from the fracture or disruption of arteries or veins. Up to 1,500 ml of blood can be lost from an isolated femur fracture. A tibial or humeral fracture can lead to a blood loss up to 750 ml.[12] Multiple fractures may result in significant blood loss, which can potentiate shock from other injuries.

Capillaries and cellular membranes can be disrupted or torn with all types of musculoskeletal injuries. Blood from vascular disruption and intracellular fluid are released into the area surrounding the injury. Edema from fluid and blood accumulation can cause compression of surrounding structures. Normal physiological mechanisms are activated to minimize damage caused by these structural disruptions:

- Initiation of the coagulation cascade to decrease bleeding

- Restoration of cellular membrane integrity to enhance fluid reabsorption

- Increased collateral blood flow to promote healing

Bone or joint displacement can compress surrounding vessels and nerves, causing pathophysiological changes distal to the injury. As arterial blood flow is obstructed, tissue oxygenation decreases resulting in tissue ischemia and cellular death. During this process, pain increases, pulses become more difficult to palpate, the limb becomes pale, cyanotic and cool, and capillary refill time increases.

Neurologic Deficits

If nerves are compressed or lacerated, conduction pathways are interrupted and the relay of nerve impulses are blocked or diminished. Nerve damage can result in diminished pain sensation. Motor and sensory functions distal to the nerve damage may result in partial or complete loss of function.

Fractures

Fractures involve a disruption of bony continuity (see Table 19).

Table 19

TYPES OF FRACTURES	
Type of Fracture	**Description**
Open	• Skin integrity over or near a fracture site is disrupted
Closed	• Skin integrity over or near a fracture site is intact
Complete	• Total interruption in bony continuity
Incomplete	• Incomplete interruption in bony continuity
Comminuted	• Splintering of bone into fragments
Greenstick	• Bone buckles or bends; fracture does not go through the entire bone
Impacted	• Distal and proximal fracture sites are wedged into each other
Displaced	• Proximal and distal fracture sites are out of alignment

Soft Tissue Injury

Disruption in the skin can result in a disturbance in water, electrolyte, or temperature homeostasis. Any skin surface wound with loss of skin integrity provides an entry for microorganisms. This can lead to infection, especially if necrotic tissue is present. The following terms are used to describe soft tissue injuries:

• Abrasion

 An epidermal and/or dermal injury caused by friction, rubbing, or scraping motion.[3,13]

233

- Avulsion

  A full thickness skin loss in which the wound edges cannot be approximated.[3,13]

- Degloving

  A serious type of avulsion injury resulting from high-energy shearing forces that tear large areas of skin and subcutaneous tissue away from the underlying vascular supply.[3]

- Contusion

  Disruption of small blood vessels and extravasation of blood into the skin and/or mucous membranes that does not interrupt the skin integrity.[13]

- Laceration

  Open wound from external forces causing a tearing or splitting of the skin, involving the dermis, epidermis, or underlying structures.

- Puncture

  Wound with a narrow opening that can penetrate deeply into the skin. Puncture wounds bleed minimally and tend to trap foreign material, that can lead to infection. Animal and human bites can be considered puncture wounds and should be treated as contaminated wounds.[9]

NURSING CARE OF PATIENTS WITH MUSCULOSKELETAL TRAUMA

Assessment

History

Refer to Chapter 3, Initial Assessment, for a description of general information that should be collected regarding every trauma victim. Only pertinent questions specific to patients with musculoskeletal injuries are described below.

- What was the mechanism of injury? Information regarding the specific injuring agents or points of contact with any extremity provide important clues in identifying the specific type and extent of extremity injury.

- Was any previous treatment or splinting done prior to arrival?

- Is there a history of previous orthopedic problems?

Physical Assessment

Refer to Chapter 3, Initial Assessment, for a description of assessment of the patient's airway and effectiveness of breathing and circulation. Certain extremity injuries may appear devastating. Since these injuries are not usually life-threatening, conduct the trauma nursing process according to the priorities outlined in Chapter 3, Initial Assessment.

INSPECTION

- Observe general appearance of extremities

    Note color, position, and obvious differences of injured extremity as compared to uninjured extremity.

- Assess integrity of the injured area

    - Note protrusion of bone or any break in the skin

    - Assess for bleeding

    - Identify soft tissue damage, including edema, ecchymosis, contusions, abrasions, avulsions or lacerations.

- Assess for deformity and/or angulation of extremity

PALPATION

Extremity assessment is often described by the five Ps: pain, pallor, pulses, paresthesia, and paralysis. This assessment relates to the neurovascular status of the injured extremity. Assess the injured extremity and compare with an assessment of the opposite, uninjured extremity.

- Assess the five Ps

    - Pain

        Carefully palpate the entire length of each extremity for pain or deformity. Determine location and quality of pain. Ischemic pain is often described as burning or throbbing.

- Pallor

  Note color and temperature of injured extremity. Pallor, delayed capillary refill (greater than two seconds), and a cool extremity indicate vascular compromise.

- Pulses

  Palpate pulses proximal and distal to the injury for comparison and then compare quality of pulses with the opposite, uninjured extremity.

- Paresthesia

  Determine presence of abnormal sensations, e.g., burning, prickling, numbness.

- Paralysis

  Assess motor function. The ability to move can be related to neurologic function.

- Note bony crepitus during palpation, which is a crackling sound produced by the grating of the ends of fractured bones.

Diagnostic Procedures

Refer to Chapter 3, Initial Assessment, for frequently-ordered radiographic and laboratory studies. Additional studies for patients with musculoskeletal trauma are listed below.

RADIOGRAPHIC STUDIES

- Anterior/posterior and lateral of injured extremity

  Some fractures can only be seen from one radiographic angle; therefore, an oblique view may be indicated.[2,10] The film should include the joints immediately above and below the injury.

- Angiography

  Angiography may be indicated to identify tears or compressions in the arterial or venous network of the injured extremity.

Nursing Diagnoses and Outcome Identification

The following nursing diagnoses are potential problems for the patient with musculoskeletal injuries. Once a patient has been assessed, diagnoses can be defined as either actual or risk. An actual nursing diagnosis is one derived from a decision based on the patient's presenting signs and symptoms. A risk nursing diagnosis is a judgment the nurse makes based on a particular patient's risk and potential for developing certain problems.

POSSIBLE NURSING DIAGNOSES AND EXPECTED OUTCOMES	
Nursing Diagnosis	**Expected Outcome**
Fluid volume deficit related to: • Hemorrhage	The patient will have an effective circulating volume as evidenced by: • Stable vital signs appropriate for developmental age • Urinary output of 1 ml/kg/hr • Strong, palpable peripheral pulses • Improved level of consciousness • Skin normal color, warm, and dry • Maintains HCT = 30 ml/dl or Hgb = 12 - 14 g/dl or greater • CVP reading of 5 - 10 cm H_2O • Capillary refill time of <2 seconds • External hemorrhage is controlled • Absence of myoglobinuria • Urine specific gravity within normal limits
Physical mobility, impaired related to: • Bone, soft tissue and/or nerve injury of extremity • Pain • Edema • External immobilization devices • Limited range of motion of affected bone	The patient will experience increased mobility as evidenced by: • Use of safety measures to minimize potential for injury • Ability to describe measures to increase mobility • Ability to tolerate movement and increased activity • Willingness to move affected part to degree allowed • Maintenance of proper body alignment

POSSIBLE NURSING DIAGNOSES AND EXPECTED OUTCOMES

Nursing Diagnosis	Expected Outcome
Infection, risk related to: • Impaired skin integrity • Contamination of wound from initial injury or instrumentation • Invasive fixation devices • Interruption in perfusion	The patient will be free from infection as evidenced by: • Core temperature measurement of 36° - 37.5°C (98° - 99.5°F) • Absence of systemic signs of infection: fever, tachypnea, tachycardia • Wounds free from redness, swelling, purulent drainage, or odor • Urinary output 1 ml/kg/hr • Negative blood cultures • WBC count within normal limits • Improved level of consciousness
Impaired skin integrity, risk related to: • Pressure, shear, friction on skin and tissue • Mechanical irritants: fixation devices, splints, and casting material • Impaired mobility	The patient will experience absence or resolution of impaired skin integrity as evidenced by: • Absence of signs of irritation: redness, ulceration, blanching, and itching • Signs of progressive healing of dermal layer • Absence of signs of infection: redness, swelling, purulent drainage, odor, and tenderness
Pain related to: • Soft tissue injury and pressure • Fractures • Tissue stretching and edema • Neurovascular compromise • Invasive procedures	The patient will experience relief of pain as evidenced by: • Diminishing or absent level of pain through patient's self-report using an objective measurement tool • Absence of physiologic indicators of pain, which include: tachycardia, tachypnea, pallor, diaphoretic skin, and increasing blood pressure • Absence of nonverbal cues of pain: crying, grimacing, inability to assume position of comfort • Ability to cooperate with care, as appropriate • Relief of pain when injury is not manipulated • Proper alignment of extremity
Tissue perfusion, altered peripheral related to: • Vessel compression secondary to edema • Vessel compression secondary to compartment syndrome • Loss of normal contour or alignment	The patient will maintain adequate peripheral tissue perfusion as evidenced by: • Absence of ischemic pain and motor paralysis • Capillary refill time of <2 seconds • Skin color normal, warm, and dry distal to injury • Strong and regular peripheral pulses • Absence of changes in mobility

238

Planning and Implementation

Refer to Chapter 3, Initial Assessment, for a description of the specific nursing interventions for patients with compromises to airway, breathing, and/or circulation.

- Splint and immobilize the affected extremity

  - Splinting is indicated when there is evidence of the following:

    - Deformity

    - Pain

    - Bony crepitus

    - Edema

    - Ecchymosis

    - Circulatory compromise

    - Open soft tissue injury

    - Impaled object

    - Paresthesia or paralysis

  - Select an appropriate splint. Three types of splints are available:

    - Rigid splints, such as cardboard, plastic devices or metal splints

    - Soft splints, such as pillows, slings, or air splints

    - Traction splints – applied for actual or suspected femur or proximal tibial fractures

  - Remove jewelry or constricting items of clothing prior to immobilization

  - Do not reposition protruding bone ends

239

- Avoid excessive movement of the fractured bone fragments. Any manipulation can increase bleeding into the tissues, increase the risk of fat emboli, or convert a closed fracture to an open fracture.

- Immobilize the joints above and below the deformity

- Modify the splint to fit the fracture, if necessary

- Reassess neurovascular status before and after immobilization. If neurovascular status is compromised, reassess, remove, adjust, or reapply the splint.

- Apply ice to reduce swelling and pain

- Elevate the extremity above the level of the heart to reduce swelling and pain. If compartment syndrome is suspected, then elevate to the level of the heart.

- Administer analgesics, as prescribed

- Administer antibiotics, as prescribed

- Prepare for definitive stabilization (Appendix 5 contains information on conscious sedation). Traction, casting, internal or external fixation may be indicated.

- Prepare for closed reduction, as indicated

- Provide psychosocial support

Evaluation and Ongoing Assessment

Refer to Chapter 3, Initial Assessment, for a description of the ongoing evaluation of the patient's airway, and effectiveness of breathing and circulation. Additional evaluations include:

- Monitoring breathing effectiveness and rate of respiration

  Tachypnea, rales, and wheezes may be indicators of fat emboli syndrome.

- Reassessing and documenting the five Ps

SELECTED MUSCULOSKELETAL INJURIES

Refer to "Nursing Care of Patients with Musculoskeletal Trauma" for a description of the phases of the trauma nursing process.

Joint Injuries

A joint may become dislocated when the normal range of motion is exceeded. Joint dislocations may be complicated by neurovascular compromise and associated fractures. Delayed reduction of a hip dislocation can lead to avascular necrosis of the femoral head and permanent disability.[10] Dislocation of the knee is considered an orthopedic emergency since peroneal nerve injury and compromises to the popliteal artery and vein may develop. Angiography is necessary to diagnose vascular trauma.

Signs and Symptoms

- Pain

- Joint deformity

- Edema

- Inability to move the affected joint

- Abnormal range of motion

- Neurovascular compromise – may have diminished or absent distal pulse; may have decreased motor or sensory function

Interventions

- Immobilize the joint

- Reassess neurovascular function

- Prepare for reduction, if indicated

Femur Fractures

Femur fractures are a result of major trauma, such as falls, motor vehicle crashes, and/or missiles causing penetrating wounds. Fractures of the proximal femur (femoral neck) are common after a fall in the elderly population. Closed femur fractures can result in a collection of 2 to 3 units of blood in the thigh.[12]

Signs and Symptoms

- Pain and inability to bear weight

- Shortening

- Rotation internally or externally depending on the location of the fracture site in the hip

- Edema of the thigh

- Deformity of the thigh

- Evidence of hypovolemic shock

Interventions

- Immobilize affected limb – a traction splint is the preferred device

- Prepare for traction pin insertion, as indicated

- Dress traction pin insertion sites per institutional protocol

Pelvic Fractures

Pelvic fractures or disruptions are stable or unstable. Two thirds of these injuries are stable.[1] Unstable fractures can be life-threatening and are often accompanied by large blood loss and injury to the genitourinary system.[1,2] A fracture of the pelvis may produce bleeding which is usually venous, due to a disruption of the veins in the pelvis. The bleeding may be significant enough to cause hypovolemic shock. Injuries to the pelvis may be open or closed. Open pelvic fractures may be associated with injuries to the perineum, genitourinary structures, or rectum. Open pelvic fractures have a significantly higher mortality rate[4] (see Figure 30).

Figure 30
Pelvic Fracture Patterns

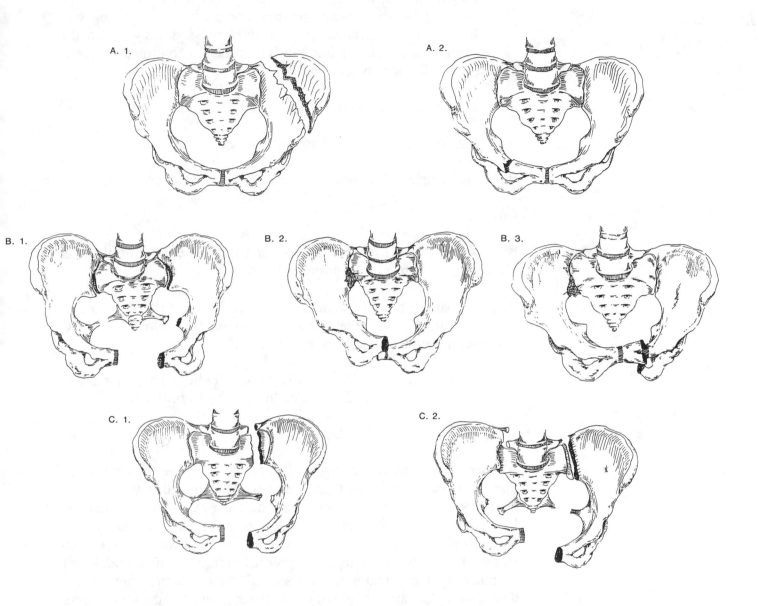

Figure Legend: A.1. – Stable fracture not involving the ring; A.2. – Stable fracture, minimal displaced fracture of the ring; B.1. – Rotationally unstable, vertically stable open book fracture; B.2. – Rotationally unstable, vertically stable lateral compression (ipsilateral); B.3. – Rotationally unstable, vertically stable lateral compression (contralateral bucket handle); C.1. – Rotationally and vertically unstable unilateral; C.2. – Rotationally and vertically unstable bilateral; C.3. – Rotationally and vertically unstable associated with acetabular fracture (not shown).

(Reprinted with permission from Kozin S, Berlet A. Pelvis and acetabulem. In: *Handbook of Common Orthopaedic Fractures.* 2nd ed. Chester, Pa: Medical Surveillance, Inc; 1992:87-93.)

Signs and Symptoms

- Pain

  Palpate the pelvis for pain or bony instability. Apply gentle pressure on the iliac crests towards the midline, noting any instability or increased pain. Gently press downward on the symphysis pubis. If a fracture is suspected, carefully palpate the pelvis. Do not rock the pelvis.

- Evidence of hypovolemic shock

- Shortening or abnormal rotation of leg

- Genitourinary or intra-abdominal injury

Interventions

- Apply PASG to splint fractures and assist in control of bleeding in hemodynamically unstable patients.[1,10]

- Prepare for application of external fixator. Unstable pelvic fractures with severe blood loss may require immediate stabilization with an external fixator.[3]

- Assist with additional diagnostic radiographs, including cystogram and/or CT scan of the pelvis, as ordered.

Open Fractures

All open fractures are considered contaminated due to the foreign materials and bacteria that can be introduced into the wound. Any open fracture may result in an infection. The risk of serious infection is greater with severe fractures. Infections can be manifested by poor tissue healing, osteomyelitis, or sepsis. Open fractures are graded from I to III according to the degree of skin and soft tissue injury surrounding the fracture site. Grade III open fractures are further described by the amount of nonviable tissue, injury to the periosteum, and vascular trauma.[2]

Signs and Symptoms

- Evidence of skin disruption, e.g., laceration or puncture, near or over the fracture

- Protrusion of bone through open wounds

- Pain

- Neurovascular compromise

- Bleeding may be minimal to severe

Interventions

- Irrigate the wound

- Facilitate a wound culture

- Cover wound with a dry, sterile dressing. Avoid frequent dressing changes. Each exposure of the wound can increase the risk of bacterial contamination.[5]

- Inspect dressings frequently for continued bleeding

- Prepare patient for operative intervention, hospital admission, or transfer, as indicated.

Amputations

Amputations may be partial or complete and usually involve the digits, distal half of the foot, the lower leg, the hand, or the forearm. The axiom of saving "life over limb" is a reminder to the trauma team to fully resuscitate the patient before managing the amputation.

The following have been cited as conditions with a favorable replantation outcome[14]:

- Multiple digits

- Thumb

- Wrist

- Forearm

- Pediatric patient (children typically have positive outcomes from replantation procedures)[14,15]

Amputations that are clean lacerations have a better chance of being successfully replanted as opposed to avulsive/tearing types of injuries. The decision to replant should be made by a surgeon or replantation team, if available.

Signs and Symptoms

- Obvious tissue loss

- Pain

- Bleeding (may be minimal to severe)

  Complete amputations will have less active bleeding than partial amputations due to retraction of the severed arteries. An exception is an avulsive type of complete amputation, which can result in extensive bleeding.

- Evidence of hypovolemic shock

Interventions

- Provide psychosocial support, especially since the loss of a limb may have psychosocial consequences

- Prepare patient for hospital admission, operative intervention, or transfer to a facility with a replantation team, as indicated.

STUMP CARE

- Control any active bleeding with pressure dressings and elevation. Avoid tourniquets or clamps.

- Elevate

- Splint as needed

- Remove gross dirt or debris[10]

AMPUTATED PART

- Keep cool, but do not freeze

- Wrap the part in a saline-moistened gauze, then place in a plastic bag, and finally place the bag in crushed ice and water. Do not allow the part to freeze.[10]

- Prepare for radiographs of both the stump and the amputated part

Crush Injuries

Certain crush injuries, depending on the location of the injury, may be life-threatening, e.g., pelvis and both lower extremities. Cellular destruction and damage to vessels and nerves make crush injuries difficult to treat. Hemorrhage from the damaged tissue, destruction of muscle and bone tissue, fluid loss resulting in hypovolemic shock, compartment syndrome, and infection are sequelae associated with crush injuries. The destruction of muscle tissue associated with release of myoglobin can result in renal failure.[1,13]

Signs and Symptoms

- Massively crushed pelvis or extremity(ies) with soft tissue swelling

- Pain

- Evidence of hypovolemic shock

- Signs of compartment syndrome

- Loss of neurovascular function distal to the injury

Interventions

- Control bleeding

- Administer an intravenous crystalloid solution to increase urinary output and facilitate excretion of myoglobin[1,13]

- Elevate the injured extremity above the heart to reduce swelling and pain

- Gently clean open wounds

- Reassess:

  - Urinary output

  - Presence of myoglobin in the urine

  - Motor and sensory function

- Prepare patient for surgical debridement, fasciotomy, and/or amputation

Compartment Syndrome

Compartment syndrome occurs as pressure increases inside a fascial compartment (see Figure 31). This occurs more frequently in the muscles of the lower leg or forearm but can involve any fascial compartment. The increased pressure may be due to an internal source, such as hemorrhage or edema, caused by open or closed fractures, or crush injuries. It can also result from an external source, such as a cast, excessive traction,[1] air splint, or PASG. Nerves, blood vessels, and muscle can be compressed. If this condition is not corrected, permanent paralysis or tissue necrosis may occur.[10]

Figure 31
Fascial Compartments of the Lower Leg

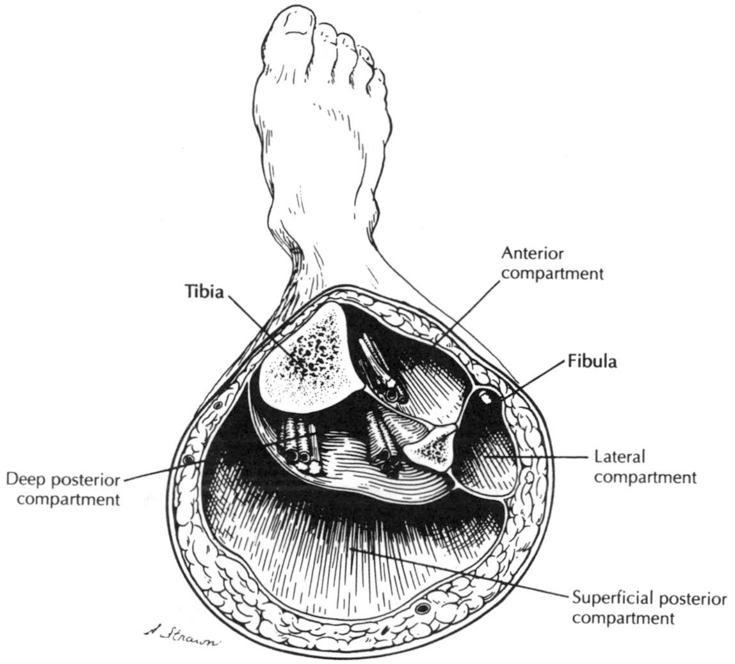

(Reprinted with permission from Bess R. Fasciotomy. In: Moore E, Eisman B, Van Way C. *Critical Decisions in Trauma*. St. Louis, Mo: CV Mosby Co; 1984:530.)

Signs and Symptoms

- Progressive increase in pain with muscle stretching or passive movement due to increased tissue pressure and ischemia.

- Sensory deficit, (e.g., numbness, tingling, total loss of sensation)

- Progressive muscle weakness

- Tense, swollen area

- Elevated muscle compartment pressures

- Loss of pulses (late sign)

Interventions

- Elevate limb to the level of the heart to promote venous outflow and prevent further swelling. Do not elevate limb above the heart as this may decrease perfusion to compromised extremity.

- Reassess and document neurovascular status on an ongoing basis. Communicate changes to the physician immediately.

- Assist with measurement of muscle compartment pressure. A reading of greater than 35 to 45 mmHg is considered elevated and indicates the need for fasciotomy.[10]

- Prepare for fasciotomy, as indicated. A fasciotomy will prevent muscle and/or neurovascular damage and loss of the limb.

Fat Embolism Syndrome

Following open or closed fractures, especially pelvic and long bone fractures, fat globules from the bone marrow can be released into nearby injured veins and become trapped in the pulmonary vasculature. It is also theorized that fat metabolism is altered after stress or trauma, increasing the release of free fatty acids. Fat globules become coated with platelets, resulting in large fat globules.[1] Obstruction of the pulmonary vasculature by fat globules damages alveoli, leading to hypoxia, confusion, and/or petechiae. This syndrome can occur within a few hours to several days after the traumatic event. While patients with fat embolism syndrome are not usually seen in the emergency department, the patient who is transferred from another facility may present with this syndrome. Immediate stabilization of fractures helps in preventing the occurrence of fat emboli.

Signs and Symptoms

- Dyspnea, tachypnea, rales, wheezes

- Tachycardia

- Elevated temperature

- Altered level of consciousness

- Decreasing PaO_2 or oxygen saturation

- Petechiae – commonly seen in upper thoracic and axillary areas

- Retinal hemorrhages

- Chest pain

Additional Diagnostic Procedures

- Serum lipase

- Urine or sputum analysis for free fat (these tests are not definitive for fat embolism syndrome)

- Arterial blood gases and pH

Interventions

Administer oxygen via a nonrebreather mask at a flow rate sufficient to keep the reservoir bag inflated; usually requires 12 to 15 L/minute. Prepare for ventilatory support, as indicated.

SUMMARY

Injuries of the extremities are usually not the first priority of care for the multiple trauma patient. However, there is a high incidence of injuries to upper and lower extremities that, although usually not life-threatening, can result in functional disability and/or loss, and long-term rehabilitation.

The proximity of vessels and nerves to musculoskeletal structures increases the risk of neurovascular damage ranging from motor, sensory, or vascular deficits to paralysis and/or hemorrhage, and shock. Disruptions and fractures of the pelvis may result in significant blood loss because of concurrent injury to the veins in the pelvic cavity. Collaborate with members of the trauma team to correct any life-threatening compromises to circulation.

During the secondary assessment, assess the extremities for indications of a fracture or dislocation. Intervene early to splint the suspected fracture and reassess neurovascular function both before and after the application of any splinting device.

Timely identification and management of suspected musculoskeletal injuries, including the use of pain control, splints, traction, and/or external fixation, contributes to improved functional patient outcomes.

REFERENCES

1. Strange JM, Kelly PM. Musculoskeletal injuries. In: Cardona VD, Hurn PD, Mason PJB, Scanlon AM, Veise-Berry SW, eds. *Trauma Nursing: From Resuscitation Through Rehabilitation.* 2nd ed. Philadelphia, Pa: WB Saunders Co; 1994:548-586.

2. Geiderman JM. Orthopedic injuries: Management principles. In: Rosen P, Barkin RM, Baker FJ, Braen GR, Dailey RH, Levy RC, eds. *Emergency Medicine: Concepts and Clinical Practice.* 3rd ed. St. Louis, Mo: Mosby-Year Book; 1992:522-544.

3. Sherman R, Ecker J. Soft tissue coverage. In: Browner BD, Jupiter JB, Levine AM, Trafton PG, eds. *Skeletal Trauma: Fractures, Dislocations, Ligamentous Injuries.* Philadelphia, Pa: WB Saunders Co; 1992;1:337-366.

4. Cwinn AA. Pelvis and hip. In: Rosen P, Barkin RM, Baker FJ, Braen GR, Dailey RH, Levy RC, eds. *Emergency Medicine: Concepts and Clinical Practice.* 3rd ed. St. Louis, Mo: Mosby-Year Book; 1992:658-683.

5. *Position Papers from the Third National Injury Control Conference.* Washington, DC: Dept Health and Human Services, Public Health Service, Centers for Disease Control, National Institute for Occupational Safety and Health, National Highway Traffic Safety Administration; 1992. US Government Printing Office 1922-634-666.

6. Mucha P. Pelvic fractures. In: Moore EE, Mattox KL, Feliciano DV, eds. *Trauma.* 2nd ed. Norwalk, Conn: Appleton & Lange; 1991:553-570.

7. Daffner RH, Lupetin AR. Patterns of high speed impact injuries in motor vehicle occupants. *J Trauma.* 1988;28:498-501.

8. Praemer MA. *Musculoskeletal Conditions in the United States.* Chicago, Ill: American Association of Orthopedic Surgeons; 1992.

9. Hipp JA, Cheal EG, Hayes WC. Biomechanics of fractures. In: Browner BD, Jupiter JB, Levine AM, Trafton PG. *Skeletal Trauma: Fractures, Dislocations, Ligamentous Injuries.* Philadelphia, Pa: WB Saunders Co; 1992;1:95-126.

10. American College of Surgeons Committee on Trauma. Extremity trauma. In: *Advanced Trauma Life Support® Course for Physicians (Student Manual)*. 5th ed. Chicago, Ill: Author; 1993:219-239.

11. American College of Surgeons Committee on Trauma. Resource document 3:Kinematics of trauma. In: *Advanced Trauma Life Support® Course for Physicians (Student Manual)*. 5th ed. Chicago, Ill: Author; 1993:319-332.

12. American College of Surgeons Committee on Trauma. Shock. In: *Advanced Trauma Life Support® Course for Physicians (Student Manual)*. 5th ed. Chicago, Ill: Author; 1993:75-94.

13. Whitney JD. Wound healing. In: Cardona VD, Hurn PD, Mason PJB, Scanlon AM, Veise-Berry SW, eds. *Trauma Nursing: From Resuscitation Through Rehabilitation*. 2nd ed. Philadelphia, Pa: WB Saunders Co; 1994:266-290.

14. Upton J. Skeletal and soft tissue injuries: Partially or totally severed parts. In: May HL, ed. *Emergency Medicine*. 2nd ed. Boston, Mass: Little, Brown, & Company: 1992;1:881-885.

15. Pederson W, Serafin D. Hand trauma. In: Moylan JA, ed. *Principles of Trauma Surgery*. New York, NY: Gower Medical Publishing; 1992:18.1-18.25.

CHAPTER TEN

BURN TRAUMA

LECTURE BEGINS ON PAGE 257.

Preface

Prior to reading this chapter, it is strongly suggested that the learner read the following section entitled "Anatomy and Physiology." Specific anatomy and physiologic concepts are presented to enhance the learner's ability to correlate such concepts with specific injuries. This material related to anatomy and physiology will not be covered during lectures, nor will it be evaluated by testing. However, knowledge of normal anatomy and physiology serves as the foundation for understanding the anatomic derangements and pathophysiologic compromises that may ensue as a result of trauma.

ANATOMY AND PHYSIOLOGY

The Skin

The skin is the elastic, self-generating, waterproof covering of the body. It functions as a protective barrier against heat and cold and is involved in the body's temperature regulating mechanisms. The two layers of skin, the epidermis and dermis, cover the subcutaneous tissue layer under the dermis (see Figure 32). The epidermis is the outermost layer and is composed of epithelial cells. The thickness of the epidermis varies, e.g., it is thickest over the palmar surfaces of the hands and the plantar surfaces of the feet. The epidermis is composed of five layers, of which the deepest layer is a single layer of cells (basal cells) capable of producing new skin cells which move to the skin's surface to replace lost cells. If, after injury, a sufficient number of basal cells survive, regeneration is possible.

Figure 32
The Skin

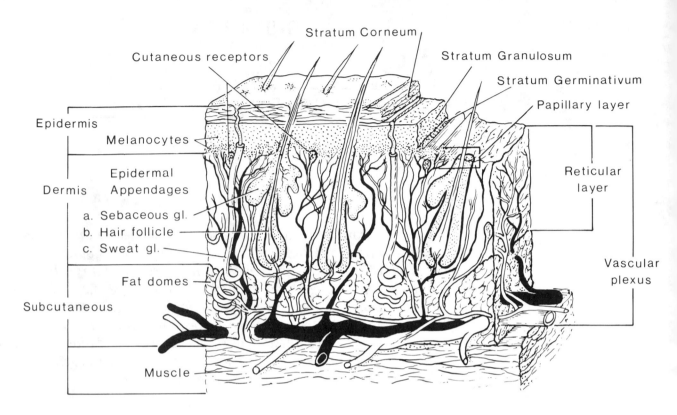

The dermis is formed by connective tissue and contains collagen and elastic fibers. The two-layered dermis contains blood vessels, nerve endings, sweat glands, sebaceous glands, lymph vessels, and hair follicles. The dermis supplies nutrition to the epidermis. Under the dermis is a layer of subcutaneous tissue composed of fat and connective tissues. The dermal layer cannot regenerate if the cells are destroyed.

The four major functions of the skin are thermoregulation, protection, secretion, and sensory reception. The sensations of pain, touch, temperature, and pressure are transmitted through the sensory nerve fibers to areas in the cerebral cortex. The sweat glands secrete sweat to maintain a normal body temperature. The sebaceous glands secrete sebum, an oily substance that contributes to lubrication of the skin, maintains the skin's texture, and contains antifungal and antibacterial properties. In terms of protection, the skin protects the body against damage from heat, cold, bacteria, fungi, and chemicals. The skin also protects the body from losing excessive amounts of fluids and electrolytes.

Burns that injure the skin may result in loss of some or all of the above functions of the skin. However, the skin not only provides these physiologic and anatomic functions, it also contributes to appearance and individual identity. Disruption of this individuality poses major readjustment problems for burn victims.

Capillary and Fluid Dynamics

The body's fluids are composed of water, electrolytes, proteins, and other substances contained in the intracellular and extracellular compartments. Since there are electrolytes and other molecular substances dissolved in body water, the fluid compartments have both electrical and chemical properties. The size of all cells is controlled by the movement of water between the compartments. Since water is in motion, the pressure that is generated is termed osmotic pressure. The osmotic activity that results is due to the number, not the size, of non-diffusible particles.[1] Water molecules, separated by a semipermeable membrane, will move from the compartment with the lesser number of nondiffusible particles to the compartment with more.

There are four forces that contribute to the fluid movement across the capillary membrane (see Table 20).

Table 20

PRESSURES CONTRIBUTING TO CAPILLARY FLOW	
Pressure	**Function**
• **Hydrostatic or Capillary Pressure** Arterial end = 30 mmHg Venous end = 10 mmHg	• Forces fluid out of the capillary at the arterial end
• **Plasma Colloid Osmotic Pressure** 28 mmHg	• Pulls fluid into the capillary at the venule end
• **Interstitial Free Fluid Pressure (IFFP)** Usually slightly less than atmospheric, -3 to -5 but can be positive, e.g., in the brain	• Pulls fluid out of the capillary (when the IFFP is negative) • Forces fluid into capillary (when the IFFP is positive)
• **Interstitial Fluid Osmotic Pressure** 8 mmHg	• Pulls fluid out of the capillary

Because the hydrostatic pressure is higher at the arterial end of a capillary than at the venule end, fluid can move out at the arterial end. At the venule end of the capillary, the hydrostatic pressure is lower. The capillary colloid osmotic pressure is the dominant pressure that pulls fluid back into the capillary at the venule end. Proteins, the only dissolved particles in the plasma that do not pass through the pores of the cell's semipermeable membrane, are responsible for generating the capillary colloid osmotic pressure. Any disruption in the integrity of the capillary membrane will lead to a reduction in the capillary osmotic pressure and a loss of intracapillary water into the interstitium.

Refer to the Anatomy and Physiology section in Chapter 7, Thoracic and Neck Injuries, for a review of respiratory anatomy and physiology.

BURN TRAUMA

OBJECTIVES

Upon completion of this chapter/lecture, the learner should be able to:

1. Identify the mechanisms of injury associated with burn trauma.
2. Analyze the pathophysiologic changes as a basis for the signs and symptoms.
3. Discuss the nursing assessment of the patient with burns.
4. Based on the assessment data, identify appropriate nursing diagnoses and expected outcomes.
5. Plan appropriate interventions for burned patients.
6. Evaluate the effectiveness of nursing interventions for patients with specific types of burn injuries.

INTRODUCTION

Epidemiology

Caring for burn victims in an emergency setting may be stressful for the trauma team because of the infrequency of such admissions. Burn victims are often faced with devastating problems, resulting not only from the initial event but subsequent hospitalizations, loss of body image and self-esteem, and lengthy periods of rehabilitation. The estimated number of burn injuries each year ranges from 1.4 to 2 million. Estimates of the number of patients who require hospitalization for burn treatment range from 54,000 to as high as 100,000.[2,3]

Overall, burns rank as the fourth leading cause of death due to unintentional injury. Approximately 6,000 persons die annually from burns with 73% dying as a result of house fires. The leading cause of death resulting from a fire in a private dwelling is inhalation of toxic substances (76%).[2]

The use of cigarettes is the most common cause of fatal house fires.[4] Alcohol is another associated factor. Over half of the adults who perish as a result of a house fire have elevated blood alcohol concentrations.[5] In those fires ignited by cigarette smoking, there is greater likelihood that alcohol was also a factor.

Scald burns are more frequent for those under the age of five years and over the age of 65. Burns due to scalds from hot liquids frequently lead to hospital admissions but, fortunately, to few deaths (approximately 100/year). Hot water from taps, showers, and bathtubs is the leading source of scald burns for children less than five years old.[2] Age is also significant in burns related to clothing ignition. Those persons aged 65 years and over account for 75% of the deaths related to clothing ignition. Clothing ignition is related to cigarette smoking and the use of stoves and space heaters.

Of the 21 reported causes of occupation-related death, the National Institute of Occupational Health and Safety lists contact with electrical current as the fifth leading cause of death, and fires and flames as the 13th.[2] Lightning accounts for about 80 deaths/year. The incidence is greatest among those between the ages of 10 and 19 years, and males have a death rate seven times greater than females. More lightning deaths occur during the summer months, and close to one third of these deaths are outdoor workers, e.g., farmers, construction workers. Lightning strikes are also more prevalent in some geographic areas.

The southeastern United States has the highest death rates (highest along coastal plains and along the Mississippi) from house fires with the use of kerosene heaters, other types of space heaters, and wood burning as key factors.[2,6]

Mechanisms of Injury and Biomechanics

The energy agents that can cause burns are:

- Thermal energy

- Chemical energy

- Electricity

- Ultraviolet radiation

- Ionizing radiation

The most common mechanism of injury leading to thermal burns are those events generating heat and/or flames.[7] Such burns can be caused by flames, flash, scalds, and contact with burning substances, objects, and chemicals. The mechanism of injury leading to pulmonary injury is related to the inhalation of heat, smoke, and toxic substances (both gases and particulate matter) released during the burning process. As natural and synthetic materials burn, the byproducts of the combustion, such as carbon monoxide, hydrogen cyanide, and other gases are released. Additionally, as oxygen is consumed for the combustion process, the atmospheric concentration of oxygen decreases, carbon dioxide levels increase, and the temperature in the environment rises.[8]

Usual Concurrent Injuries

Although the burn to the skin may be the first injury observed, the potential for injury to the pulmonary system requires immediate assessment and intervention. Additional injuries may be a direct result of explosive forces that caused the initial fire or may result from falls or jumps to safety. Fractures, head injuries, abdominal injuries, and/or chest injuries may occur.

PATHOPHYSIOLOGY AS A BASIS FOR SIGNS AND SYMPTOMS

Skin and Soft Tissue Injury

Heat, or thermal energy, which the body cannot dissipate, can burn the layers of the skin and underlying structures. (Chemical and electrical injuries will be discussed later in the chapter.) Severe burns on the skin present zones of injury.

- Zone of coagulation

  The affected cells form an area of coagulation at the center where the tissue is not viable.

- Zone of stasis

  Surrounding the zone of coagulation is the area where capillary occlusion, diminished perfusion, and edema occur 24 to 48 hours after the burn.

- Zone of hyperemia (increased blood flow)

  This is the area around the zone of stasis. The increased flow is just one of the consequences of the resulting inflammatory response.

A number of vasoactive chemicals are released from mast cells, white blood cells, and platelets as a result of the injury process. The seriousness of a thermal burn is related to the degree of systemic problems, such as hypovolemia and/or respiratory or renal failure. In the presence of severe injury to the skin, systemic pathophysiologic changes can be anticipated.[3]

Plasma Loss and Other Vascular Responses

The burn victim may present in shock due to intravascular volume loss and diminished tissue perfusion. As a result of both the direct injury to capillaries and the release of vasoactive substances, the semipermeability of the capillary is lost, leading to movement of proteins and other dissolved substances out of the intravascular spaces into the interstitium. The hyperemia (increased blood flow) increases the capillary pressure at the arterial end of the capillary. The loss of proteins decreases the capillary colloid osmotic pressure. Both of these pressure changes contribute to hypovolemia and edema. Edema formation postburn is due to the hyperosmolar state of the interstitium from the presence of [7]:

- Sodium and osmotically active cellular debris

- Protein leakage

The rate of fluid loss from intravascular spaces depends on:

- Patient's age

- Burn size and depth

- Intravascular pressures

- Time elapsed since the burn

The pathophysiologic response to the burn leads to the following changes in the vascular system:

- Hemoconcentration of the blood as manifested by an elevated hematocrit

- Increased blood viscosity. Since the percentage of red blood cells is higher, the friction between cells is greater. The friction of cells is what influences the ability of the cells to move. The more the friction, the greater the viscosity and resistance to flow.

- Increased peripheral resistance due to the increased viscosity

- Although the percentage of red blood cells is greater, the actual number of red blood cells is diminished due to direct hemolysis and thrombi formation.

Hypoxemia/Asphyxia

The process of combustion consumes oxygen. Therefore, victims of fires who are in closed spaces, such as a house or a car, inhale air that has a concentration of oxygen less than 21%. The reduction in the fraction of inspired oxygen (FiO_2) leads to arterial hypoxemia. Asphyxia occurs when the blood has a decreased amount of oxygen and there is an increase in carbon dioxide in the blood and tissues of the body.[9,10] Asphyxiation or deprivation of oxygen may be from the lack of oxygen in the environment or the inhalation of toxic substances. The inhalation of substances, most commonly carbon monoxide, has been cited as the leading cause of death resulting from house fires.[10]

Carbon Monoxide Poisoning

Carbon monoxide (CO) is a tasteless, odorless, and colorless gas that is present in the smoke of the combustion of organic materials, such as wood, coal, and gasoline. Carbon monoxide is also released when the available oxygen to support combustion is consumed and incomplete combustion occurs. Carbon monoxide, when inhaled, crosses the alveolar-capillary membrane and binds to the oxygen binding sites on hemoglobin molecules. Because CO has a 200 to 300 times greater affinity and tenacity to stay bound to hemoglobin than does oxygen, the oxygen-carrying capacity of hemoglobin is reduced. CO can also affect cardiac muscle by binding with myoglobin (the oxygen-transporting pigment of muscle), leading to such changes as hemorrhage and necrosis of cardiac muscle.

The oxygen remaining on the hemoglobin molecule is not readily released to the tissues. Thus, tissue hypoxia is even more serious for those patients who have pre-existing cardiac and/or pulmonary conditions. The presence of carbon monoxide on hemoglobin does not affect the patient's partial pressure of oxygen (PaO_2) but does affect the oxygen content (oxygen content = oxygen combined with hemoglobin in physical solution).[11] The patient will have a below normal oxygen saturation (SaO_2) as calculated from an arterial blood gas sample. The SpO_2 obtained by pulse oximetry may be inaccurate since the pulse oximeter cannot accurately discriminate between oxy and carboxyhemoglobin. Since the PaO_2 stays normal, the chemoreceptors are not stimulated to increase ventilation, and the patient sustains tissue hypoxia.[7,12] In fires, the inhalation of toxic substances is not limited to carbon monoxide.

Pulmonary Injury

Combustion and incomplete combustion of organic materials produces byproducts, some of which can be toxic when inhaled (see Table 21).

Table 21

TOXIC CHEMICALS FROM COMBUSTION	
Burning Source	**Toxic Substance**
• Organic materials	• Carbon Monoxide
• Polyurethane	• Hydrogen Cyanide Ammonia, Halogen Acids
• Rubber	• Sulfur Dioxide
• Upholstery	• Hydrogen Chloride
• Wool, silk	• Hydrogen Cyanide, Hydrogen Sulfide
• Polyvinyl chloride	• Phosgene

Smoke is the mixture of gases and particulate matter produced during the decomposition and combustion of natural or synthetic materials. The actual composition of the smoke depends on the[10]:

- Substance burning

- Temperature and rate at which it is being generated

- Amount of oxygen present in the burning environment

As the victim inhales, smoke and soot particles will enter the respiratory tract. The size of the particles and the anatomic location of their deposit will be reflected in the severity of the lung injury. Larger particles may affect the upper airways but will be somewhat filtered and prevented from entering the lower airways. Some gases when inhaled produce harmful acids and/or alkalies, resulting in edema of the membranes with subsequent ulcer formation and necrosis. Other gases destroy the cellular membrane and interfere with the cell's ability to use oxygen. Steam, which has 4,000 times more heat-carrying capacity than dry air, when inhaled can directly injure the airways by direct thermal (heat) damage.

Airway obstruction, atelectasis, and impaired ciliary clearance occur due to the accumulation of debris and secretions. Smoke inhalation may extend to the alveoli, leading to edema and collapse. Additionally, there may be a loss of surfactant, which normally lines the interior surface of the alveoli and reduces surface tension. Without surfactant the alveoli collapse and pulmonary compliance is reduced.

Pulmonary edema may be seen in patients who have sustained severe thermal injury to the skin with or without inhalation injury. Pulmonary edema and adult respiratory distress syndrome (ARDS) are two of the major complications of severe burns.

Hypermetabolism

An increase in the metabolic rate after major trauma and burns is related to the autonomic nervous system response and subsequent release of hormones from the adrenal glands, hypothalamus, and pituitary gland. The degree of increase in the metabolic rates of patients postburn is related to the extent of the burn, percentage of body surface area burned, and the degree of hyperemia.[13] Other influences on the body's response to the burn and rate of metabolism are[13]:

- Age

- Ambient temperature

- Pain

- Anxiety

- Patient activity

- Infection (late complication)

Hypermetabolism is demonstrated in the patient by:

- Tachypnea, due in part to increased oxygen consumption

- Tachycardia, due in part to increased sympathetic response

- Low-grade fever

NURSING CARE OF PATIENTS WITH THERMAL BURNS

Assessment

History

Refer to Chapter 3, Initial Assessment, for a description of general information that should be collected regarding every trauma victim. Only pertinent questions specific to patients with burn injuries are described below.

- Does the patient have any clothing or jewelry that must be immediately removed to stop the burning process?

- What are the patient's complaints?

- Is the patient hoarse?

- What caused the burn?

- Where was the patient located in the environment?

  An inhalation injury should be suspected if the fire was in an enclosed space, in association with heated air, steam, or the burning of potentially toxic materials. An explosion increases the chances of other life-threatening injuries, including penetrating trauma.

- What was the causative agent of the burn? What caused the burn, e.g., flash fire, direct contact with flame, scald from steam or a hot liquid, hot object contact, a chemical, or an electrical source?

- What was the patient's approximate weight prior to burn?

- Is the patient a chronic smoker?

Physical Assessment

Refer to Chapter 3, Initial Assessment, for a description of the assessment of the patient's airway and effectiveness of breathing and circulation.

INSPECTION

- Determine airway patency and effectiveness of breathing

    - Inspect nasopharynx and oropharynx

        Look for evidence of soot, carbonaceous sputum, irritation of mucous membranes, and/or increased secretions. Determine presence or absence of cough, hoarseness, and swallow reflex.

    - Inspect for singed nasal, facial, and eyebrow hairs

- Inspect for burns and edema, especially around the face and neck

- Count respiratory rate, determine breathing pattern, and watch expansion of chest during inspiration

    Increased respiratory rate may indicate hypercarbia, pulmonary injury, shock, anxiety, pain, and/or hypermetabolism. Circumferential burns of the thorax may prevent total inflation of the lungs and lead to respiratory compromise.

- Determine depth of burn injury (see Table 22)

    - Superficial (first-degree) burns are dry, erythematous areas with no bullae (blisters). The burned area blanches and is tender, and the epidermis is intact.

    - Partial thickness (second-degree) burns usually appear hyperemic in color, are moist, and have blisters. The patient will complain of pain. There are two classifications of partial thickness burns:

        - Superficial partial thickness burns involving the upper portion of the dermis.

        - Deep partial thickness burns involving the deeper portions of the dermis.

    - Full thickness (third-degree) burns range in color from pale yellow to cherry red, brown, or carbon black. These burns have a dry, leathery appearance. The burned tissue is inelastic and lacks sensation. This depth of burn can be limb and/or life-threatening.

- Depth of burn injury may not be completely determined in the emergency department. Depth can only be determined after careful examination, debridement, and cooling of the heated area.

Table 22

DEPTH AND DEGREE OF BURN		
Depth	**Degree**	**Characteristics**
Superficial	First	• Dry, red, blanches, tender
Partial Thickness • Superficial Partial Thickness • Deep Partial Thickness	Second	• Hyperemic, moist, bullae, painful • Involves upper dermis • Involves deeper dermis
Full Thickness	Third	• Dry • May be leathery looking or translucent • Color varies from yellow to red to brown or black • Not painful

- Determine the extent of the burn injury

  - The extent of the burn is the percent of total body surface area (TBSA) burned. Fluid amounts for intravenous infusion are calculated using the percent of TBSA burned for patients with partial and full thickness burns.

  - The Rule of Nines divides the TBSA into areas comprising 9% or multiples of 9%, except for the perineum which is equal to 1% of TBSA. The Rule of Nines is an estimate and is most useful for adults and children over the age of 10 (see Figure 33).

  - The Lund and Browder chart provides a more accurate calculation of the TBSA burned because body proportions change during childhood growth. The percentages are related to the patient's age and represent a more accurate estimate of the proportions of specific body surfaces (see Table 23).

Figure 33
The Rule of Nines

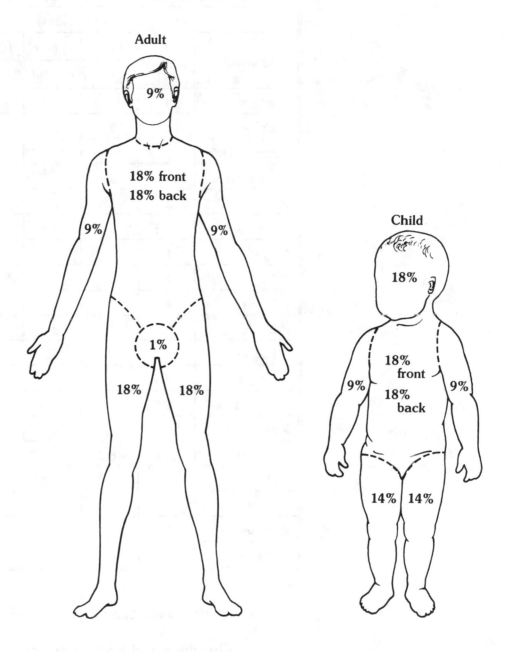

■ To measure the extent of irregular burns, the percentage of burned surface can be estimated by considering the palm of the patient's hand as equal to 1% of the total body surface and then estimating the TBSA burned in reference to the palm.

Table 23

MODIFIED LUND AND BROWDER CHART						
Age (years)						
Burned Area	*1*	*1 to 4*	*5 to 9*	*10 to 14*	*15*	*Adult*
	Total Body Surface (%)					
Head	19	17	13	11	9	7
Neck	2	2	2	2	2	3
Anterior trunk	13	13	13	13	13	13
Posterior trunk	13	13	13	13	13	13
Right buttock	2.5	2.5	2.5	2.5	2.5	2.5
Left buttock	2.5	2.5	2.5	2.5	2.5	2.5
Genitalia	1	1	1	1	1	1
R.U. arm	4	4	4	4	4	4
L.U. arm	4	4	4	4	4	4
R.L. arm	3	3	3	3	3	3
L.L. arm	3	3	3	3	3	3
Right hand	2.5	2.5	2.5	2.5	2.5	2.5
Left hand	2.5	2.5	2.5	2.5	2.5	2.5
Right thigh	5.5	6.5	8	8.5	9	9.5
Left thigh	5.5	6.5	8	8.5	9	9.5
Right leg	5	5	5.5	6	6.5	7
Left leg	5	5	5.5	6	6.5	7
Right foot	3.5	3.5	3.5	3.5	3.5	3.5
Left foot	3.5	3.5	3.5	3.5	3.5	3.5

- Determine the location of the burn injuries

  - Circumferential burns of the chest may lead to respiratory compromise. Circumferential burns of the extremities may contribute to neurovascular compromise.

  - Certain locations of thermal burns present specific patient problems. Burns of the face and neck may cause respiratory problems if edema is present. Burns in this area may also interfere with the patient's ability to talk, swallow, eat, or drink. Burns of the hands inhibit the ability to perform a number of activities, including those of daily living. Burns of the feet interfere with ambulation. Patients with burns of the perineum are at increased risk of infection, difficulties with urinary and bowel elimination, and sexual activity.

- Determine the severity of the burn

  - Based on the depth, extent, and location of the burn, the severity of the thermal injury can be determined.

  - Age, general pre-existing health status, presence of other injuries, and mechanism of injury contribute to overall severity.

AUSCULTATION

- Auscultate breath sounds

  Burn victims may have inhaled the byproducts of combustion. If the victim has a circumferential burn of the thorax, increased inspiratory pressure may be noted during mechanical ventilation as the chest is auscultated.

- Auscultate pulses in burned digits (fingers and toes) with a Doppler Ultrasonic Flow Meter, if available

PALPATION

- Palpate peripheral pulses to detect any vascular compromise associated with circumferential burns to the extremities and any direct injury to vessels.

- Palpate extremities to determine sensory function and to detect any neurologic compromise. Full thickness burns, which destroy nerve endings, will not be paintul. Areas around the full thickness burn that are not as severely burned will still have sensation and be painful.

- Feel the temperature of the skin to determine peripheral perfusion status. Burn tissue feels cold due to decreased perfusion and fluid loss.

Diagnostic Procedures

Refer to Chapter 3, Initial Assessment, for frequently-ordered radiographic and laboratory studies. Additional studies for patients with a burn are listed below.

RADIOGRAPHIC STUDIES

- Chest radiograph – important because of possible pulmonary injury

LABORATORY STUDIES

- Arterial blood gases, pH, and SaO_2

  - An arterial blood sample can be used for extended testing of oxyhemoglobin, carboxyhemoglobin, and methemoglobin.

  - The normal level of carboxyhemoglobin is 0 to 13%; the toxic level is considered greater than 25%; and the lethal level is over 60%.[14]

- Urinalysis and test for hemoglobin and myoglobin

OTHER

- Pulse oximetry

  Pulse oximeters cannot differentiate between carboxyhemoglobin and oxyhemoglobin, yet oximetry still may be useful to measure SpO_2 in certain patients.[15]

- Fiberoptic, flexible bronchoscopy – may be performed to determine the degree of inhalation injury

Nursing Diagnoses and Outcome Identification

The following nursing diagnoses are potential problems for the patient with burns. Once a patient has been assessed, diagnoses can be defined as either actual or risk. An actual nursing diagnosis is one derived from a decision based on the patient's presenting signs and symptoms. A risk nursing diagnosis is a judgment the nurse makes based on a particular patient's risk and potential for developing certain problems.

POSSIBLE NURSING DIAGNOSES
AND EXPECTED OUTCOMES

Nursing Diagnosis	Expected Outcome
Airway clearance, ineffective related to: • Edema of the airway, vocal cords, epiglottis, and upper airway • Irritation of the respiratory tract • Laryngeal spasm • Altered level of consciousness secondary to hypoxia • Pain	The patient will maintain a patent airway as evidenced by: • Regular rate, depth, and pattern of breathing • Bilateral chest expansion • Effective cough/gag reflex • Absence of signs and symptoms of airway obstruction: stridor, dyspnea, and hoarse voice • Clear sputum of normal amount without abnormal color or odor • Absence of signs and symptoms of retained secretions: fever, tachycardia, and tachypnea

Gas exchange, impaired related to:
• Alveolar damage
• Fluid shifts
• Decreased transport, release, and utilization of oxygen secondary to carbon monoxide inhalation
• Shock
	The patient will experience adequate gas exchange as evidenced by:
	• ABG values within normal limits:
	  ▪ PaO_2 80 - 100 mmHg (10.0 - 13.3 KPa)
	  ▪ SaO_2 >95%
	  ▪ $PaCO_2$ 35 - 45 mmHg (4.7 - 6.0 KPa)
	  ▪ pH between 7.35 - 7.45
	• Improved mental status
	• Vital signs within normal limits for developmental age
	• Decreasing carboxyhemoglobin level
	• Skin normal color, warm, and dry

Breathing pattern, ineffective related to:
• Respiratory distress secondary to alveolar damage
• Pain
• Circumfrential burns to thoracic cavity or neck
• Altered level of consciousness secondary to elevated carboxyhemoglobin level
	The patient will have an effective breathing pattern as evidenced by:
	• Normal rate, depth, and pattern of breathing
	• Symmetrical chest wall expansion
	• Absence of stridor, dyspnea, or cyanosis
	• Breath sounds present and equal bilateral
	• ABG values within normal limits:
	  ▪ PaO_2 80 - 100 mmHg (10.0 - 13.3 KPa)
	  ▪ SaO_2 >95%
	  ▪ $PaCO_2$ 35 - 45 mmHg (4.7 - 6.0 KPa)
	  ▪ pH between 7.35 - 7.45

POSSIBLE NURSING DIAGNOSES AND EXPECTED OUTCOMES	
Nursing Diagnosis	**Expected Outcome**
Fluid volume deficit related to abnormal fluid losses secondary to: • Increased capillary permeability • Protein shifts • Inflammatory processes • Evaporation losses	The patient will have an effective circulating volume as evidenced by: • Stable vital signs appropriate for developmental age • Urinary output 1 ml/kg/hr • Strong, palpable peripheral pulses • Improved level of consciousness • Serum electrolyte, hematocrit, and hemoglobin within normal limits • Absence of myoglobinuria • Urine specific gravity within normal limits • CVP reading of 5 - 10 cm H_2O
Hypothermia, risk related to: • Impairment in skin integrity • Resuscitative procedures • Exposure	The patient will maintain a normal core body temperature as evidenced by: • Core temperature measurement of 36° - 37.5°C (98° - 99.5°F) • Absence of shivering
Infection, risk related to: • Impaired skin integrity • Presence of invasive lines • Immobility • Break in sterile technique	The patient will be free from infection as evidenced by: • Core temperature measurement of 36° - 37.5°C (98° - 99.5°F) • Absence of systemic signs of infection: fever, tachypnea, and tachycardia • Wounds free from redness, swelling, purulent drainage, or odor • Urinary output 1 ml/kg/hr • Negative blood cultures • WBC within normal limits • Normal level of consciousness

Planning and Implementation

Refer to Chapter 3, Initial Assessment, for a description of the specific nursing interventions for patients with compromises to airway, breathing, and/or circulation.

Interventions

• Stop the burning process, if still active

   If there are sufficient trauma team members, remove <u>all</u> clothing and jewelry, e.g., rings, watches, necklaces, in anticipation of edema formation.

- Ensure patent airway

Prepare for early intubation as needed, especially if signs of inhalation injury are present. Intubation of the trachea may be difficult due to edema. Summon someone skilled in difficult intubations and surgical airway techniques. It is important that a large tube be used to facilitate adequate ventilation and pulmonary clearing, especially in patients with inhalation injury. If facial burns are present, consider using umbilical tape to secure the endotracheal tube.

- Administer oxygen via a nonrebreather mask at flow rate sufficient enough to keep the reservoir bag inflated; usually requires 12 to 15 L/minute

- Assist ventilation, if needed

Positive end expiratory pressure (PEEP) or continuous positive airway pressure (CPAP) may be used to maintain alveolar inflation and to prevent respiratory distress. Ventilators should be equipped to administer oxygen that is warmed and humidified.

- Cannulate two veins with large-bore, 14- or 16-gauge catheters, and initiate infusion of an intravenous solution

  - Avoid burned areas, if possible

  - Infuse a crystalloid solution such as lactated Ringer's solution according to a pre-established fluid protocol. Patients with more than 25% of the TBSA burned require fluid resuscitation.[13] A number of formulas are available for calculating an estimate of fluid requirements for the first 24 hours postburn. However, fluid resuscitation is based on the individual patient's response to the injury. Patients who may require more fluid than predicted are those patients who have[13]:

    - An inhalation injury

    - A high voltage electrical injury

    - Consumed alcohol

    - Delayed fluid resuscitation since the time of injury

  - The patient's weight and the extent (percent of TBSA) are the determining factors of the fluid resuscitation needs. Pre-existing medical conditions should also be considered.

- The American Burn Association recommends replacing 2 to 4 ml/kg/% of total body surface area burned in the first 24 hours postburn.[16] Of this calculated amount, one half should be infused in the first eight hours postburn. The 24-hour time period begins from the time of the actual burn, not the time of arrival to the emergency department. The following is an example:

24-HOUR BURN FLUID CALCULATION

- 40% total body surface area burn
- 60 kg patient
- Burn occurred at 10:00 pm
- Order reads – Give 2 ml per kg per % TBSA burned

- 2 x 60 x 40 = 4,800 ml in first 24 hours postburn event
- 2,400 ml infused by 6:00 am (first eight hours since burn event)
- 2,400 ml or 150 ml/hour infused from 6:00 am to 10:00 pm

- Administer analgesic medications, as prescribed

  Narcotics, e.g., morphine, should be administered intravenously. Absorption may be altered if the intramuscular route is used. The intravenous route also allows a more accurate titration of medication to control the pain.

- Insert a gastric tube

  If patient has TBSA more than 25%, nausea and vomiting are present, or patient has other body system injuries gastric intubation is indicated.

- Apply cool, saline-moistened, sterile dressings to TBSA burns less than 10%

  - Do not use ice

  - Keep the area cool will help to relieve pain

  - Apply cool dressings within 10 minutes of the burn to reduce the heat content of the tissues and the depth of the burn injury[13]

- Keep the patient warm

  Since a burn victim cannot maintain body heat, keep the room warm to prevent hypothermia. Keeping the ambient temperature warm is also important since the patient may be in a hypermetabolic state. For those patients with burns >50%, increasing the ambient temperature above 30°C (86°F) can reduce their hypermetabolism.[13]

- Assist with escharotomies of chest wall, extremities, or digits as needed to facilitate chest wall expansion or adequate arterial flow. An escharotomy is an incision made into the eschar or burned tissue to relieve circumferential tension.

- Elevate extremities, if not contraindicated, to facilitate venous return

- Treat or assist with care of the burn wound

  Wound care is a low priority in the initial care of a severely burned patient. Direct wound care should not be attempted until the patient's airway, breathing, and circulatory status have been addressed.

- General care of the burned wound includes[13]:

  - Administering an analgesic medicine before wound care

  - Cleaning the wound gently with a soap solution

  - Debriding nonviable epidermis

  - Excising bullae (blisters) is recommended by some. The American College of Surgeons' ATLS Program recommends leaving blisters intact.[17]

  - Shaving hair around wound. Never shave eyebrows.

  - Applying a topical antimicrobial agent, such as:

    - Sulfamylon (Mafenide acetate cream) applied 1/8 inch layer

    - Silvadene (Silver sulfadiazine cream) applied same as above

    - Silver nitrate (0.5% solution) applied in multilayer occlusive dressings

- Provide psychosocial support to the patient and family, especially since burn wounds may be difficult for the patient and family to view.

- Prepare patient for operative intervention, hospital admission, or transfer, as indicated. If the patient is to be transferred, consult with the receiving facility for instructions on wound care. If wound care is to be done before transfer, wash wounds, debride loose tissue, and cover with a dry, sterile dressing.

- Prepare for transfer to burn facility

The American Burn Association and the American College of Surgeons have recommended that the following patients be considered for transfer to a burn center.[17] Patients with:

- Partial thickness and full thickness burns greater than 10% of body surface area (BSA) in patients under 10 or over 50 years of age

- Partial thickness and full thickness burns greater than 20% BSA in other age groups

- Deep partial thickness and full thickness burns that involve the face, hands, feet, genitalia, perineum, and overlying major joints

- Full thickness burns greater than 5% BSA in any age group

- Significant electrical burns including lightning injuries

- Significant chemical burns

- An inhalation injury

- Pre-existing medical conditions that could complicate management, prolong recovery, or affect mortality

- Concomitant trauma, which poses an increased risk of morbidity or mortality, and who have been initially stabilized in a trauma center

- Children with burns seen in hospitals without qualified personnel or equipment necessary to care for such children should be transferred to a facility with these capabilities

- Need for special social, and emotional, or long-term rehabilitative support, including those patients suspected of child maltreatment

- Assist with transfer to a facility with a chamber for hyperbaric oxygen therapy (HBO)

  Oxygen (100%) is delivered to the patient under high pressure to reduce the half-life of carboxyhemoglobin and to reduce cerebral edema and cerebral pressure.[18] HBO may also be considered for patients who have been poisoned with cyanide, hydrogen sulfide, or carbon tetrachloride.[19]

- Administer medications, as prescribed, to treat hydrogen cyanide poisoning

  The burning of polyurethane, wool, silk, and paper can be a source of hydrogen cyanide.[10] Cyanide has the ability to inactivate cytochrome oxidase, which is an important enzyme in cellular production of ATP.[20] The administration of amyl nitrite by inhalation and sodium nitrite by intravenous injection converts the iron in hemoglobin to form methemoglobin, which cannot combine with oxygen but can attract the cyanide molecules. This frees the cyanide from cytochrome oxidase, allowing it to participate in cellular activities. Sodium thiosulfate is also given to enhance excretion of cyanomethemoglobin.[20]

Evaluation and Ongoing Assessment

Refer to Chapter 3, Initial Assessment, for a description of the ongoing evaluation of the patient's airway, and effectiveness of breathing and circulation. Additional evaluations include:

- Monitoring urinary output

- Assessing peripheral circulation by palpating peripheral pulses and using a Doppler Ultrasonic Flow Meter

- Assessing progression of edema formation

SELECTED BURN INJURIES

Refer to "Nursing Care of Patients with Thermal Burns" for a description of the phases of the trauma nursing process.

Electrical Burns

Burns from electricity, as compared to burns from heat, result in different types of injuries. It is difficult to assess the true extent of damage since electricity enters the body at the point of contact and travels the path of least resistance. The path may traverse internal

277

structures and deeper tissues before eventually exiting. The skin may be intact except for the entrance and exit wounds, while underlying tissues may be injured to the point of necrosis. The electricity may injure any type of tissue and depends on the tissue's resistance, the intensity (voltage divided by resistance), and the length of contact. Electrical current follows the path of certain tissues in the order of their ability to conduct the current; nerves are the first structures that current will pass through, followed by blood vessels, muscles, skin, tendons, fat, and then finally bone.[21] More important than tissue resistance is current density. The smaller the area that comes in contact with the electricity, the greater the tissue damage. Electrical injuries cause significant damage to the extremities and less damage to the torso and viscera.[13]

The damage to vessels and muscles is an important aspect of electrical injury. Vascular disruption, hemorrhage, and/or thrombi may result from damage to blood vessels. Hemoglobin may be released and appear in the urine. Muscle damage may lead to edema formation and subsequent elevation of compartment pressures. If striated muscle fibers are destroyed (rhabdomyolysis), then myoglobin, the protein pigment in muscle that transports oxygen, may be released and excreted in the urine.

Alternating current (AC) is more dangerous than direct current.[21] AC current may cause tetany, so that a person's grip on an electrical source tightens, which lengthens the exposure to the current. The electrical current in the United States used in most dwellings is 110 volt, alternating current. During assessment, it is important to determine the:

- Voltage

- Type of current

- Location of electrical source

- Duration of contact with the electrical source

Signs and Symptoms

- Entrance and/or exit wounds

- Altered level of consciousness

- Cardiac dysrhythmias, including atrial or ventricular fibrillation and asystole

278

Interventions

- Infuse intravenous fluid at a rate to maintain urinary output between 75 to 100 ml/hour. Fluid resuscitation estimates cannot be calculated since TBSA cannot be calculated.

- Observe color of urine

  If dark, pink, or red, myoglobin may be present. If urine color does not return to normal, anticipate administration of mannitol (hyperosmolar diuretic) to promote diuresis and excretion of myoglobin. The administration of sodium bicarbonate may be considered to facilitate excretion of these substances since they are excreted more readily in alkaline urine. Myoglobin, if not excreted, can precipitate in the renal tubules which may result in renal failure.[13]

- Monitor cardiac rate and rhythm

- Monitor for signs and symptoms of compartment syndrome and prepare for fasciotomies, as indicated

- Monitor pH, PaO_2, $PaCO_2$, SaO_2, SpO_2, and serum bicarbonate levels. Assure ventilation and fluid replacement are adequate.

Chemical Burns

Chemical burns occur when the victim comes in direct contact with caustic chemical agents, such as acids, alkalies, and/or petroleum-based products. Alkaline chemicals, e.g., soda and anhydrous ammonia, are generally responsible for more serious burns since alkalies penetrate the contact area more deeply than acids. Damage to the skin in any type of chemical burn is influenced by the length of contact and the concentration and amount of the chemical. In most cases, damage is limited to the local area and does not involve a systemic response. During the assessment phase of nursing care, it is imperative to identify the causative agent. Contact with a regional poison center may be needed to identify the characteristics of certain substances and to identify neutralization methods.

Signs and Symptoms

- Erythema, edema, blisters, or tissue necrosis may be apparent

- Pain

Interventions

- Assure protection of the trauma team from contamination by using gloves, gown, mask, and goggles

- Irrigate burned area with water or normal saline; alkalies require longer irrigation times to neutralize and remove.

- Flush with copious amounts of water. Do not waste time identifying a neutralizing agent. Surface burns due to lime or lime-containing compounds, such as concrete, should NOT be initially irrigated with water since the combination of water and lime produces a corrosive substance that will cause further burning. After brushing off the lime powder with a dry towel, the area can then be irrigated thoroughly.

- Surface burns due to phenol contamination (carbolic acid) should NOT be irrigated with water since phenol is not water-soluble. Irrigate with a lipid-soluble solvent, e.g., polyethylene glycol. Phenol absorption can produce serious systemic sequelae such as CNS depression.[13]

- Hydrofluoric acid burns (used in glass etching, dental laboratories, industry, and electronic plants) are extremely serious and may be life-threatening. Inhalation of this acid may lead to pulmonary edema. Local contact on the skin leads to deep penetration, causing tissue necrosis. The time from exposure to tissue damage can be seconds. Since this acid depletes serum calcium levels, subcutaneous local injections of 5% calcium gluconate may be required.[22]

- For patients with moderate to large tar or asphalt burns, cool the area first and use petroleum products, e.g., neomycin sulfate or mineral oil to dissolve the substance.

SUMMARY

The leading cause of death from being involved in a fire in a dwelling is inhalation of toxic substances. Regardless of the extent and depth of a thermal burn, adhere to the principles outlined in the initial assessment to correct any life-threatening compromises to airway, breathing, and/or circulation. Determine the severity of a burn by determining the depth, extent, location of the burn, and the age, as well as general pre-existing health status of the patient.

After intervening to assure airway clearance and adequate ventilation, initiate intravenous fluid replacement if the extent of the patient's burn is greater than 25% TBSA. Follow the guidelines of the American Burn Association for considering transfer of certain patients to a comprehensive burn center.

The burn victim may be facing a long, painful, and stressful recovery with devastating consequences to self-esteem, image, and equilibrium. The trauma nursing process, initiated in the emergency department, will affect the patient's response to the burn injury. The nursing process in collaboration with others is intended to prevent or correct those pathophysiologic changes, which could lead to serious sequelae, such as shock, pulmonary failure, and/or infection.

REFERENCES

1. Porth CM. *Pathophysiology Concepts of Altered Health States*. 4th ed. Philadelphia, Pa: JB Lippincott Co; 1994.

2. Baker SP, O'Neill B, Ginsburg MJ, Guohua LM. *The Injury Fact Book*. 2nd ed. New York, NY: Oxford University Press; 1992.

3. McManus W, Pruitt B. Thermal injuries. In: Moore EE, Mattox KL, Feliciano DV, eds. *Trauma*. 2nd ed. Norwalk, Conn: Appleton & Lange; 1992:751-764.

4. McLoughlin E, McGuire A. The causes, cost, and prevention of childhood burn injuries. *AJDC*. 1990;144:677-683.

5. Mierley M, Baker S. Fatal house fires in an urban population. *JAMA*. 1983;249:1466-1468.

6. *Injury Mortality Atlas of the United States 1979-1987*. Atlanta, Ga: Centers for Disease Control, US Department of Health & Human Services, Public Health Service. 1992.

7. Dimick A, Wagner R. Burns. In: Schwartz GR, Cayton CG, Mangelsen MA, Mayer TA, Hanke BK, eds. *Principles and Practice of Emergency Medicine*. 3rd ed. Philadelphia, Pa: Lea & Febiger; 1992:1200-1209.

8. Einhorn I, Grunnet M. The toxicology of combustion products. *Emerg Care Q*. 1985;1:60-80.

9. Orlando R. Smoke inhalation injury. *Emerg Care Q*. 1985;1:22-30.

10. Miles RH, Dries DJ, Gamelli RL. Inhalation injury: Pathophysiology and treatment. In: Miles RH, Dries DJ, Gamelli RL, eds. *Trauma 2000: Strategies for the New Millennium*. Austin, Tex: RG Landes Co; 1992:44-63.

11. Nunn JF. *Nunn's Applied Respiratory Physiology*. 4th ed. London, England: Butterworth Heinemann; 1993.

12. Safar P, Bircher N. The pathophysiology of dying and reanimation. In: Schwartz GR, Cayton CG, Mangelsen MA, Mayer TA, Hanke BK, eds. *Principles and Practice of Emergency Medicine*. Philadelphia, Pa: Lea & Febiger; 1992:3-42.

13. Mozingo DW, Cioffi WG, Pruitt BA. Burns. In: Bongard F, Sue D, eds. *Current Critical Care Diagnosis and Management*. Norwalk, Conn: Appleton & Lange; 1994:657-685.

14. Benzer T, Slomenbaum N. The poisoned patient. In: Schwartz GR, Cayton CG, Mayer T, Mangelsen MA, Mayer TA, Hanke BK, eds. *Principles and Practice of Emergency Medicine*. Philadelphia, Pa: Lea & Febiger; 1992:2918-2925.

15. Severinghaus JW, Kelleher JF. Recent developments in pulse oximetry. *Anesthesiology*. 1992;75:1018-1038.

16. DeMuth MW, Dimick A, Gillespie RW, et al. *Advanced Burn Life Support Provider Manual*. Lincoln, Neb: Advanced Burn Life Support; 1992.

17. American College of Surgeons Committee on Trauma. Burn care. In: *Resources for Optimal Care of the Injured Patient: 1993*. Chicago, Ill: Author; 1993:63-66.

18. Price DP, Silverman H, Schwartz GR. Smoke inhalation. In: Schwartz GR, Cayton CG, Mangelsen MA, Mayer TA, Hanke BK, eds. *Principles and Practice of Emergency Medicine*. 3rd ed. Philadelphia, Pa: Lea & Febiger; 1992:2862-2869.

19. Schwartz GR. Overview and general considerations of the poisoned patient. In: Schwartz GR, Cayton CG, Mangelsen MA, Mayer TA, Hanke BK, eds. *Principles and Practice of Emergency Medicine*. 3rd ed. Philadelphia, Pa: Lea & Febiger; 1992:2926-2945.

20. McKenry LM, Salerno E. *Mosby's Pharmacology in Nursing*. St. Louis, Mo: Mosby-Year Book; 1992.

21. McCabe C, Browne B. Electrical and chemical burns. *Emerg Care Q*. 1985;1:31-40.

22. Upfal M, Doyle C. Medical management of hydrofluoric acid exposure. *Occupational Med*. 1990;32:726-731.

CHAPTER ELEVEN

TRAUMA AND PREGNANCY

OBJECTIVES

Upon completion of this chapter/lecture, the learner should be able to:

1. Identify the mechanisms of injury associated with trauma in the pregnant trauma patient.
2. Analyze the pathophysiologic changes as a basis for signs and symptoms.
3. Discuss the nursing assessment of the pregnant trauma patient.
4. Based on the assessment data, recall appropriate nursing diagnoses and expected outcomes.
5. Plan appropriate interventions for the pregnant trauma patient.
6. Evaluate the effectiveness of nursing interventions for the pregnant trauma patient with specific types of injuries.

INTRODUCTION

Epidemiology

Trauma is the leading cause of death in women during the reproductive years. It is also the leading nonobstetric cause of death and disability in pregnant women.[1] As a result of economic changes, more women are employed and participating in events outside the home. The pregnant woman is no exception to these changes. It is common for pregnant women to continue to travel, work, drive and remain physically active throughout pregnancy. This exposure has increased the frequency of injury. The actual incidence of injury is unknown, but it is estimated that seven percent of pregnant women will be injured during pregnancy.[1]

Biomechanics and Mechanisms of Injury

The resuscitation priorities for the injured pregnant patient are identical to those of the nonpregnant patient. The pregnant trauma victim presents a challenge to the resuscitation team because members are faced with the simultaneous management of two patients. Because of the low incidence of injury to pregnant women, the trauma team may not be as familiar with the physiologic changes of pregnancy and fetal development, which complicate the resuscitation process.

285

Similarly, obstetric consultants who should be consulted early may be unfamiliar with the effects of trauma on the mother and fetus. Diagnostic and therapeutic procedures need to benefit both patients; yet the risk-benefit of such procedures must be considered. Do not delay resuscitation if pregnancy is suspected or confirmed.

Injury to the pregnant patient can result from forces causing blunt or penetrating trauma. The uterus has elastic fibers and, therefore, is not as susceptible to rupture as the placenta, which has no elastic fibers and is more susceptible to shearing forces. Energy applied to the abdomen of the pregnant patient is absorbed in part by the uterus, amniotic fluid, and the fetus. Therefore, other abdominal organs are somewhat protected from energy loads. Blunt trauma is the most frequent cause of maternal and fetal injury. Motor vehicle injuries are the leading cause of death for women in the child-bearing years. Falls are the second most common cause of injury during pregnancy.[2] Fatigue, pelvic ligamentous laxity, and the protuberant abdomen contribute to gait instability.[2,3] The incidence of intentional injury from domestic violence rises during pregnancy.

Penetrating trauma during pregnancy is most commonly due to gunshot wounds.[2,4] The incidence of uterine injury increases with each trimester. The enlarged uterus shields most of the abdominal organs from injury, making the uterus the most likely organ to be injured.

Stab wounds are less common than gunshot wounds and have a better prognosis for both the mother and fetus. Stab wounds to the lower abdomen are more likely to injure the enlarged uterus.

Types of Injury

Head injury is the major cause of maternal death.[2,4,5] A pelvic fracture with subsequent hemorrhage from laceration of engorged pelvic vessels, is the most common injury to the mother that results in fetal death.[5] The physiologic and anatomic changes of pregnancy affect the pattern and severity of other injuries.

- The risk of diaphragmatic tears increases as the uterus enlarges with the pregnancy.

- Upward displacement of the bladder from the normally protected position within the pelvis increases the chances of bladder injury.

- Uterine injury is common, particularly in the second and third trimester as the uterus becomes larger and more protruding.[2,3]

- Fetal demise may result from placental lacerations and placental separation.

- Fetal injury is more common during the third trimester when the head is relatively fixed in the pelvis, and less amniotic fluid is present to buffer energy transfer.[5,7] The fetus can also sustain skull fractures, intracranial injuries, hepatic, splenic, and clavicular injuries.[6,7]

- By the third trimester of pregnancy, the veins of the pelvis become congested. Pelvic fractures can result in severe hemorrhage.[8,9]

ANATOMIC AND PHYSIOLOGIC CHANGES DURING PREGNANCY AS A BASIS FOR SIGNS AND SYMPTOMS

Cardiovascular

The pregnant woman is normally in a hypervolemic and hyperdynamic state. The mechanism of hypervolemia is unclear, but as early as the 10th week of pregnancy, a slight increase in pulse rate and stroke volume increases cardiac output by 1 to 1.5 L/minute.[10] The perfusion of the uterus is increased to 25% of the total cardiac output.[3,8]

The "anemia of pregnancy" is a result of the increase in plasma volume, which is proportionately greater than the increase in erythrocyte volume. In late pregnancy, a hematocrit of 31 to 34% is common.[3,8]

The hypervolemia allows the maternal circulation to compensate for a gradual loss of maternal blood volume up to 30%, and an acute blood loss of 10 to 15%. The uterine vessels cannot autoregulate their blood vessel size in response to variations in blood pressure.[3] Uterine perfusion decreases as the uterine artery vasoconstricts during the initial response to shock, with little or no change in maternal vital signs.[3,9]

As the pregnancy progresses, the mother's heart is elevated and rotated forward to the left. The heart rate increases gradually throughout pregnancy and reaches a rate of 15 to 20 beats per minute higher than in the nonpregnant state. During the second trimester, the systolic and diastolic blood pressure falls 5 to 15 mmHg.[10] Hypertension in the pregnant patient may indicate an obstetrical complication.

The fetus is compromised with a maternal blood loss of 15 to 30%. The first evidence of decreased uterine perfusion may be demonstrated by the fetus. Signs and symptoms include changes in fetal movement and either fetal tachycardia or bradycardia.[11]

The enlarged uterus may compress the inferior vena cava and aorta, impeding venous return and decreasing cardiac output. As a result, the pregnant patient may experience hypotension, or vena caval syndrome, when placed in the supine position. Symptoms include dizziness, discomfort, and/or nausea.

The leukocyte count is normally elevated during pregnancy and even further elevated during labor. A leukocyte count as high as 15,000/mm^3 is considered normal during pregnancy.[3]

The levels of fibrinogen and other clotting factors are elevated, resulting in hypercoaguability. The injured pregnant patient is predisposed to disseminated intravascular coagulation (DIC) if placental abruption or amniotic fluid embolus occurs.[5,8]

Respiratory

Tidal volume (amount of air moved in and out of the lungs with each breath) increases by 40%, and vital capacity (maximum amount of air exhaled from point of maximum inspiration) increases by 100 to 200 ml. Respiratory rate usually increases slightly. Arterial blood gases reflect hyperventilation and compensated respiratory alkalosis. PaCO$_2$ may decrease to 30 mmHg (4.0 KPa).[10] PaO$_2$ will increase to 101 to 104 mmHg (13.5 - 13.9 KPa) (see Table 24).

The elevated diaphragm decreases functional residual capacity (volume of air in the lungs at end of expiration) and reduces the patient's tolerance of hypoxia. Upper respiratory passages are engorged due to increased vascularity, predisposing the patient to nasopharyngeal bleeding.

Abdominal

Throughout pregnancy, a physiologic ileus may exist due to a decrease in gastric motility and an increase in emptying time.[1] Hormonal changes relax the gastroesophageal sphincter, predisposing the patient to vomiting and aspiration.[3]

The normal responses to peritoneal membrane irritation are changed due to stretching of the abdominal wall. Because of the gradual compression of the viscera and stretching of the abdominal wall by the uterus, rebound tenderness and abdominal guarding may be decreased.[5,8]

Table 24

MATERNAL CARDIOVASCULAR AND RESPIRATORY CHANGES DURING PREGNANCY			
Cardiovascular		**Respiratory**	
• Cardiac output	• ↑ 30%	• Tidal volume	• ↑ 40%
• Heart rate	• ↑ by 15 to 20 beats/min	• Vital capacity	• ↑ by 100 to 200 ml
• Blood pressure	• ↓ by 5 to 15 mmHg	• Respiratory rate	• ↑ Slightly
• Venous pressure	• CVP varies • Increased in lower extremities	• $PaCO_2$	• ↓ to 30 mmHg (4.0 KPa)
		• PaO_2	• ↑ to 101 to 104 mmHg (13.5 - 13.9 KPa)
• Hematocrit	• ↓ to 31 to 34%	• Arterial pH • Serum HCO_3	• ↑ Slightly • ↓
• White blood count	• Increased to 15,000/mm³ • Normal differential		
• Electrocardiogram	• Flattened or inverted T waves in III, AVF, AVL		
• Fibrinogen and clotting factors VII, VIII, IX	• ↑ Increased		

Urinary

Urinary frequency is common in pregnancy due to an increased glomerular filtration rate and the pressure of the uterus on the bladder. In late pregnancy, the bladder is elevated anteriorly, out of the protective ring of the pelvis, into the abdomen. Glycosuria is common, yet proteinuria is not.

Neurologic

Pregnancy induced hypertension (PIH), protein in the urine, and edema may cause seizures and symptoms that can mimic a head injury.

Musculoskeletal

Hormonal changes cause a softening of most joints and relaxation of the sacroiliac joint. By the third trimester, the symphysis pubis is widened by 4 to 8 mm.[8,10] Because of these changes, the pelvis is less susceptible to fractures.

NURSING CARE OF THE PREGNANT TRAUMA PATIENT

Assessment

History

Refer to Chapter 3, Initial Assessment, for a description of general information that should be collected regarding every trauma victim. Only pertinent questions specific to pregnant patients with injuries are described below.

- What was mechanism of injury?

- Was the patient wearing a safety restraint device?

- When was the last menstrual period (LMP)?

  Consider the possibility of pregnancy in any female of childbearing age. If the last menstrual period was more than 4.5 weeks ago, consider the patient possibly pregnant. If pregnant, the date of the last menstrual period is a crude means of determining gestational age.

- When is the expected date of confinement (EDC)?

  To estimate the EDC, count back three months from the LMP and add seven days.

- What problems or complications have occurred during this or other pregnancies?

- Are uterine contractions or abdominal pain present?

- Is there fetal activity?

  An early sign of fetal distress may be a marked decrease in fetal activity.

Physical Assessment

Refer to Chapter 3, Initial Assessment, for a description of the assessment of the patient's airway, and effectiveness of breathing and circulation.

INSPECTION

- Inspect the perineum

  Determine if there is any vaginal bleeding or presence of amniotic fluid. The patient may describe having had a sudden gush of fluid. This may be an indication of a spontaneous bladder void or premature rupture of amniotic membranes.

- Inspect the vaginal opening for crowning or any abnormal fetal presentation

  Prolapse of the umbilical cord is rare. Relieve cord compression immediately, if present.

- Observe the shape and contour of the abdomen

  A change in shape may indicate uterine rupture or concealed hemorrhage.

- Observe the abdomen for signs of fetal movement

AUSCULTATION

Auscultate fetal heart tones and rate

- Fetal heart tones may be heard with a fetoscope at approximately 20 weeks gestation and by ultrasound device at 10 to 14 weeks gestation. Auscultate for two minutes.[3] The fetal heart rate is normally 120 to 160 beats per minute. A sustained fetal heart rate (FHR) of less than 110 is considered bradycardia.[9] A sustained fetal heart rate of 160 is considered tachycardia.[8]

- During auscultation discriminate between the mother's pulse rate and the pulse rate of the fetus.

PALPATION

- Palpate and determine the height of the fundus

Fundal height is an indicator of gestational age. The fundus is measured in centimeters from the symphysis pubis to the top of the fundus and approximates the number of weeks of gestation. The fundal height reaches the symphysis at 12 weeks, the umbilicus at 20 weeks, and costal margin at 36 weeks[6] (see Figure 34).

Figure 34
Uterine Size and Location Reflecting Gestational Age

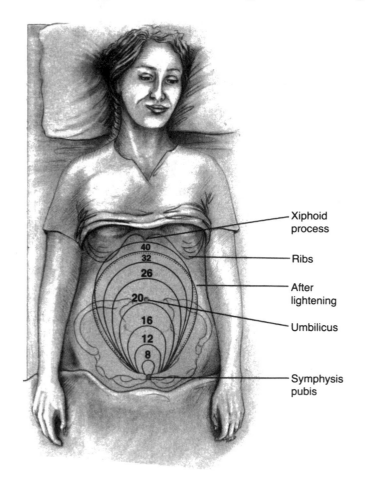

(Reprinted with permission from Gorrie TM, McKinney ES, Murray SS. Physiological adaptations to pregnancy. In: *Foundations of Maternal Newborn Nursing*. Philadelphia, Pa: WB Saunders; 1994:118.)

- Palpate the uterus

Note any uterine tenderness or contractions.

Diagnostic Procedures

Refer to Chapter 3, Initial Assessment, for frequently-ordered radiographic and laboratory studies. Additional studies for the pregnant trauma patient are listed below.

RADIOGRAPHIC STUDIES

Do not withhold radiographic studies. However, avoid unnecessary studies and duplication of films. Shield the fetus from unnecessary exposure with a lead apron.[8]

- Intravenous pyelogram (IVP) and cystogram

  From the 10th week of gestation through six weeks postpartum, a physiologic dilation of the renal calyxes, renal pelvis, and ureters may be seen on IVP.

- Computerized tomography[3,7]

- Ultrasonography

  Determines:

  - Gestational age – very accurate up to 22 weeks of age.

  - Fetal weight, heart rate, and viability (a fetus older than 25 weeks or weighing over 750 grams is potentially viable).[3,8,12]

  - Placental abruption.

LABORATORY STUDIES

- Serum blood sample for typing

- Serum bicarbonate and lactate

  Altered serum bicarbonate levels correlate with fetal outcome more significantly than other variables reflective of shock and hypoxia.

- PT and PTT

  Incoagulable blood is the hallmark of placental separation.

- Beta Human Chorionic Gonadotropin (HCG)

  HCG in blood confirms pregnancy as early as one to two weeks after conception, and in urine two to four weeks after conception.

- Kleihauer-Betke Assay

  Detects fetal red cells in the maternal circulation, indicating hemorrhage of fetal blood through the placenta into the mother's circulation. This is particularly important for the woman who is Rh negative and the fetus who is Rh positive. Under these circumstances, hemorrhage can cause Rh sensitization requiring treatment with $Rh_O(D)$ immune globin (Rhogam).[5,8]

- Kleihauer-Betke Staining

  Detects whether blood in the vagina is fetal in origin. A cesarean section may be indicated if the stain is positive, the fetus is alive, and the gestation is at least 25 weeks.[6]

OTHER PROCEDURES

- Assist with diagnostic peritoneal lavage

  Since the physical exam of the abdomen is unreliable, consider a DPL, which can be done safely in the pregnant trauma patient.[6] Insert a gastric tube and indwelling urinary catheter prior to the procedure. After determining fundal height, the open technique with supraumbilical incision is recommended.[6]

- Assist with a pelvic exam

  Assess if the cervix is open or closed and if the membranes are intact. Test any obvious vaginal fluid. The pH of amniotic fluid is 7.5; the pH of urine is 4.6 to 6. If amniotic fluid is observed, use a sterile speculum for exam.

- Monitor fetal heart tones and rate

  If fetal heart tones cannot be heard with a fetoscope, consider using an external ultrasound device designed for obstetrical purposes.[3] Using this device, continually monitor the fetal heart rate. An abnormal fetal heart tracing may indicate maternal hypovolemia, possible placental separation, or uterine rupture.

- Monitor uterine contractions, as indicated, e.g., premature labor

Assist with the placement of a device to monitor uterine contractions. A cardiotocograph, which monitors both fetal heart rate and uterine contractions with an externally placed sensor, is often used as an assessment tool.

- Assist with amniocentesis, as indicated

Amniocentesis is rarely indicated in trauma. An amniocentesis positive for blood may indicate the need for urgent operative intervention if the fetus has fetal heart tones and is at least 28 weeks gestation.

Nursing Diagnoses and Outcome Identification

The following nursing diagnoses are potential problems for the obstetrical patient with trauma. Once a patient has been assessed, diagnoses can be defined as either actual or risk. An actual nursing diagnosis is one derived from a decision based on the patient's presenting signs and symptoms. A risk nursing diagnosis is a judgment the nurse makes based on a particular patient's risk and potential for developing certain problems.

POSSIBLE NURSING DIAGNOSES AND EXPECTED OUTCOMES	
Nursing Diagnosis	**Expected Outcomes**

Aspiration, risk related to:
• Reduced level of consciousness secondary to injury, concomitant substance abuse
• Impaired cough and gag reflex
• Structural defect to head, face, and/or neck
• Secretions and debris in airway
• Increased risk of vomiting secondary to gastro-intestinal changes of pregnancy
	The patient will not experience aspiration as evidenced by:
	• A patent airway
	• Clear and equal bilateral breath sounds
	• Regular rate, depth, and pattern of breathing
	• ABG values within normal limits:
	  ▪ PaO_2 101 - 104 mmHg (13.5 - 13.9 KPa)
	  ▪ SaO_2 >95%
	  ▪ $PaCO_2$ 25 - 30 mmHg (3.3 - 4.0 KPa)
	  ▪ pH between 7.35 - 7.45
	• Clear CXR without evidence of infiltrates
	• Ability to handle secretions independently

POSSIBLE NURSING DIAGNOSES AND EXPECTED OUTCOMES	
Nursing Diagnosis	**Expected Outcomes**

Gas exchange, impaired related to:
• Ineffective breathing pattern: loss of integrity of thoracic cage and impaired chest wall movement secondary to injury, deterioration of ventilatory efforts
• Ineffective airway clearance
• Aspiration
• Increased oxygen consumption, decreased tidal volume secondary to pregnancy
• Shock
	The patient will experience adequate gas exchange as evidenced by:
	• ABG values within normal limits:
	  ▪ PaO_2 101 - 104 mmHg (13.5 - 13.9 KPa)
	  ▪ SaO_2 >95%
	  ▪ $PaCO_2$ 25 - 30 mmHg (3.3 - 4.0 KPa)
	  ▪ pH between 7.35 - 7.45
	• Skin normal color, warm, and dry
	• Improved level of consciousness
	• Regular rate, depth, and pattern of breathing
	• Fetal heart tones maintained between 120 - 160 beats/min

Fluid volume deficit related to: • Hemorrhage secondary to maternal injury, uterine rupture, abruptio placenta • Fluid shifts • Alteration in capillary permeability • Alteration in vascular tone • Myocardial compromise • Vena cava compression by enlarged uterus	The patient will have an effective circulating volume as evidenced by: • Stable vital signs appropriate for stage of pregnancy • Urinary output of 1 ml/kg/hr • Improved level of consciousness • Skin normal color, warm, and dry • Maintains HCT = 30 ml/dl or Hgb = 12 - 14 g/dl or greater • CVP reading of 5 - 10 cm H_2O • External hemorrhage is controlled
Infection, risk related to: • Impaired skin integrity • Presence of invasive lines • Immobility • Break in aseptic technique • Premature rupture of membranes secondary to injury during pregnancy	The patient will be free from infection as evidenced by: • Core temperature measurement of 36° - 37.5°C (98° - 99.5°F) • Absence of systemic signs of infection: fever, tachypnea, tachycardia • Wounds free from redness, swelling purulent drainage or odor • Urinary output 1 ml/kg/hr • Negative blood cultures • WBC count within normal limits • Normal level of consciousness • Uterus will be nontender to palpation

POSSIBLE NURSING DIAGNOSES AND EXPECTED OUTCOMES	
Nursing Diagnosis	**Expected Outcomes**
Anxiety/Fear (patient, family) related to: • Actual or perceived threat of death • Separation from support systems • Unfamiliar environment • Invasive procedures and therapeutic treatments • Threat of fetal injury or death	The patient/family will experience decreasing anxiety/fear as evidenced by: • Absence of fear-related behavior, e.g., crying, shouting, agitated behavior, noncommunicative behavior, blank stare. Facial expressions, voice tone, and body posture within normal for patient (family). • Acknowledging fear and stating decreasing fear • Absence of physiologic indicators of fear, e.g., palpitations, increased blood pressure, diaphoresis, tachycardia • Patient/family voicing concerns and fears
Grieving related to: • Actual or anticipated losses associated with recent injury (patient, family) • Actual or potential loss of significant other (family) • Actual or anticipated injury of death of fetus	The patient and/or family will begin the grieving process as evidenced by: • Expressing signs of the grieving process • Participating in decision-making • Recognizing reasons for feelings • Sharing feelings of grief with significant other(s)

Planning and Implementation

Refer to Chapter 3, Initial Assessment, for a description of the specific nursing interventions for patients with compromises to airway, breathing, and/or circulation.

• Position the patient on her left side, if greater than 20 weeks gestation

  If on a backboard, tilt the backboard 15 to 20 degrees to the left. If this is not possible, manually displace the uterus to the left side.[3,8]

• Initiate intravenous fluid replacement, as ordered

• Insert a gastric tube

- Determine potential effects of medications on the fetus

    The potential risks of medications must be weighed against expected therapeutic benefits. Determine the pregnancy safety category for all medications administered to pregnant patients.

- Consider obtaining an obstetric consult

- Prepare patient for operative intervention, hospital admission, or transfer, as indicated

- Provide psychosocial support

    Provide realistic reassurance related to the well-being of the fetus. Allay any maternal fears related to fetal safety during diagnostic procedures.

Evaluation and Ongoing Assessment

Refer to Chapter 3, Initial Assessment, for a description of the ongoing evaluation of the patient's airway, and effectiveness of breathing and circulation. Additional evaluations include:

- Monitoring maternal cardiovascular status for evidence of changes consistent with shock

- Assessing the abdomen and uterine activity

- Monitoring fetal activity and heart rate

SELECTED OBSTETRIC INJURIES

Refer to "Nursing Care of the Pregnant Trauma Patient" for a description of the phases of the trauma nursing process.

Premature Labor

Premature labor is the most frequent complication in the pregnant trauma patient. Premature labor usually can be detected in alert patients, but may go unnoticed in an unconscious or intubated patient.

Signs and Symptoms

- Uterine contractions more than six per hour

  Patient may or may not sense the contractions.

- Back pain

- Clear or bloody vaginal discharge

- Cervical dilation or effacement

Interventions

- Position patient on either side

- Monitor uterine contractions for duration and frequency

- Administer fluid volume replacement to prevent dehydration, which can cause uterine irritability and subsequent contractions

- Administer medications to inhibit uterine contractions, as prescribed

  If premature labor is diagnosed, and the mother is stable without rupture of membranes, medications may be given to inhibit uterine contractions.[13,14]

Abruptio Placentae

Abruptio placentae is the partial or total separation of the normally implanted placenta from the uterine wall. It is a common cause of fetal death following motor vehicle crashes. Suspect separation of the placenta if the patient presents with vaginal bleeding. The signs and symptoms can be vague, particularly with a partial separation. Changes in fetal heart rate may be the only indication. Abruptio placentae can develop as late as 48 hours after trauma.

Signs and Symptoms

- Vaginal bleeding (may be present or absent if the blood remains retroplacental)

- Premature labor

- Abdominal pain or cramps

- Uterine tenderness, tetany, or rigidity

- Maternal hemorrhage and evidence of hypovolemic shock

- Fetal distress

- Increasing fundal height[3,8]

Interventions

- Monitor maternal vital signs frequently

- Monitor amount of uterine and/or vaginal blood loss

- Measure and record fundal height every 30 minutes

- Assess serial coagulation studies

    Incoagulable blood is the hallmark of placental separation.

- Prepare the patient for immediate operative intervention, as indicated

Uterine Rupture

Uterine rupture is rare and may occur in those patients with extreme compression injury, or with a history of cesarean sections. Uterine rupture may be associated with bladder rupture, indicated by blood or meconium in the urine. Uterine rupture often results in fetal demise. It is rarely repairable and generally requires a hysterectomy. Early detection and repair of minor lacerations or tears can prevent maternal hemorrhage and fetal compromise.

Signs and Symptoms

- Abdominal pain

    Patient may have a history of acute pain followed by no pain.

- Uterine tenderness

- Difficulty identifying the fundal height

- Change or loss of normal contour of the uterus. Fetal body parts may be more palpable.

300

- A palpable mass outside the uterus (may be the fetus)[3]

- Vaginal bleeding

- Maternal hemorrhage and evidence of hypovolemic shock

- Absent fetal heart tones

Interventions

Prepare the patient for surgical intervention

Severe Fetal Distress

The alert patient may describe the disappearance of fetal movements. Additional evaluation of the fetus may indicate fetal demise. Infant survival is dependent on severity of maternal and fetal injuries.

Signs and Symptoms

- Changes in fetal movement

- Fetal tachycardia or bradycardia

Interventions

- Maintain maternal oxygenation, ventilation, and circulation

- Anticipate the need for emergency cesarean section

Maternal Cardiopulmonary Arrest/Fetal Delivery

The following conditions have been reported to contribute to the successful outcome of delivering a fetus by cesarean section from a pregnant trauma victim in cardiopulmonary arrest[15]:

- Procedure performed within 15 minutes of maternal arrest

- Viable fetal gestational age

- Continuation of cardiopulmonary resuscitation throughout the cesarean section

- Availability of a neonatal resuscitation team

- Correction of maternal metabolic acidosis

SUMMARY

Since the pregnant woman continues to work outside the home and participate in numerous activities, she is susceptible to injury. The pregnant trauma patient imposes a unique challenge and responsibility for health care professionals. The resuscitation priorities for the injured pregnant patient are identical to those of the nonpregnant patient. Maintaining maternal well-being is the principle that guides the management of the injured mother. Fetal well-being is dependent on an adequate blood flow to the uterus and placenta, as well as satisfactory tissue oxygenation. The best chance for fetal survival is maternal survival.[3,8]

ENA believes that care of the obstetrical patient should take place in the area best prepared to handle the needs of the patient. When a fetal monitor is used in the ED, the nurse responsible for monitoring will be educated and credentialed, and will meet institutional standards for fetal monitoring.[16]

REFERENCES

1. Baker D. Trauma in the pregnant patient. *Surg Clin North Am.* 1982;62:275-289.

2. Crosby WI. Traumatic injuries during pregnancy. *Clin Obstet Gynecol.* 1988;26:902-912.

3. Gerber-Smith L. The pregnant trauma patient. In: Cardona VD, Hurn PD, Mason PJB, Scanlon AM, Veise-Berry SW, eds. *Trauma Nursing: From Resuscitation Through Rehabilitation.* 2nd ed. Philadelphia, Pa: WB Saunders Co; 1994:667-692.

4. Timberlake GM, McSwain NE. Trauma in pregnancy: a ten year perspective. *Am J Surg.* 1989;55:151-155.

5. Pearlman MD, Tintinalli JE, Lorenz RP. Current concepts: blunt trauma during pregnancy. *N Eng J Med.* 1990;323:1609-1613.

6. Maull KI, Pedigo RE. Injury to the female reproductive system. In: Moore EE, Mattox KL, Feliciano DV, eds. *Trauma.* 2nd ed. Norwalk, Conn: Appleton & Lange; 1991:587-595.

7. Esposito TM, Gens DB, Gerber-Smith L, Scorpio R. Evaluation of blunt abdominal trauma occurring during pregnancy. *J Trauma.* 1989;29:1628-1632.

8. Neufeld JD, Marx JA. Trauma in pregnancy. In: Rosen P, Baker FJ, Barkin RM, Braen GR, Dailey RH, Levy RC, eds. *Emergency Medicine: Concepts and Clinical Practice.* 3rd ed. St. Louis, Mo: Mosby-Year Book; 1992:287-302.

9. Rozycki GS, Champion HR, Drass MJ. Traumatic injuries in the pregnant patient. *Hosp Phys.* 1989:20-27.

10. American College of Surgeons Committee on Trauma. Trauma in pregnancy. In: *Advanced Trauma Life Support® Course for Physicians (Student Manual).* 5th ed. Chicago, Ill: Author; 1993:283-292.

11. Manley LK. Trauma in pregnancy. In: Neff JA, Kidd PS, eds. *Trauma Nursing: The Art and Science.* St. Louis, Mo: Mosby-Year Book; 1993:499-525.

12. Esposito TJ, Gens MD, Smith LG, Scorpio R, Buchman T. Trauma during pregnancy: a review of 79 cases. *Arch Surg.* 1991;126:1073-1078.

13. Drost TF, Rosemurgy AS, Sherman HF, Scott LM, Williams JK. Major trauma in pregnant women: maternal/fetal outcome. *J Trauma.* 1990;30:574-578.

14. Kulb NW. Preterm labor. In: Buckley K, Kulb NW, eds. *High Risk Maternity Nursing Manual.* Baltimore, Md: Williams & Wilkins; 1990:311-325.

15. Gatrell CB. Trauma in pregnancy. In: Schwartz GR, Cayton CG, Mangelsen MA, Mayer TA, Hanke BK, eds. *Principles and Practice of Emergency Medicine.* 3rd ed. Philadelphia, Pa: Lea & Febiger; 1992:1142-1151.

16. Emergency Nurses Association. *The Obstetrical Patient in the ED.* Position statement. Park Ridge, Ill: Author; 1993.

CHAPTER TWELVE

PEDIATRIC TRAUMA

OBJECTIVES

Upon completion of this chapter/lecture, the learner will be able to:

1. Identify mechanisms of injury associated with pediatric trauma.
2. Analyze the anatomic and pathophysiologic differences in children as a basis for signs and symptoms.
3. Discuss the nursing assessment of a pediatric trauma patient.
4. Based on the assessment data, identify appropriate nursing diagnoses and expected outcomes.
5. Plan appropriate interventions for the pediatric trauma patient.
6. Evaluate the effectiveness of nursing interventions for the pediatric trauma patient.

INTRODUCTION

Epidemiology

Injuries are the number one cause of death and disability of children over one year of age in the United States. While there has been a dramatic reduction in child mortality due to natural causes, no corresponding reduction has occurred in deaths due to injuries.

More than 28,000 children, 19 years and younger, die annually from injuries.[1] Considerably more children sustain nonfatal injuries, which may result in permanent disability. Approximately 75% of deaths are caused by unintentional injury, such as motor vehicles crashes.[2] The other 25% of deaths are caused by intentional injuries from violence, homicide, and suicide. Homicide victims under the age of five have a higher incidence of child maltreatment. Whereas, adolescents are more frequently victims of gang and peer violence.[2] For all causes of injury, males are at a consistently higher risk for death due to injury than females.[1-3]

Mechanisms of Injury and Biomechanics

The age and developmental stage of a child influences the mechanisms of injury. In the toddler and preschool age group, burns, drownings, being struck by a motor vehicle, motor vehicles crashes, and child maltreatment are the primary causes of death. The four leading causes of death in school-age children are being struck by a motor vehicle, motor vehicle crashes, burns, and drownings. Middle school-age children die as a result of motor vehicle crashes, pedestrian versus motor vehicle events, and homicide. Motor vehicle crashes are the leading cause of death for high school-age youth. Other causes of death in this group include homicide and suicide.[1,2]

Classic patterns of injury are associated with specific mechanisms of injury in children. Waddell's Triad describes a combination of head, trunk, and extremity injuries sustained when a child is struck by a motor vehicle.[4-6] (see Figure 35).

Figure 35
Waddell's Triad

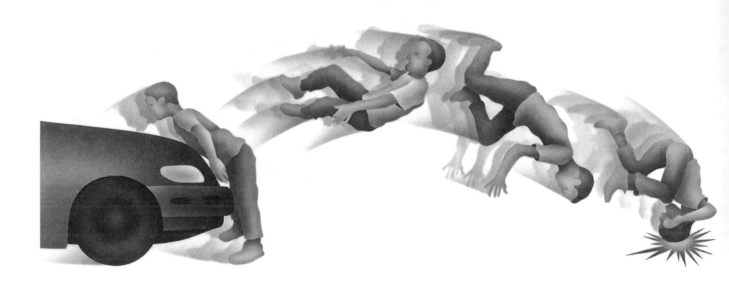

(Redrawn by permission from Whaley, Lucille F., and Wong. Donna L.: *Nursing Care of Infants and Children*, ed. 4, St. Louis, 1991, Mosby-Year Book, Inc.)

Lap Belt Complex describes injuries sustained by children restrained only by lap belts.[7,8] Because the anterior iliac crest of the child is less prominent, the lap restraint may slide up above the pelvis. Upon rapid deceleration against the seatbelt, there is flexion of the lumbar spine and a sudden rise in intra-abdominal pressure, that may result in rupture of the small bowel and/or injury to the lumbar spine. Duodenal and pancreatic injuries may occur during bicycle crashes when the child is thrown against the handlebars.[9]

Child maltreatment is associated with head injuries, burns, abdominal injuries, and fractures. One characteristic of child maltreatment is an inconsistency between the stated mechanism of injury and the actual injury observed. Often there is a significant time lapse between the injury and presentation in the emergency department.

Types of Injuries

Blunt trauma accounts for 80 to 95% of pediatric injuries, the remaining are penetrating.[3-6] In order of frequency, the most commonly injured body areas are the head, musculoskeleton, thorax, and abdomen.[3]

Head injuries contribute to a high percentage of traumatic deaths. Focal injury is less common in children,[10] but if present, suspect maltreatment. Bony facial injuries are less common in children due to the resilience and elasticity of their facial tissues. Facial fractures are usually associated with significant trauma and underlying head injury.

Thoracic injuries are usually associated with head injuries in the pediatric population.[6] The most common thoracic injuries are a pneumothorax, pulmonary contusion, pulmonary laceration, and hematoma.[6] Pneumothorax and pulmonary contusion are often present in the absence of rib fractures.

The most commonly injured abdominal organ is the spleen, followed by the liver.[7] Pelvic fracture is uncommon in pediatric trauma. Depending on the height of the child, the pelvis may be fractured when the child is struck by a motor vehicle. These fractures can be associated with bladder rupture.

ANATOMIC AND PHYSIOLOGIC DIFFERENCES IN CHILDREN AS A BASIS FOR SIGNS AND SYMPTOMS

The trauma nursing process associated with the care of a pediatric trauma patient is based on knowledge of pediatric anatomy, physiology, and the child's response to injury. Inherent in this process is the recognition of the distinct anatomic and physiologic differences between the pediatric and adult patient.

Respiratory

- The tongue and the pharyngeal tissue are softer and relatively larger when compared to the size of the oral cavity.[4,5,10] Edema of these structures is a cause of airway obstruction.

- Small amounts of mucus, blood, or edema may occlude the airway due to its smaller diameter.

- Infants, during the first several months of their lives, are obligatory nose breathers. Any nasal obstruction can cause respiratory distress.

- Airway cartilage is soft, particularly the larynx in infants and small children. Flexion or hyperextension of the neck may cause airway compression.

- The larynx is higher and more anterior, increasing the risk of aspiration. The anterior position of the vocal cords makes direct visualization during intubation more difficult.

- In children under eight years of age, the cricoid cartilage is the narrowest portion.[10] An uncuffed endotracheal tube is indicated in children less than eight years of age.

- The trachea is shorter, increasing the possibility of intubation of the mainstem bronchus.

- Children under eight years of age rely primarily on movement of the diaphragm for breathing because of their immature intercostal muscles. Excessive gastric air from crying or assisted ventilations may affect the child's ability to ventilate adequately.

- The chest wall in infants and young children is more pliable because the sternum and ribs are cartilaginous. A significant force may result in an injury to an underlying structure without concomitant rib fracture. In the presence of a rib fracture, suspect underlying thoracic injury.

- Normal respiratory rates vary according to the child's age. Generally, the younger the child, the faster the rate[11] (see Table 25). A respiratory rate greater than 60 per minute is abnormal for any child.

Table 25

VITAL SIGNS BY AGE			
Age	Respiratory Rate/min	Pulse Beats/min	Blood Pressure (Systolic) mmHg
Birth to 1 week	30 to 60	100 to 160	50 to 70
1 to 6 weeks	30 to 60	100 to 160	70 to 95
6 months	25 to 40	90 to 120	80 to 100
1 year	20 to 30	90 to 120	80 to 100
3 years	20 to 30	80 to 120	80 to 110
6 years	18 to 25	70 to 110	80 to 110
10 years	15 to 20	60 to 90	90 to 120

(Adapted from: Seidel J, Henderson D, eds. *Prehospital Care of Pediatric Emergencies.* Los Angeles Pediatric Society; 1987:10. Reprinted with permission.)

- Children have lower glucose stores despite having increased metabolic demands. In addition, they may have less elastic tissue to keep the pulmonary alveoli expanded, lower tidal volumes, and less residual capacity. Due to these factors, and the underdevelopment of intercostal muscles, children may become fatigued during increased work of breathing. Respiratory failure may ensue.

Cardiovascular

- Normal blood pressure varies according to the child's age (see Table 25).

- Children can compensate for up to a 40 to 45% blood loss by increasing the heart rate and peripheral vascular resistance, which maintains a normal systolic blood pressure. Therefore, blood pressure is an unreliable indicator of shock.[12-15]

- Normal heart rates vary according to the child's age. Generally, the younger the child, the faster the heart rate (see Table 25). Tachycardia is one of the first signs of shock, but it can also be caused by many other factors, including anxiety and agitation. Increased heart rate caused by agitation and crying should return to normal when the child becomes calm. To maintain the cardiac output during shock, the heart rate rather than the stroke volume increases.

- Blood volume is dependent on the size of the child. The circulating blood volume of an infant and child is approximately 80 ml/kg.[4,10,14] Small blood losses can stimulate compensatory mechanisms. A closed femur fracture can cause a blood loss of 300 to 400 ml in a small child.[5]

Temperature Regulation

Children have a less effective thermoregulatory mechanism, a greater ratio of body surface area to body mass, and less subcutaneous tissue for heat insulation. Hypothermia is not well tolerated. Infants and small children lose a significant amount of heat from their heads.

Other Anatomic and Physiologic Characteristics

- The metabolic demands of children are twice those of adults, and anxiety alone can increase the metabolic rate significantly.[4]

- The anterior and posterior fontanelles are open in infants.

- The head is heavier and larger in relation to the rest of the body, predisposing the child to head and neck trauma.

- The cranium is thinner and more pliable in young children.

- Children sustaining head injury are susceptible to increases in intracranial pressure due to cerebral vasodilation and hyperemia.

- The myelin sheaths around nerves are less developed.

- The neck muscles and ligaments are weaker.

- The bony spine is more flexible, spinal ligaments are lax.

- The abdominal muscles are thinner, weaker, and less developed.

- The liver is more anterior and less protected by the ribs.

- The kidney is mobile and not protected by fat.

- The bones of the extremities are more pliable and resilient to injury.

- Injuries to, or adjacent to, growth plates can potentially retard normal bone growth or alter bone development.[10]

NURSING CARE OF THE PEDIATRIC TRAUMA PATIENT

Assessment

History

Refer to Chapter 3, Initial Assessment, for a description of general information that should be collected regarding every trauma victim. Only pertinent questions specific to pediatric patients are described below.

- Who is the caregiver accompanying the child?

  If the child is a minor, obtain permission for treatment according to institutional protocols.

- Is the child's immunization status up-to-date?

- What was the child's weight prior to the injury?

- Was an air bag deployed at the time of the crash?

Physical Assessment

Refer to Chapter 3; Initial Assessment, for a description of the assessment of the patient's airway, and effectiveness of breathing and circulation.

INSPECTION

- Assess breathing for nasal flaring and/or intercostal retractions

- Assess circulation for mottled skin or differences in central versus peripheral color. Cyanosis is a late sign of decreased oxygenation.

- Inspect the abdomen for abrasions or ecchymosis, which may indicate injury from an inappropriately placed lapbelt

AUSCULTATION

- Auscultate breath sounds, especially at the anterior axillary lines

Since the child's chest wall is thin, breath sounds may be ausculated in all areas of the lung, even in the presence of a pneumothorax.

- Auscultate the apical heart rate

  Bradycardia is an ominous sign of impending cardiopulmonary arrest.[16]

- Auscultate blood pressure

  Hypotension is a late sign of shock and represents uncompensated hypovolemia. Use noninvasive, automated, oscillometric blood pressure monitors in critically injured children with caution. Some models are not accurate in children, and accuracy decreases in extremely high and low blood pressure ranges.[15]

PALPATION

- Palpate the fontanelles for fullness or bulging

  Full fontanelles in a supine position are not necessarily clinically significant.

- Palpate capillary refill

- Palpate the abdomen for distention

  Children swallow large amounts of air especially when crying. Distention may reflect gastric dilation from air.

The neurological assessment is tailored to the age and developmental stage of the child. For an example of a Pediatric Coma Scale, see Table 26.[17]

Table 26

PEDIATRIC COMA SCALE			
Eye Opening			
Score	>1 Year		<1 Year
4	Spontaneously		Spontaneously
3	To verbal command		To shout
2	No pain		To pain
1	No response		No response
Best Motor Response			
Score	>1 Year		<1 Year
6	Obeys		Spontaneous
5	Localizes pain		Localizes pain
4	Flexion-withdrawal		Flexion-withdrawal
3	Flexion-abnormal (decorticate rigidity)		Flexion-abnormal (decorticate rigidity)
2	Extension (decerebrate rigidity)		Extension (decerebrate)
1	No response		No response
Best Verbal Response			
Score	>5 Years	2 to 5 Years	0 to 23 Months
5	Oriented and converses	Appropriate words/phrases	Smiles, coos appropriately
4	Disoriented and converses	Inappropriate words	Cries, consolable
3	Inappropriate words	Persistent crying and screaming	Persistent inappropriate crying and/or screaming
2	Incomprehensible sounds	Grunts	Grunts, agitated, restless
1	No response	No response	No response
TOTAL = 3 to 15			

(Adapted from Simon J, Goldberg A. *Prehospital Pediatric Life Support*. St. Louis, Mo: CV Mosby; 1989:11. Reprinted with permission.)

Diagnostic Procedures

Refer to Chapter 3, Initial Assessment, for frequently-ordered radiographic and laboratory studies.

RADIOGRAPHIC STUDIES

- Significant spinal cord injury can occur with no evidence of bony damage or fracture on radiographic film.[10] Suspected spinal cord injury without radiographic abnormality (SCIWORA) necessitates further evaluation in addition to routine cervical spine studies.

- Extremity radiographic studies may need to include comparative views of the uninjured extremity

LABORATORY STUDIES

Small children have lower hemoglobin levels than adults

OTHER

Diagnostic peritoneal lavage (DPL) is not commonly performed in children. If a DPL is used, 10 to 15 ml/kg of warmed isotonic crystalloid solution is infused over 10 to 15 minutes through the peritoneal catheter.[10]

Nursing Diagnosis and Outcome Identification

The following nursing diagnoses are potential problems for the pediatric trauma patient. Once the child has been assessed, diagnoses can be defined as either actual or risk. An actual nursing diagnosis is one derived from a decision based on the child's presenting signs and symptoms. A risk nursing diagnosis is a judgment the nurse makes based on a particular child's risk and potential for developing certain problems.

POSSIBLE NURSING DIAGNOSES AND EXPECTED OUTCOMES	
Nursing Diagnosis	**Expected Outcomes**

Aspiration, risk related to:
• Reduced level of consciousness secondary to injury
• Impaired cough and gag reflex
• Structural defect to head, face, and/or neck
• Secretions and debris in airway
	The patient will not experience aspiration as evidenced by:
	• A patent airway
	• Clear and equal bilateral breath sounds
	• Regular rate, depth, and pattern of breathing
	• ABG values within normal limits:
	  ■ PaO_2 80 - 100 mmHg (10.0 - 13.3 KPa)
	  ■ SaO2 >95%
	  ■ $PaCO_2$ 35 - 45 mmHg (4.7 - 6.0 KPa), or 25 - 30 mmHg (3.3 - 4.0 KPa) with hyperventilation
	  ■ pH between 7.35 - 7.45
	• Clear CXR without evidence of infiltrates
	• Ability to handle secretions independently

Gas exchange impaired related to:
• Ineffective breathing pattern: loss of integrity of thoracic cage and impaired chest wall movement secondary to injury, deterioration of ventilatory efforts
• Ineffective airway clearance
• Aspiration
• Shock
	The patient will experience adequate gas exchange as evidenced by:
	• ABG values within normal limits:
	  ■ PaO_2 80 - 100 mmHg (10.0 - 13.3 KPa)
	  ■ SaO_2 >95%
	  ■ $PaCO_2$ 35 - 45 mmHg (4.7 - 6.0 KPa), or 25 - 30 mmHg (3.3 - 4.0 KPa) with hyperventilation
	  ■ pH between 7.35 - 7.45
	• Skin normal color, warm, and dry
	• Improved level of consciousness: Pediatric Coma Scale = ability to recognize caregivers, behavior normal for developmental age
	• Regular rate, depth, and pattern of breathing
	• Clear CXR without evidence of infiltrates
	• Ability to handle secretions independently

POSSIBLE NURSING DIAGNOSES AND EXPECTED OUTCOMES	
Nursing Diagnosis	**Expected Outcomes**
Fluid volume deficit related to: • Hemorrhage • Fluid shifts • Alteration in capillary permeability • Alteration in vascular tone • Myocardial compromise	The patient will have an effective circulating volume as evidenced by: • Stable vital signs appropriate for developmental age • Urinary output of 1 - 2 ml/kg/hr • Strong, palpable peripheral pulses • Improved level of consciousness: Pediatric Coma Scale = ability to recognize caregivers, normal behavior for developmental age • Skin normal color, warm, and dry • Maintains normal HCT or Hgb for age • Capillary refill <2 seconds • External hemorrhage is controlled
Hypothermia related to: • Rapid infusion of intravenous fluids • Decreased tissue perfusion • Exposure	The patient will maintain a normal core body temperature as evidenced by: • Core temperature measurement of 36° - 37.5°C (98° - 99.5°F) • Absence of shivering, cool skin, pallor • Skin normal color, warm, and dry
Infection, risk related to: • Impaired skin integrity • Contamination of wound from initial injury or instrumentation • Invasive fixation devices • Interruption in perfusion	The patient will be free from infection as evidenced by: • Core temperature measurement of 36° - 37.5°C (98° - 99.5°F) • Absence of systemic signs of infection: fever, tachypnea, tachycardia • Wounds free from redness, swelling, purulent drainage or odor • Urinary output 1 - 2 ml/kg/hr • Negative blood cultures • WBC count within normal limits • Improved level of consciousness
Pain related to: • Soft tissue injury and edema • Fractures • Pleural irritation • Stimulation of nerve fibers • Invasive procedures	The patient will experience relief of pain as evidenced by: • Diminishing or absent level of pain through patient's self-report using an objective measurement tool appropriate for developmental age. • Absence of physiologic indicators of pain which include: tachycardia, tachypnea, pallor, diaphoretic skin, increasing blood pressure, restlessness • Absence of nonverbal cues of pain: crying, grimacing, inability to assume position of comfort, and/or guarding • Ability to cooperate with care as appropriate

POSSIBLE NURSING DIAGNOSES AND EXPECTED OUTCOMES	
Nursing Diagnosis	**Expected Outcomes**
Altered health maintenance, risk for altered (caregiver) related to: • Insufficient knowledge of care of wounds, casting material, immobilization devices, ambulatory aids • Restrictions to activity • Signs and symptoms of complications • Follow-up care	The caregiver is knowledgeable about self-care and follow-up as evidenced by: • Recognizing and promptly reporting signs and symptoms that indicate serious complications • Stating necessity and planning for ongoing medical care • Describing and demonstrating proper use and care of ambulatory aids • Identifying how to reduce the risk of infection • Relaying an intent to comply with agreed restrictions
Anxiety/Fear (patient, caregiver) related to: • Unfamiliar environment • Unpredictable nature of condition • Invasive procedures • Possible disfigurement, scarring	The patient/caregiver will experience decreasing anxiety/fear as evidenced by: • Oriented to surroundings • Ability to describe reasons for equipment and procedures used in treatment • Utilizing effective coping skills • Caregivers spending time with child
Powerlessness (patient, caregiver) related to: • Loss of function • Uncontrolled pain • Lack of privacy • Lack of knowledge	The patient/caregiver will experience an increasing feeling of control over the situational crisis as evidenced by: • Caregivers' participation in decision-making activities • Questioning by caregivers and patient, if age appropriate, regarding treatment and course of care

Planning and Implementation

Refer to Chapter 3, Initial Assessment, for a description of the specific nursing interventions for patients with compromises to airway, breathing, or circulation.

• Administer oxygen via a pediatric nonrebreather mask at a flow rate sufficient to keep the reservoir bag inflated; usually requires 12 to 15 L/minute

Oxygen demands are greater due to increased metabolic need.

- Assist with endotracheal intubation

  Select an appropriately-sized endotracheal tube. Tube size depends on the age and size of the child. An uncuffed endotracheal tube is indicated in children less than eight years of age. Commercial pediatric resuscitation tapes used to measure the length of the child provides information regarding appropriately-sized tubes. Tube size can also be estimated by matching the diameter of the child's little finger with the diameter of the tube. Another method involves calculating the size using the formula: [16 + age (in years)] divided by 4.[18]

- Verify placement and secure endotracheal tube

  Stabilize the child's head to prevent hyperextension, which could cause the tube to descend into the right mainstem bronchus. Prevent flexion, which could increase the possibility of extubation and/or esophageal intubation.

- Hyperventilate

  If the child has a head injury, hyperventilation ($PaCO_2$ of approximately 25 mmHg; 3.3 KPa) is the most effective means to control increased intracranial pressure and maintain CPP.

- Stabilize and/or immobilize the cervical spine

  Since infants and young children have a large occiput, positioning them supine on a backboard causes their cervical vertebrae to flex and move anteriorly (see Figure 36). This flexion may contribute to airway compromise and/or decreased effectiveness of the jaw thrust or chin lift maneuvers. Place padding under the child's shoulders to bring the shoulders into horizontal alignment with the external auditory meatus. This position provides neutral alignment of the cervical spine[12,19,20] (see Figure 37).

- Initiate cardiopulmonary resuscitation, as indicated

  CPR is indicated if the child is pulseless or bradycardic with evidence of poor perfusion.

- Insert a gastric tube

  Decompression of air from the stomach will improve the child's ability to ventilate.

Figure 36
Child on a Standard Backboard

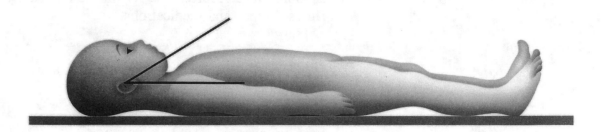

Figure 37
Proper Positioning of Child on a Backboard

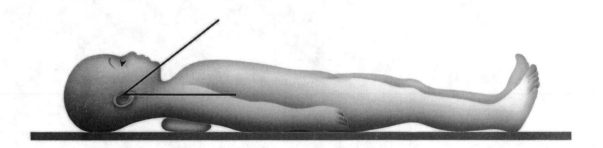

- Cannulate two veins with 22-gauge or larger catheters, and initiate infusion of warmed lactated Ringer's solution

  - Infuse a bolus of 20 ml/kg

  - Reassess circulation and initiate a second bolus, if indicated

  - Anticipate blood replacement

    If the child remains hemodynamically unstable after two boluses, blood transfusions of 10 ml/kg may be indicated.[10]

- Initiate intraosseous access for fluid replacement

  If peripheral venous access cannot be established within three attempts or 90 seconds, initiate intraosseous (IO) access with a 16- or 18-gauge bone marrow needle. In children under six

319

years of age, use the proximal tibia (see Figure 38) since it is flat and free of major vessels and nerves.[10] Verify placement by aspiration of bone marrow. Secure the IO needle since movement of the needle erodes the entry site allowing fluid extravasation. Once secured, the IO line can be safely used to infuse fluids, blood, and medications.

Figure 38
Site for Intraosseous Infusion

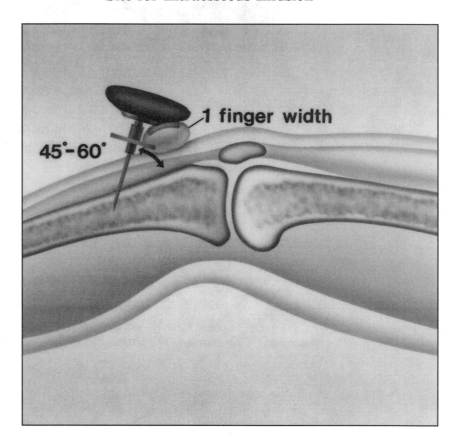

(Reprinted with permission from American College of Surgeons Committee on Trauma. Pediatric trauma. In: *Advanced Trauma Life Support Course® for Physicians (Student Manual)*. 5th ed. Chicago, Ill: Author; 1993:270.)

● Insert an indwelling urinary catheter

■ Normal urinary output for infants is 2 ml/kg/hr. For small children, it is 1 ml/kg/hr.

■ Infuse intravenous fluids for the child who has sustained a thermal or electrical burn as follows:

◆ Maintain a urinary output of 2 to 3 ml/kg/hr in the child weighing less than 30 kg

- ◆ Maintain a urinary output of 30 ml/hr in the older child

- Keep child warm

  Use warming lights, warm blankets, and apply a stockinette to the heads of infants and small children.

- Get a complete set of vital signs, including temperature

- Obtain a pediatric consult

- Provide psychosocial support

  - Undressing the awake child can be a very frightening experience

  - Speak softly and provide reassurance

  - Provide psychosocial support to help the child cope with the change in body image and fear of treatment procedures[21]

  - Utilize anxiety-reducing techniques, e.g., stuffed animal, tape recorded music

  - Provide family members with information frequently

  - Include the family in the child's care by asking them to provide information regarding the child's medical history and events surrounding the injury

  - Consider allowing the family members in the treatment area, as guided by institutional protocols

  - Refer family members to available trauma support or bereavement programs

  - Utilize available Critical Incident Stress Management programs for debriefing and follow-up for health care providers

- Report suspected child maltreatment according to institutional protocols and state laws

- Prepare child for operative intervention, hospital admission or transfer, as indicated. It is recommended that children under 12 years of age with a concussion be admitted.[22]

321

- Determine need for injury prevention teaching to caregivers, e.g., use rear-facing car seat in the front seat of a car equipped with air bags

SUMMARY

The leading cause of death for all children over the age of one is trauma. Youth violence is increasing at an alarming rate. The National Center for Injury Prevention and Control at the CDC has made prevention of youth violence a national priority. For information regarding community activities to promote child safety, refer to *The Prevention of Youth Violence A: Framework for Community Action*, which is an extensive manual outlining principles and descriptions of prevention programs across the United States.[23]

The foundation of the trauma nursing process used to care for pediatric patients is the knowledge the nurse needs related to the anatomic and physiologic characteristics of children, related to their age, size, and developmental stage. The assessment of airway, breathing, and circulation are guided by an awareness of the anatomic differences in the airways of infants and children, the reliance on the diaphragm for the work of breathing, and their relatively small blood volumes compared to body size (80 ml/kg). It is recommended that nurses who care for pediatric patients consider completing the Emergency Nurses Association *Emergency Nursing Pediatric Course* (ENPC).

When caring for children, first follow the principles of correcting airway, breathing, and circulatory compromises before proceeding to the management of specific injuries. The psychosocial aspects of trauma care are heightened when the patient is a child, especially a critically-ill or injured child. The family's need for information, compassionate care, and a perception of hope are guiding principles. Consider transfer of the critically-ill pediatric patient to a trauma center with comprehensive resources to care for the special needs of children.

REFERENCES

1. *Vital Statistics of the United States, 1989, Vol 2, Mortality Part B.* Washington, DC: National Center for Health Statistics, Public Health Service:1992:192. US Government Printing Office publication DHHSTUB, THS 92-1102.

2. *A Data Book of Child and Adolescent Injury.* Washington, DC: National Center for Education in Maternal and Child Health; 1991:7.

3. Dandrinos-Smith S. The epidemiology of pediatric trauma. *Crit Care Clin North Am.* 1991;3:387-389.

4. Semonin-Holleran R. Pediatric trauma. In: Neff JA, Kidd PS, eds. *Trauma Nursing: The Art and Science.* St. Louis, Mo: Mosby-Year Book; 1993:527-553.

5. Keen T. Nursing care of the pediatric multitrauma patient. *Nurs Clin North Am.* 1990;25:131-141.

6. Dickinson CT. Thoracic trauma in children. *Crit Care Clin North Am.* 1991;3:324-332.

7. Lebet R. Abdominal and genitourinary trauma in children. *Crit Care Clin North Am.* 1991;3:433-444.

8. Slater M, Coran A. Appendiceal transection in a child associated with lap belt restraint. *J Trauma.* 1992;33:765-766.

9. Grosfeld J, Rescorda F, West K, Vane DW. Gastrointestinal injuries in childhood, analysis of 53 patients. *J Pediatr Surg* 1989;24:580-583.

10. American College of Surgeons Committee on Trauma. Pediatric trauma. In: *Advanced Trauma Life Support Course® for Physicians (Student Manual).* 5th ed. Chicago, Ill: Author; 1993:261-281.

11. Seidel J, Henderson D, eds. *Prehospital Care of Pediatric Emergencies.* Los Angeles, Ca: Los Angeles Pediatric Society; 1987:10.

12. Nypaver M, Treloar DF. Neutral cervical spine positioning in children. *Ann Emerg Med.* 1994;23:208-211.

13. Graneto JD, Soglin D. Transport and stabilization of the pediatric trauma patient. *Pediatr Clin North Am.* 1993;40:365-380.

14. American Heart Association. Anticipating cardiopulmonary arrest. In: *Pediatric Advanced Life Support (Provider) Manual.* 3rd ed. Dallas, Tx: Author; 1990:3-9.

15. Derrico D. Comparison of blood pressure measurement methods in critically ill children. *Dimensions in Crit Care Nurs.* 1993;12:31-39.

16. Emergency Nurses Association. Triage and initial assessment. In: *Emergency Nursing Pediatric Course (Provider) Manual.* Park Ridge, Ill: Author; 1993:51.

17. Simon J, Goldberg A. *Prehospital Pediatric Life Support.* St. Louis, Mo: CV Mosby; 1989:11.

18. American Heart Association. Airway management. In: *Pediatric Advanced Life Support (Provider) Manual.* 3rd ed. Dallas, Tx: Author; 1990:21-36.

19. Mellick LW, VanStralen D, Perkin RS. Emergency transport and positioning in young children who have an injury of the cervical spine. *Pediatr Emerg Care.* 1993;9:128.

20. Herzenberg JE, Hensinger RN, Dedrick DK, Phillip WA. Emergency transport and positioning of young children who have an injury to the cervical spine. *J Bone Joint Surg.* 1989;71A:15-22.

21. Emergency Nurses Association. Crisis intervention. In: *Emergency Nursing Pediatric Course (Instructor) Manual.* Park Ridge, Ill: Author; 1993:209-223.

22. American College of Surgeons Committee on Trauma. Head trauma. In: *Advanced Trauma Life Support Course® for Physicians (Student Manual).* 5th ed. Chicago, Ill: Author; 1993:159-183.

23. *The Prevention of Youth Violence: A Framework for Community Action.* Atlanta, Ga: Centers for Disease Control and Prevention; 1993. US Department of Health and Human Services, Public Health Service Centers for Disease Control and Prevention, National Center for Injury Prevention and Control, Office of the Assistant Director for Minority Health.

CHAPTER THIRTEEN

PSYCHOSOCIAL ASPECTS
OF TRAUMA CARE

OBJECTIVES

Upon completion of this chapter/lecture, the learner should be able to:

1. Define stress, crisis, grief, and attempted suicide.
2. Define three specific psychosocial needs of a trauma patient and family.
3. Discuss the psychosocial assessment of a trauma patient and/or family experiencing crisis, grief, and/or attempted suicide.
4. Based on assessment data, recall appropriate nursing diagnoses associated with patients experiencing crisis, grief, or an attempted suicide.
5. Plan appropriate interventions for a trauma patient and/or family experiencing crisis, grief, and/or attempted suicide.
6. Define a critical incident.
7. Discuss the assessment of trauma team members experiencing a reaction to a critical incident.
8. Plan appropriate interventions for trauma team members experiencing a reaction to a critical incident.

INTRODUCTION

Injury often happens without warning and usually changes the lives of the patient and family. "Family" defines an individual's support system and may include, but is not limited to, relatives, friends, and significant others. Usual coping methods employed on a daily basis frequently do not enable a person to handle the intense emotional, physical, social, and spiritual needs produced by a trauma event. Understanding the concepts of stress, crisis, and grief will assist the emergency nurse in caring for the trauma patient and family. A patient who attempts suicide requires care according to the trauma nursing process outlined in Chapter 3, Initial Assessment. Additional assessments and interventions focused on the psychosocial implications of the attempt requires consideration by the trauma team.

Stress

Stress is "the body's arousal response to any demand, change, or perceived threat. A stressor is the circumstance or event that elicits this response."[1] The definition of stress connotes "a relationship between a person and the environment that is appraised by the person as taxing or exceeding his or her resources and endangering his or her well-being."[2] Stress may contribute to health by providing an individual with a challenge for personal growth. Conversely, stress may be harmful when the response leads to functional problems. Whether a particular event or circumstance leads to stress depends on the individual's perception of the stressor.[3] The response to stress has been described biologically as a general adaptation syndrome with three stages: alarm reaction, resistance, and exhaustion.[3] Adaptation or the healthy response to stress prevents advancing to stage III.[4]

Crisis

Crisis is not synonymous with stress. A crisis is a state of disequilibrium that occurs when usual coping strategies are inadequate and immediate interventions are required. It is not the event(s) that constitutes the crisis, but how the person perceives the event(s). The person in crisis perceives a loss of control and feelings of helplessness, and is usually more vulnerable and open to assistance.

People who have experienced previous crises may be able to cope with less intervention, due to behaviors learned and used in the past. A crisis is also an opportunity to strengthen positive coping mechanisms.[5] Often through these experiences, new coping mechanisms are mastered. Crisis may occur at any time, depending on the perception of the event. Trauma patients and their families may experience crisis when usual methods of coping and problem-solving are unavailable or inadequate to resolve the situation. Other potential factors contributing to this crisis situation are the overwhelming stimuli of the event and the personal experiences and perceptions brought by each individual person. For example, some patients may be more concerned about loss of function, while others may be more concerned about their appearance.[6]

Crisis may occur:

- Immediately after the injury

    The patient may be concerned for his or her own life or the potential death of others involved in the incident. The lack of information or inappropriate perception of information may produce crisis.

326

- When usual methods of coping and problem-solving are unavailable or inadequate to resolve the situation

  This is of particular significance if the patient or family are from out-of-town, alone, or have no previous experience with such events.

- As time passes, pain and discomfort increase, and physical and mental energy are depleted

Additionally, crisis states tend to have the following characteristics:

- Response state can be nonspecific and varies from individual to individual

- May produce dangerous, self-destructive, or socially un-acceptable behaviors if not resolved

- Sudden onset – no warning for most trauma events

- Short-lived and self-limiting – a period of vulnerability is amen-able to interventions, and acute escalation of crisis can be prevented

- Opportunity to increase emotional strength when the crisis has been successfully resolved[5]

Grief

Grief is the physical, emotional, spiritual, cognitive, social, and behavioral response to loss. It is often precipitated by the death of someone close, but can be caused by loss of function or change in body image. Various theoretical models have proposed that the responses to loss include the following stages: grieving (shock, disbelief, anger, protest), mourning (depression, isolation, sadness, frustration), and bereavement (awareness and acceptance).[7] The final adaptation to loss is restitution, whereby the individual renews and invests in new relationships.[7] Although the stages appear to be sequential, few people pass through them in an orderly fashion. Grief reactions related to injury and loss are experienced not only by patients and families, but also by the trauma team members.

CONCEPTS OF PSYCHOSOCIAL NEEDS

The psychosocial needs of trauma patients and their families are centered around three concepts:

- Need for information

- Need for compassionate care

- Maintenance of hope

Providing accurate and understandable information to the patient and family in a timely and frequent manner is essential. When information is not provided, the patient and family may have inaccurate perceptions. The family will benefit from seeing the patient in the treatment environment as soon as possible.

Patients and families need to feel that care is being rendered in a compassionate manner. Touch, tone of voice, personal reference to the patient by name, words, and behaviors of the nurse contribute to this perception. In addition, some people attribute the nurse's presence, amount of information provided, and amount of time spent with the patient as indicators of care. Pain control is another indicator of caring. Families often feel a nurse who is gentle and caring with them will also exhibit similar behaviors to the patient.[8,9]

No matter how critical the situation, the patient and family need to maintain a sense of hope. Hope may be for recovery, for the individual as a spiritual and physical whole, or for an after-life. The nurse should allow the patient and/or family to realistically hold on to hope. It may be the only positive emotion they feel while listening to discouraging and frightening facts.[8,10]

NURSING CARE OF INDIVIDUALS EXPERIENCING CRISIS

Assessment

Refer to Chapter 3, Initial Assessment, for a description of general information that should be collected regarding every trauma victim. Only pertinent questions specific to psychosocial alterations are described below.

History

After physiologic stability is ensured, the following additional information should be obtained from the patient or family.

- What is their perception of the precipitating event or present situation?

  Ask the patient to recount the event and the present situation. Has anything else happened in the recent past to trigger this crisis? The injury may have been triggered by another event, e.g., recent job loss, change in marital status, quarrel, financial stress. Determine stressors or critical incidents that may have preceded the present situation or are currently present.

- Is there a concurrent maturational crisis, e.g., birth, marriage, separation, death, retirement?[5]

- What was their previous level of functioning and ability to problem-solve?

  Has anything like this ever happened before, and if so what happened? How did they react and handle the situation? Determine problem-solving or coping strategies usually used unsuccessfully or successfully in the past.

- Is there any recent, actual or perceived, loss or change in body appearance?

- Are there any persistent stressors, e.g., frequent injuries, chronic illness, change in job or family status?

Physical Assessment

Conduct a cursory mental status exam to initially rule out psychiatric disturbances. If the patient exhibits the need for definitive psychiatric care, especially after crisis intervention steps have been taken, obtain a psychiatric consult. Always rule out organic causes of psychologic disequilibrium.

- The physical signs often seen as an emotional response to trauma range from anxiety to withdrawal and include:

  - Talks fast, loudly, profanely

  - Paces, is demanding, restless

- Poor eye contact

- Is withdrawn, isolates self

- Denies obvious injury or emotions

- Is overly compliant or noncompliant with instructions

- Tachycardia, sweaty palms, dry mouth, and/or hyperventilation due to sympathetic nervous system activation

- Helplessness

  Cannot identify resources and solutions. Cannot state how to notify spouse, family, or friends about incident. May not be able to make necessary arrangements for transportation, child or elder care, if needed.

- Diminished ability to problem-solve, e.g., states "I don't know what to do about the baby sitter at home, the children, groceries in the car."

- Increased frustration, decreased coping and decision-making ability

  Says "I can't make these decisions, quit asking me."

- Expression of negative feelings about self

  Feels responsibility for negative things happening. Says "I can't do anything right."

- Self-destructive behavior

  This is a higher risk if the patient has a history of suicidal behavior or recent suicidal thoughts.

- Positive findings for a patient with ongoing ineffective coping include:

  - Lack of concern about appearance

    Lack of concern about appearance, removal of dried blood, dirt from uninjured parts of body, or need for privacy or modesty

- Behavior

  Altered mood or affect, flat affect, denies obvious pain, tense and rigid, compulsive, agitated, or restless after pain medications

- Garbled or irrational thought pattern

- Diminished impulse control, e.g., pulls out intravenous catheters, aggressive or assaultive behavior

- Self-destructive behavior

Nursing Diagnoses and Outcome Identification

The following nursing diagnoses are potential problems for the patient or family with a psychosocial alteration. Once a patient has been assessed, diagnoses can be defined as either actual or risk. An actual nursing diagnosis is one derived from a decision based on the patient's presenting signs and symptoms. A risk nursing diagnosis is a judgment the nurse makes based on a particular patient's risk and potential for developing certain problems.

| POSSIBLE NURSING DIAGNOSES AND EXPECTED OUTCOMES ||
Nursing Diagnosis	Expected Outcome
Family processes, altered related to: • Situational crisis secondary to patient's injury	The family unit will experience supportive family interactions as evidenced by: • Acknowledging the severity/extent of the injury • Engaging in open communication and mutual support with each other • Utilizing successful coping skills. Absence of prolonged despair, guilt, blame or hostility towards each other. • Verbalizing feelings to nurse and other members of the health care team • Participating in care of the trauma patient when possible • Accepting appropriate external resources

POSSIBLE NURSING DIAGNOSES AND EXPECTED OUTCOMES	
Nursing Diagnosis	**Expected Outcome**
Anxiety (patient, family) related to: • Situational crisis • Knowledge deficit • Actual or perceived threat of death	The patient/family will experience decreasing anxiety as evidenced by: • Questioning expected routines and treatments • Participating in decision-making and self-care whenever possible • Relating a decrease in anxiety • Absence in physiologic indicators of anxiety: increased heart rate, increased respiratory rate, increased arousal
Fear (patient, family) related to: • Actual or perceived threat of death • Separation from support systems • Unfamiliar environment • Invasive procedures and therapeutic treatments	The patient/family will experience decreasing fear as evidenced by: • Absence of fear-related behavior, e.g., crying, shouting, agitated behavior, noncommunicative behavior, blank stare. Facial expressions, voice tone, and body posture within normal for patient (family). • Acknowledging fear and stating decreasing fear • Absence of physiologic indicators of fear, e.g., palpitations, increased blood pressure, diaphoresis, tachycardia
Grieving related to: • Actual or anticipated losses associated with recent injury (patient, family) • Actual or potential loss of significant other (family)	The patient and/or family will begin the grieving process as evidenced by: • Expressing signs of the grieving process • Participating in decision-making • Recognizing reasons for feelings • Sharing feelings of grief with significant other(s)
Body image disturbance related to: • Perceived negative effects of changed appearance, loss of body functions(s), role performance	The patient will have minimal disturbance in body image as evidenced by: • Willingness to discuss limitation, deformity, or disfigurement • Willingness to participate in care • Realistic appraisal of situation

POSSIBLE NURSING DIAGNOSES AND EXPECTED OUTCOMES	
Nursing Diagnosis	**Expected Outcome**
Violence, risk related to: • Fear and anxiety secondary to crisis event • Compromised neurologic function (head injury) • Concomitant substance abuse	The patient or family member will not be violent toward persons or objects as evidenced by: • Exhibiting behavior that demonstrates increased trust of health care providers • Verbally expressing feelings of frustration • Responding to limit setting interventions • Demonstrating control of behavior with assistance from others • Absence of indicators of aggressive behavior, e.g., clenched fists, pacing, shouting

Planning and Implementation

Refer to Chapter 3, Initial Assessment, for a description of the specific nursing interventions for patients with compromises to airway, breathing, and/or circulation.

Crisis intervention is immediate help for a person to re-establish equilibrium. It is short-term and focuses on solving immediate problems to restore the patient's previous level of functioning. The long-term goal is functional equilibrium higher than the precrisis level.[11]

- Encourage coping skills used successfully in the past but not being used now, e.g., allow individual to cry, use the phone to call for help, use healthy denial, and provide the opportunity to talk or remain quiet[5]

- Identify friends or relatives who can provide support[5]

- Encourage the patient to express feelings that may decrease tension, explore new coping mechanisms, and re-establish social interactions[5]

- Clarify any misconceptions the patient or family may perceive[5]

- Do not discourage expressions of anger[5]

- Actively listen and provide opportunities for verbalization and privacy

333

- Establish a trusting relationship

- Promote the patient's sense of self-esteem

- Give the patient as many choices as possible, e.g., what name to be called, choice of positioning, when to see family

- Structure the environment

  Set approximate time frames. Give patient instructions on how to comply with recommendations and what to report to nurse, e.g., increased level of pain.

- Explain procedures and diagnosis in clear and understandable language

  Give realistic information without taking away hope.

- Identify the most pressing psychosocial needs in collaboration with the patient

- Assist in establishing realistic short-term goals

  It may be necessary to frequently repeat information, explanations, and encouragement as the patient's attention span may be short and/or recollection of information may be limited.

- Assist the patient to establish an actual plan for coping or resolving the crisis[5]

  Reinforce strengths and previously used coping strategies.

- Facilitate implementation of the plan

  Give positive feedback for compliance with the plan.

Additional interventions for the family include:

- Notify the family

  If the family was present at the scene, the police may have already given them some information and transported them to the hospital. Generally, it is not appropriate to notify the family over the phone that the patient has expired unless the family has to travel a long distance. In this case, tell the family the exact time of death to decrease potential guilt they may feel for not being present.[10,12] If the family is notified by telephone:

334

- Verify the identity and relationship of the person being notified

- Provide clear, concise information, including a general description of the patient's condition, injuries, and hopeful findings, e.g., "He is able to move both arms and legs, patient is alert."

- Provide hospital name, address, phone number, and directions

- Obtain unknown patient information, e.g., allergies, immunization status, current medications, medical history. Providing this information might make the family feel more useful and alleviate some of the helplessness feelings.

- Before ending the conversation, ask if there are any questions and determine their understanding of the patient's condition. Confirm the name, address, and phone number. Provide directions to the hospital, and confirm their transportation plans to the hospital.[13]

When family arrives at the hospital:

- Have a health care team member meet the family

- Determine whether any family member wishes to be present in the resuscitation area, based on institutional protocols

- Take other family members to a private place

  - Identify each family member and their relationship to the patient, and then refer to patient and family by name.

  - Sit comfortably next to the closest relative and make eye contact. Touch may be appropriate. Speak in quiet soothing tones.

  - Introduce oneself and describe the role of other trauma team members

  - Determine what information is already known. Verify and provide an update on the patient's condition, including diagnostic and therapeutic interventions. Advise the family what the patient will look like when they enter the room.

335

- Allow periods of silence to allow the family time to grasp information that may be distressing

- Encourage the family to express their feelings; do not discourage crying

- Assure the family that someone is currently with the patient providing care

- Give the family a realistic time of when they can expect more information and from whom

- Ask if there are any more questions and answer them in short, clear, and factual answers

- Encourage the family to visit the patient when feasible

- Allow the family to touch and talk to the patient

- Identify potential coping skills. If family reports few coping skills, identify potential support systems, e.g., friends, clergy, journaling (recording reactions to specific experiences).

- Provide periodic updates regarding patient condition

- Encourage the family to seek periodic fresh air and rest breaks, nutrition, and hydration to help them focus and concentrate

- Continually assess maladaptive behaviors exhibited by the family

- Seek assistance from security personnel, if necessary, to provide a safe environment

NURSING CARE OF FAMILIES EXPERIENCING GRIEF

Physical Assessment

People who are grieving may exhibit a variety of reactions. Patient and family reactions should be supported and not thwarted. Usually these reactions help to begin the grieving process. The family's reactions may include[14]:

- Shock/disbelief

- Numbness

- Denial

- Anger

- Hostility

- Physical complaints

- Guilt

- Panic

Interventions

In addition to the interventions listed under the Planning and Implentation section of Crisis, the following are aimed at supporting the grieving process:

- Reinforce reality, e.g., use words such as dead, death, or has died. Avoid the use of the word expired.

- Be supportive and use silence immediately after notification of death to allow the family to react

- Avoid statements negating or minimizing their feelings and thoughts. Do not use statements such as "It was really for the best." Instead of offering solutions, simply say you are sorry.

- Do not reinforce denial

- Prepare the family for the condition of the room and the patient. It may not be necessary to totally clean the room before the family sees the patient.

- Allow the family to see the patient and suggest touching and holding

- Show acceptance of the body, even if severely injured

- Request organ or tissue donation when death is imminent, according to hospital policy

- Assist any family member who feels sick or faint, i.e., have a chair and ammonia inhalants available

- Provide the family with the opportunity to leave the emergency department

NURSING CARE OF INDIVIDUALS ATTEMPTING SUICIDE

In the United States, suicide accounts for close to 31,000 deaths each year. The highest incidence of suicide occurs in persons between 25 and 34 years of age. Seventy-three percent of all suicidal deaths occur in white males. In comparison to 1986, the suicide death rate has declined for every age group except for those persons over the age of 85.[15] In Australia, there are more deaths from suicide than motor vehicle crashes.

Suicide, the taking of one's own life, is at the end of a spectrum between hope and hopelessness. According to Rawlins, hope includes ". . . confidence, faith, inspiration, and determination. At the other end of the continuum is hopelessness, despair, helplessness, doubt, grief, apathy, sadness, depression, and suicide."[16] Suicidal actions include[17]:

- Suicidal ideation or thoughts about harming oneself

- Suicidal threat – when one verbalizes suicidal ideations

- Suicidal gesture – when one performs a certain act designated to cause self-injury but does not cause a life-threatening result

- Suicidal attempt – when one causes self-injury and expects the result to be death

Physical Assessment

For the patient who has attempted suicide, the first priority is completing an assessment according to those principles of the trauma nursing process outlined in Chapter 3, Initial Assessment. After any compromises to airway, breathing, and circulation have been corrected, or when the patient's suicidal attempt has not resulted in any physiological compromises, the patient requires a thorough assessment of his or her mental status. Depending on the resources available, the patient may be referred to a psychiatrist, mental health professional, or mental health clinical specialist. Determine the patient's suicidal risk:

- Does the patient have a chronic or terminal disease?

- Does the patient have a history of drug or alcohol abuse?

- Has the patient had previous suicide attempts or gestures?

- Does the patient have feelings of depression, despair, guilt, or hopelessness?

- Are the patient's thoughts disorganized?

- Is there a history of other mental health disorders, e.g., schizophrenia or bipolar disorder?

- Has there been a recent change or loss in the patient's life, e.g., death in the family, loss of a job, or relational disturbance?

- Is there a family history of suicide?

- Does the patient have feelings of inferiority, poor self-esteem, or inadequacy?

Nursing Diagnosis and Outcome Identification

The following nursing diagnoses are potential problems for the patient who has attempted suicide. Once a patient has been assessed, diagnoses can be defined as either actual or risk. An actual nursing diagnosis is one derived from a decision based on the patient's presenting signs and symptoms. A risk nursing diagnosis is a judgment the nurse makes based on a particular patient's risk and potential for developing certain problems.

POSSIBLE NURSING DIAGNOSIS AND EXPECTED OUTCOMES	
Nursing Diagnosis	**Expected Outcomes**
Violence, self-directed related to: • Threats of suicide • Suicidal gestures • Inability to problem solve • Inability to control negative behavior	The patient will not be violent towards self as evidenced by: • Stating no thoughts of harm • Stating has a will to live • Demonstrating coping skills

Planning and Implementation

Refer to Chapter 3, Initial Assessment, for a description of the specific nursing interventions for patients with compromises to airway, breathing and/or circulation.

- Assign a trauma team member to maintain close observation of the patient at all times

- Keep the patient in an environment where there are no items or equipment that could potentially produce self-harm, e.g., knives, glass objects, windows. Inspect the patient's personal items and clothing.

- Engage the patient in expression of thoughts and feelings related to the suicidal gesture or attempt

- Promote hope and discourage hopelessness

- Ensure your own safety if a patient attempts further harm while in the emergency department

- Refer the patient to appropriate mental health resources

NURSING CARE OF TRAUMA TEAM MEMBERS

A critical incident is any situation experienced by trauma team members causing them to feel unusually strong emotional reactions that have the potential to interfere with their ability to function. Some common examples of critical incidents that may trigger these reactions are[18]:

- Any event with significant emotional power to overwhelm usual coping mechanisms

- Death of a child or a child injured by malicious or careless adults

- Victims who are relatives or friends of the trauma team member

- Events that threaten the safety or life of trauma team members

- Events that attract excessive media attention

- Incidents with unusual circumstances and/or distressing sights, sounds, or smells

- Mass casualty situations

The trauma team members may also need help in identifying potential coping skills during or after caring for trauma patients. Ongoing peer support and understanding, along with the opportunity to discuss difficult situations, are effective coping skills. If the situation has been a critical incident for the nurse, intervention from a critical incident stress management (CISM) team may by helpful. The CISM team consists of mental health professionals and peer support personnel. The major purposes of the CISM team are to:

- Prepare the staff to manage their job-related stress

- Provide assistance for those staff who are experiencing the negative effects of stress

- Provide education and prevention programs

Physical Assessment

Critical incidents may produce a characteristic set of physical, cognitive, emotional, and behavioral symptoms.[18] Reactions to a critical incident may appear immediately, within a few hours, within days, several weeks, or months later. Reactions may last an indefinite period of time. These reactions reflect a normal reaction to an abnormal event (see Table 27).

Table 27

SIGNS AND SYMPTOMS OF STRESS	
Physical	**Cognitive**

• Fatigue
• Nausea
• Muscle tremors
• Twitching
• Chest pain
• Dyspnea
• Elevated blood pressure
• Tachycardia
• Thirst
• Headaches
• Visual difficulties
• Dizziness
	• Confusion
	• Intrusive images
	• Nightmares
	• Cognitive deficits in:
	  ■ Decision-making
	  ■ Concentration
	  ■ Memory
	  ■ Problem-solving
	  ■ Abstract thinking

Emotional	**Behavioral**
• Anxiety • Guilt • Grief • Denial • Fear • Uncertainty • Loss of emotional control • Depression • Apprehension • Intense anger • Irritability • Agitation	• Withdrawal • Emotional outbursts • Suspiciousness • Alcohol consumption • Inability to rest • Pacing • Nonspecific bodily complaints • Change in sexual functioning • Changes in activity and speech

Interventions

Critical Incident Stress Management (CISM) may include utilization of defusing or debriefing techniques. Defusings are gatherings after a stressful situation and are primarily informational.[19] They provide an opportunity to discuss the impact of a difficult event. Defusings are much shorter, less formal and less structured than debriefings. They allow for ventilation of feelings regarding the incident.[19]

Debriefings provide an early opportunity (within 24 to 72 hours of the incident) for the nurse to be a part of an organized debriefing group that will deal with these stress responses. The goal is to provide an opportunity for trauma team members to effectively deal with their intense emotions in a supportive environment, thus enabling them to return to a productive level of functioning. Debriefings provide staff with time to express anger, frustrations, and grief, thereby facilitating closure of incident.[19] The following are debriefing interventions:

- Promote the ventilation of feelings

- Provide support and reassurance

- Mobilize resources. Additional support may be required after a debriefing.[18]

- Do not criticize anyone's performance

- Conduct the debriefing with specially trained facilitators

There are seven steps in a debriefing[19]:

- Initial phase: the people in attendance are introduced and the rules of debriefing are discussed. Only those involved in the event are allowed to attend. Issues discussed are considered confidential.

- Fact phase: each individual involved discusses his or her role in the event and describes what was seen, done, heard, and smelled.

- Thought phase: persons willing to speak are asked to share what they felt during the incident and how they personalized the experience.

- Reaction phase: participants describe their reactions to the worst part of the incident and how they reacted. This allows a safe environment to discuss the psychologic and physiologic effects of the incident.

- Symptom phase: the participants discuss any reactions to stress they have experienced since the incident. Mental health professionals determine the need for additional help for any of the group members.

- Teaching phase: team members talk about stress management strategies and methods to support one another during a crisis.

- Re-entry phase: the group is given an opportunity to ask any additional questions. The events of the crisis are summarized, and referrals are made for additional help, if needed.

SUMMARY

The psychosocial aspects of trauma include but are not limited to stress, grief, and crisis. Sustaining an injury is a stressor not only to the patient but also for family and/or significant persons related to the patient. Whether a particular event or circumstance leads to stress depends on the individual's perception of the stressor. Only in rare circumstances would a patient not perceive any degree of trauma as a stressor. Adaptation is the healthy response to stress.

Relating to families of trauma victims poses additional responsibilities for the trauma nurse. Conduct in-person or telephone communication in a manner that recognizes the patient's and family's needs for accurate and understandable information, compassion, care, and hope.

Interventions to reduce the effects of a crisis are aimed at restoring one's previous level of function and, in the long term, may also enhance functional equilibrium to a level higher than the precrisis level.

Trauma team members may perceive certain environmental events or circumstances as stressors. CISM, which includes debriefing, is a method to assist trauma team members in coping with the effects of stress and/or crisis.

343

REFERENCES

1. Landrum PA, Beck K, Rawlins RP, Williams SR. The person as a client. In: Rawlins RP, Williams SR, Beck K, eds. *Mental Health – Psychiatric Nursing A Holistic Life-Cycle Approach.* 3rd ed. St. Louis, Mo: Mosby-Year Book; 1993:31.

2. Townsend MC. An introduction to the concept of stress. In: Townsend MC. *Psychiatric/Mental Health Nursing: Concepts of Care.* Philadelphia, Pa: FA Davis; 1993:10.

3. Selye H. *The Stress of Life.* 2nd ed. New York, NY: McGraw-Hill; 1978.

4. Townsend MC. An introduction to the concept of stress. In: Townsend MC. *Psychiatric/Mental Health Nursing: Concepts of Care.* Philadelphia, Pa: FA Davis; 1993:4.

5. Aguilera DC. *Crisis Intervention Theory and Methodology.* St. Louis, Mo: CV Mosby Co; 1990.

6. Lenahan GP. Emotional impact of trauma. *Nurs Clin North Am.* 1986;21:729-740.

7. Newman AM. Loss. In: Rawlins RP, Williams SR, Beck K, eds. *Mental Health – Psychiatric Nursing A Holistic Life-Cycle Approach.* 3rd ed. St. Louis, Mo: Mosby-Year Book; 1993:239-256.

8. Belinger JE. Coping tasks in critical care. *Dimen of Crit Care Nurs.* 1983;2:80-88.

9. Brown L. The experience of care: patient perspectives. *Topics in Clin Nurs.* 1986;8:56-62.

10. Hickey M. What are the needs of families of critically ill patients? *Focus on Crit Care.* 1985;12:41-43.

11. Williams SR. Crisis intervention. In: Rawlins RP, Williams SR, Beck K, eds. *Mental Health – Psychiatric Nursing A Holistic Life-Cycle Approach.* 3rd ed. St. Louis, Mo: Mosby-Year Book; 1993:542-560.

12. McLaughlan C. Handling distressed relatives and breaking bad news. *Br Med J.* 1990;301:1145-1150.

13. Robinson MA. Telephone notification of relatives of emergency and critical care patients. *Ann Emerg Med.* 1982;11:616-618.

14. McFarland G, McFarlane E. *Nursing Diagnosis and Interventions; Planning Patient Care*. 2nd ed. St. Louis, Mo: Mosby-Year Book; 1993.

15. Advance report of final mortality statistics, 1992. *Monthly Vital Statistics Report*. National Center for Health Statistics. Hyattsville, Md: 1994;43:1-36.

16. Rawlins RP. Hope-hopelessness. In: Rawlins RP, Williams SR, Beck K, eds. *Mental Health – Psychiatric Nursing A Holistic Life-Cycle Approach*. 3rd ed. St. Louis, Mo: Mosby-Year Book; 1993:257-284.

17. Badger JM. Reaching out to the suicidal patient. *AJN*. 1995;95:24-32.

18. Mitchell JT, Bray GP. *Emergency Services Stress*. Englewood Cliffs, NJ: RJ Brady/Prentice Hall; 1990.

19. Emergency Nurses Association. Crisis intervention. In: *Emergency Nursing Pediatric Course (Instructor) Manual*. Park Ridge, Ill: Author; 1993:209-223.

CHAPTER FOURTEEN

STABILIZATION, TRANSFER, AND TRANSPORT

OBJECTIVES

Upon completion of the chapter/lecture, the learner should be able to:

1. Describe the trauma system components related to the stabilization and transfer of critical trauma patients.
2. Identify indications for transfer of trauma patients to a designated or verified trauma center.
3. Discuss the specific interventions to stabilize trauma patients prior to transfer.
4. Explain the precautions to be observed during intrahospital transport of trauma patients.

INTRODUCTION

Research done in the late 1970s and the early 1980s reported that survival is improved if severely injured patients are cared for in trauma facilities with dedicated resources and staff to meet their special needs.[1-3] More recent studies continue to support this concept.[4,5] In Canada, researchers reported a 38% reduction in the odds of dying when treated at a Level I Trauma Center.[6] They also reported a statistically significant trend towards lower mortality when a higher level of trauma care was rendered in the receiving facility.[7] Early resuscitation and transfer are critical factors in reducing morbidity and mortality.[8] The American College of Surgeons, Committee on Trauma (ACS-COT) recommends that "no longer should the trauma patient be transferred to the closest hospital, but rather to the closest appropriate hospital, preferably a designated trauma center."[9]

To evaluate whether a facility has the necessary resources to care for a trauma patient, consider not only those resources for initial care, but also those needed for subsequent hospitalization. If the initial receiving hospital does not have the necessary resources, or it takes a significant amount of time to mobilize them, resuscitate, stabilize, and consider transfer to a more comprehensive facility.

UNITED STATES (For presentation in the US only)

Federal Transfer Law

Legally there is an obligation to transfer a patient following emergency stabilization if the facility cannot provide adequate definitive care.[10] Never consider the financial status of the patient when providing initial care or withholding transfer to another facility. Federal legislation, mandated through the Consolidated Omnibus Budget Reconciliation Act of 1986 (COBRA), regulates the safe and appropriate transfer of patients between hospitals[11] (see Table 28).

Table 28

COBRA REQUIREMENTS	
A patient with an emergency medical condition* must be either stabilized or transferred to another facility if:	
Receiving Facility	**Transferring Facility**
• Has available bed • Has qualified personnel • Has agreed to accept patient	• Provides copy of medical records • Arranges transfer to occur with qualified personnel and life support equipment

* An emergency medical condition exists, if lack of medical attention:
  • Poses a serious threat to the patient's health
  • Threatens impairment of bodily functions, or
  • Threatens function of body organs or part	

(Adapted with permission from: Southard PA. COBRA legislation: complying with ED provisions. *JEN.* 1989;15:23-25.)

One section of the COBRA legislation is the Emergency Medical Treatment and Active Labor Act (EMTALA). Hospitals that are Medicare-participating facilities are required to provide medical screening for any person who comes to the emergency department. Once an emergency medical condition has been determined, the patient must be stabilized. There are two circumstances under which an unstabilized patient may be transferred:

- The patient requests a transfer

- The physician documents that the benefit of transferring the patient outweighs the risk of not transferring

More detailed requirements under EMTALA are available in the June 22, 1994 issue of the Federal Register.

If it is determined that the patient would benefit from transfer to a facility with more comprehensive resources, the following four requirements must be met prior to transfer:

- A physician at the receiving facility must accept the patient

- The receiving facility must be appropriate with qualified personnel to accept the patient

- The interhospital transport team and transport mode must be appropriate for the patient's condition

- All relevent medical records must accompany the patient to the receiving facility

TRAUMA SYSTEMS

A systematic and organized approach to trauma care has proven effective in decreasing death and disability due to injury.[13,14] Established plans and protocols that ensure rapid access to care by personnel with expertise in trauma care, at facilities with dedicated resources, help to protect the public from premature death and disability.[15] A trauma system addresses the continuum of care from injury prevention, to acute care, through rehabilitation and reintegration into society.[16] Different states and countries may utilize trauma system guidelines developed by the ACS-COT or by other national and statewide agencies.

The ACS-COT has defined a trauma system as one consisting of four groups of providers. They are involved in system management, prehospital care, acute care facilities, and rehabilitation services. The components of a comprehensive trauma system are:

- Medical direction

- Prevention

- Communication

- Training

- Triage

- Prehospital care

- Transportation

- Hospital care

- Public education

- Rehabilitation

- Medical evaluation

The development and legislation of a comprehensive trauma system is a major challenge for the community. To legislate trauma systems, public support and clinical expertise from health professionals are required.[15] A model plan is available, as well as federal funds, to aid states in planning and implementing trauma systems.[17] This is usually the responsibility of state EMS agencies. Unfortunately, only 25% of the states in the US have a trauma system.[4]

Levels of Trauma Centers

Trauma centers are distinguished from other hospitals by a strong commitment to provide 24-hour availability of dedicated resources for trauma care. Nurses, physicians, and ancillary personnel with specialized knowledge in trauma care must be immediately available. Hospital resources such as surgical services, critical care units, and diagnostic services must also be readily available.[15]

The ACS-COT identifies four levels of trauma facilities[15] (see Table 29).

Table 29

SELECTED CHARACTERISTICS OF TRAUMA CENTER FACILITIES				
	LEVEL			
	I	**II**	**III**	**IV**
• Trauma service	E	E	E	–
• Trauma Director	E	E	E	–
• In-house 24-hour surgeon availability	E	E	E	D
• Multi-specialties	E	E	L	–
• Emergency resuscitation equipment for all ages	E	E	E	E
• Operative suite in-house staff 24 hours\day	E	E	D	–
• Comprehensive diagnostic and rehabilitation services	E	E	L	L
• Cardiopulmonary bypass capability	E	E	–	–
• Quality improvement program	E	E	E	E
• Prevention/public education	E	D	–	–
• Trauma research program	E	D	–	–
• Outreach program	E	E	–	–
• Dedicated Trauma Coordinator	E	E	D	D
E = Essential; D = Desirable; L = Limited; – = Not Required				

(Adapted with permission from: American College of Surgeons Committee on Trauma. Hospital criteria. In: *Resources for Optimal Care of the Injured Patient: 1993*. Chicago, Ill: Author; 1993:29-34.)

INTERFACILITY TRANSFER

Indications for Transfer

The American College of Surgeons-Committee on Trauma (ACS-COT) has guidelines to identify those patients to be considered for early transfer[18] (see Table 30). These criteria are based on specific injuries that should prompt the trauma team to consider transfer to a facility with comprehensive resources.

Table 30

HIGH-RISK CRITERIA FOR CONSIDERATION OF EARLY TRANSFER
(These guidelines are not intended to be hospital-specific)

CENTRAL NERVOUS SYSTEM
  • Head injury
    ■ Penetrating injury or open fracture (with or without cerebrospinal fluid leak)
    ■ Depressed skull fracture
    ■ Glasgow Coma Scale (GCS) Score less than 14 or GCS deterioration
    ■ Lateralizing signs
  • Spinal cord injury
    ■ Spinal column injury

CHEST
  • Major chest wall injury
  • Wide mediastinum or other signs suggesting great vessel injury
  • Cardiac injury
  • Patients who may require prolonged ventilation

PELVIS
  • Unstable pelvic ring disruption
  • Unstable pelvic fracture with shock or other evidence of continuing hemorrhage
  • Open pelvic injury

MAJOR EXTREMITY INJURIES
  • Fracture/dislocation with loss of distal pulses
  • Open long-bone fractures
  • Extremity ischemia

MULTIPLE-SYSTEM INJURY
  • Head injury combined with face, chest, abdominal, or pelvic injury
  • Burns with associated injuries
  • Multiple long-bone fractures
  • Injury to more than two body regions

HIGH-RISK CRITERIA FOR CONSIDERATION OF EARLY TRANSFER
COMORBID FACTORS • Age >55 years • Children • Cardiac or respiratory disease • Insulin-dependent diabetics, morbid obesity • Pregnancy • Immunosuppression
SECONDARY DETERIORATION (LATE SEQUELAE) • Mechanical ventilation required • Sepsis • Single or multiple organ system failure (deterioration in central nervous, cardiac, pulmonary, hepatic, renal, or coagulation systems) • Major tissue necrosis

(Reprinted with permission from: American College of Surgeons Committee on Trauma. Interhospital transfer. In: *Resources for Optimal Care of the Injured Patient:* 1993. Chicago, Ill: Author; 1993:71.)

Protocols and Procedures

Interfacility transfer of trauma patients involves both administrative and clinical aspects. Policies, procedures, protocols, and interfacility transfer agreements must be in place and operational prior to the need for transfer. The decision to transfer and preparation for transfer, occur simultaneously during patient stabilization.

Protocols and procedures include:

• The criteria to identify those patients who should be transferred

• Identification of the medical authority responsible for the transfer

• Identification of facilities with specific clinical resources, e.g., burn centers, pediatric trauma centers

• Type of available transport services

• Necessary personnel and equipment to accompany the patient

• Clinical protocols and/or standing orders for transport

• Steps to arrange transfer

• Guidelines to include the family and significant others in the transfer process

- Transfer forms and required documentation

- Identification of medical reports and clinical records that should accompany the patient

- Recommendations for handling special situations during the transport, e.g., vehicle breakdown, long detours, patient deterioration or death

Transfer Agreements

Written transfer agreements facilitate effective communication, establish treatment protocols, and define a patient follow-up process. Transfer agreements are established between transferring and receiving facilities. Transfer agreements that outline specific treatment and transfer protocols are suggested for the following clinical categories:

- Burns

- Head injuries

- Spinal cord and vertebral column injuries

- Multiple system trauma

- Limb and digit amputations

- Children, pregnant women, elderly patients, or patients with pre-existing disease (cardiac, pulmonary or other chronic disease)

Transferring Hospital

The transferring hospital is responsible for performing those treatment and diagnostic studies requested by the receiving facility. The physician in the transferring facility is responsible for activating the transfer process by first obtaining approval from a physician willing to accept the patient at the receiving facility.[9] The transferring facility is responsible for assuring the appropriate personnel and equipment are available to maintain care en route.

The transferring and receiving facility must make a collaborative decision regarding the most appropriate transport service. When choosing between ground and air transport, consider the following factors:

- Equipment availability

- Workspace

- Qualifications of transport personnel

- Weather and road conditions or obstacles

- Patient's response to mode of transport

Ground ambulances, because of their increased availability, are the most commonly used interhospital transport service. Basic life support (BLS) ambulances are typically not equipped for the complex care necessary for the severely injured trauma patient. Advanced life support (ALS) ambulances are staffed by personnel trained to perform more definitive care, such as endotracheal intubation, intravenous therapy, and drug administration. The transferring facility must send appropriate personnel with equipment to provide the patient with advanced life support, if a BLS ambulance is used.

Two types of aircraft are used for air transport: helicopters and fixed-wing planes. Flight teams are composed of some combination of a nurse, physician, respiratory therapist, and/or paramedic. Helicopters can be used in most communities without a significant delay in overall transfer time. Fixed-wing aircraft may be utilized for transfer of the trauma patient when the transport distances exceed the fuel and distance range of a helicopter (usually transport greater than 150 miles).[19]

NURSING INTERVENTIONS PRIOR TO INTERFACILITY TRANSFER

Refer to Chapter 3, Initial Assessment, for a description of the assessment and interventions for airway, breathing, and circulation.

- Secure a patent airway

- Immobilize the vertebral column

  It is safer to transport the trauma patient with full spinal immobilization.

- Ensure adequate breathing

  - Have a bag-valve-mask or portable ventilator available. Ensure there is an adequate supply of supplemental oxygen available in the transport vehicle.

  - Assist with chest tube insertion prior to transport, as indicated

    Connect the chest tube to a chest drainage system or Heimlich valve. Avoid chest drainage systems that use glass bottles. Ensure an additional suction device is available in the transport vehicle.

  - Attach a pulse oximeter

- Ensure adequate circulation

  - Use plastic intravenous fluid bags

  - Ensure additional intravenous fluids are available in the transport vehicle

  - Connect extension sets to intravenous tubing to allow more flexibility during patient movement

  - Consider positioning an uninflated PASG under the patient. Inflate if indicated

- Insert indwelling urinary catheter and attach to a closed urinary drainage system

- Insert a gastric tube

- Administer methylprednisolone to suspected spinal cord injured patient, as prescribed

- Splint suspected fractures

  Do not use air splints.

- Cover wounds with sterile dressings

- Do not suture superficial lacerations

- Cover large burns with a dry sterile sheet. Follow wound care as described in Chapter 10, Burn Trauma.

- Administer tetanus and antibiotic prophylaxis, as prescribed

- Administer analgesic and antianxiety medications, as prescribed

- Obtain those radiographic and laboratory studies outlined in Chapter 3, Initial Assessment, as time permits

- Prepare copies of medical records, results of diagnostic studies, and x-rays[11]

- Obtain consent for transfer

  After discussing the need for transfer with the patient and family, obtain consent for the transfer. Use clear and simple explanations to describe the need to transfer, as well as the risks.

- Complete a transfer checklist, according to institutional protocol

- Explain to the patient special circumstances surrounding the transfer, e.g., use of a helicopter

- Call the receiving facility and give a brief report

- Allow the family to see the patient

  If the patient's prognosis is poor, it may be the last time the family will see the patient alive.

- Suggest that the family stay at the initial hospital until the patient has left

- Provide written directions or maps to the receiving facility

  Reinforce the need for family and others to observe all traffic laws. Caution the family not to attempt to follow the ambulance.

- Provide psychosocial support to the patient and family

NURSING INTERVENTIONS DURING INTERFACILITY TRANSFER

- Monitor vital signs

  Normal assessment techniques, such as auscultation, may be difficult due to noise and vibration levels.

- Assign a designated person to direct the movement of the patient into the transport vehicle

- Maintain airway and ventilatory support

- Administer supplemental oxygen

- Maintain circulation

- Monitor any air or fluid-filled devices, e.g., PASG

- Adhere to clinical protocols, as indicated

- Communicate the patient's status to the receiving facility

- Document all assessments, interventions, and patient responses

INTRAFACILITY TRANSPORT

Transport of the trauma patient out of the emergency department is inevitable. Intrafacility transport of trauma patients may occur between the following treatment areas:

- Radiology/special procedures department

- Operating suite

- Critical care unit

- Stepdown unit

- Medical/surgical unit

Several factors place the patient at risk for instability during intra-hospital transport[20]:

- Inadequate airway maintenance

- Dysrhythmias

- Physiologic instability

- Rapid, rough, or disorganized transport

- Inadequate monitoring or reassessment

- Long distances between treatment areas

- Discontinuance of the effects of sedation or anesthesia

- Patient position

Written policies and procedures usually outline the qualifications of personnel accompanying the patient during intrahospital transport, the minimal equipment needed for transport, communication protocols, and monitoring guidelines.[21]

Select the type of personnel to conduct the transport based on the patient's clinical status, distance, and destination. A registered professional nurse, with trauma care knowledge and skills, is an appropriate person to accompany all actual and potentially unstable patients during the transport.

Recommended nursing interventions to increase safety prior to intrahospital transport include[22]:

- Suction airway and endotracheal tube, as indicated

- Maintain ventilation

- Assess neurologic status

- Explain the logistics of the transport to the patient and family

- Give a report regarding the patient to the receiving nurse to include:

  - Mechanism of injury

  - Prehospital history

- Patient assessment and interventions

- Results of diagnostic procedures

- Vital signs

- Planned interventions or procedures

SUMMARY

Stabilization, Transfer, and Transport

The majority of trauma victims (80%) are not critically injured. However, approximately 15% of all trauma victims are seriously injured, with another 5% being critically injured. Trauma systems that coordinate prehospital and hospital services into an integrated regional program for the optimal care of the more critically and seriously injured victims, have proven to be effective in reducing mortality and morbidity.

Staff in any hospital that receives a trauma victim must decide whether to stabilize and admit the patient, or stabilize and transfer the patient to a facility with more comprehensive resources. Once a decision is made to transfer a patient, the administrative policies, procedures, and protocols to facilitate the transfer must be activated. Resuscitation and stabilization of the patient is carried on simultaneously with implementing the transfer.

Predetermined protocols, written transfer agreements with tertiary facilities, and advance identification of qualified personnel for interfacility transfers will enhance the transfer process once it is initiated by the transferring physician. Intrafacility transfers require adherence to standards of care previously identified by institutional protocols and procedures.

REFERENCES

1. Cales RH. Trauma mortality in Orange County: the effect of implementation of a regional trauma system. *Ann Emerg Med.* 1984;13:1-10.

2. West JG, Trunkey D, Lim RC. Systems of trauma care: a study of two counties. *Arch Surg.* 1979;114:455-459.

3. West JG, Cales RH, Gazzaniga AB. Impact of regionalization: the Orange County experience. *Arch Surg.* 1983;118:740-744.

4. Eastman AB. Blood in our streets: the status and evolution of trauma care systems. *Arch Surg.* 1992;127:677-681.

5. Champion HR, Sacco WS, Copes WS. Improvement in outcome from trauma center care. *Arch Surg.* 1992;127:333-338.

6. Sampalis JS, Lavoie A, Williams J, Mulder D, Kalina M. Impact of on-site care, prehospital time, and level of in-hospital care on survival in severely injured patients. *J Trauma.* 1993;34:252-261.

7. Sampalis JS, Lavoie A, Williams J, Mulder D, Kalina M. Standardized mortality ratio analysis on a sample of severely injured patients from a large Canadian city without regionalized trauma care. *J Trauma.* 1992;33:205-212.

8. Hicks TC, Danzl DF, Thomas DM, Flint LM. Resuscitation and treatment of trauma patients: a prospective study. *Ann Emerg Med.* 1982;11:269-299.

9. American College of Surgeons Committee on Trauma. Stabilization and transport. In: *Advanced Trauma Life Support® Course for Physicians (Student Manual).* 5th ed. Chicago, Ill: Author; 1993:293-304.

10. Frew SA. *Patient Transfers: How to Comply with the Law.* Dallas, Tex: American College of Emergency Physicians; 1991.

11. Southard P. COBRA legislation: complying with ED provisions. *JEN.* 1989;15:23-25.

12. Department of Health and Human Services. Health care financing administration interim final rule. *Federal register.* 1994;59:32086.

13. Mullins RJ, Veum-Stone J, Helgfand M, et al. Outcome of hospitalized injured patients after institution of a trauma system in an urban area. *JAMA*. 1994;271:1919-1924.

14. Kane G, Wheeler N, Cook S, Englehardt R, Pavey B, Green K, Clark O, Cassou J. Impact of the Los Angeles County trauma system on the survival of seriously injured patients. *J Trauma*. 1992;32:576-583.

15. American College of Surgeons Committee on Trauma. The trauma care system. In: *Resources for Optimal Care of the Injured Patient: 1993*. Chicago, Ill: Author; 1993:7-12.

16. Esposito TJ, Nania J, Maier RV. State trauma system evaluation: a unique and comprehensive approach. *Ann Emerg Med*. 1992;21:351-357.

17. *Model trauma care system plan*. Rockville, Md: US Department of Health and Human Services, Public Health Service, Health Resources and Services Administration; September 30, 1992.

18. American College of Surgeons Committee on Trauma. Interhospital transfer. In: *Resources for Optimal Care of the Injured Patient: 1993*. Chicago, Ill: Author; 1993:69-72.

19. Association of Air Medical Services. Appropriate use of emergency air medical services. *J Air Med Transport*. 1990;9:29-37. Position paper.

20. Gavin-Fought S, Nemeth L. Intrahospital transport: a framework for assessment. *Crit Care Nurs Q*. 1992;15:87-90.

21. Guidelines Committee, American College of Critical Care Medicine, Society of Critical Care Medicine and the Transfer Guidelines Task Force, American Association of Critical Care Nurses. Guidelines for the transfer of critically ill patients. *Am J Crit Care*. 1993;2:189-195.

22. Tice P. Intrahospital transport of critically ill adults: potential physiologic changes and nursing implications. *Focus Crit Care*. 1991;18:424-428.

CHAPTER FIFTEEN

DEMONSTRATION OF THE TRAUMA NURSING PROCESS STATION

OBJECTIVES

Upon completion of this demonstration, the learner should be able to:

1. Demonstrate a primary assessment.
2. Identify life-threatening conditions recognized during the primary assessment.
3. Identify the interventions to manage life-threatening conditions recognized during the initial assessment.
4. Demonstrate a secondary assessment.
5. Based on data from the secondary assessment, identify appropriate diagnostic studies and interventions.

INTRODUCTION

The phases of the Trauma Nursing Process are integrated into a scenario-driven psychomotor skill station in the *Trauma Nursing Core Course*.

Assessment, diagnosis, outcome identification, planning, and implementation are the first five steps in the nursing process. Evaluation, the last step, is an ongoing process once the patient arrives in the emergency department.

During actual patient care, all personnel who anticipate direct patient contact or contact with the patient's body fluids must wear personal protective equipment. (NOTE: Since TNCC skill stations are simulated situations, the use of personal protective equipment is optional.)

Assessment

Primary Assessment

All elements assessed during the primary assessment are of such a critical nature, that major deviations from normal require immediate intervention. Do not proceed until all major life-threatening conditions have been treated. The primary assessment addresses airway (A), breathing (B), circulation (C), and disability or neurologic status (D).

Secondary Assessment

The secondary assessment is completed after the primary assessment. It includes E - I as described in Table 31. The focus of the secondary assessment is to identify ALL injuries, in order to determine the priorities for the planning and implementation phases of the nursing process.

Table 31

TRAUMA ASSESSMENT MNEMONIC
A = Airway and cervical spine stabilization
B = Breathing
C = Circulation
D = Disability (neurologic status)
E = Expose patient
F = Fahrenheit – Keep patient warm
G = Get vital signs
H = History/Head-to-toe examination
I = Inspect posterior surfaces

During the Trauma Nursing Process skill station learners should state they would obtain additional information from prehospital providers, patient-generated information, and past medical history, if available. The learner must demonstrate and describe the head-to-toe assessment by describing appropriate inspection techniques, (e.g., noting lacerations, abrasions, contusions, ecchymosis, etc.), demonstrating appropriate palpation techniques, and demonstrating appropriate auscultation techniques.

Nursing Diagnoses, Outcome Identification, Planning, and Implementation

The severity of the patient's condition may require simultaneous assessment, diagnosis, and intervention. Appropriate nursing diagnoses are based on assessment findings. Specific patient outcomes are then identified, and a plan is developed to achieve them. For the purposes of this station, the learner will **NOT** be asked to identify nursing diagnoses or outcomes. The priorities for intervention will depend on the complexity of the patient's injuries, and the availability and qualifications of the emergency department staff and/or trauma nurse. Priority is given to those injuries that have the greatest potential to compromise airway, breathing, circulation, and/or disability.

Ongoing Evaluation

Evaluate the patient's responses to any interventions to determine the need for further interventions. Evaluate the effectiveness of any intervention expected to have an immediate effect on the patient. Any abnormalities identified in the primary assessment, and the vital signs must be re-evaluated at the completion of the secondary assessment.

DEMONSTRATION

Two instructors will demonstrate through role-play, how to perform a trauma nursing assessment, and will identify examples of interventions for each step of the assessment. During the skill station rotation, learners will have the opportunity to practice these skills based on specific case scenarios. For further explanation of specific assessments and interventions, refer to each clinical chapter in the manual. The following tables serve as guidelines to conduct the assessment and identify appropriate interventions (see Tables 32 to 34).

During the learner's evaluation in the Trauma Nursing Process stations the learner will be asked to identify five additional diagnostic studies and/or interventions based on the case scenario. Be specific with regards to the radiographic studies.

Evaluate the effectiveness of those interventions that are expected to have an immediate effect on the patient, e.g., auscultation of breath sounds after intubation. Re-evaluate all primary assessment interventions and vital signs at the completion of the secondary assessment.

Table 32

PRIMARY ASSESSMENT	
Assessments	**Interventions**
A = Airway And Cervical Spine Stabilization	
While maintaining spinal stabilization: ● Vocalization ● Tongue obstruction ● Loose teeth or foreign objects ● Bleeding ● Vomitus or other secretions ● Edema	● Position the patient ● Jaw thrust or chin lift ● Suction or remove foreign objects ● Oro/nasopharyngeal airway ● Cervical spine stabilization ● Endotracheal intubation ● Needle or surgical cricothyroidotomy
B = Breathing	
● Spontaneous breathing ● Chest rise and fall ● Skin color ● General rate and depth of respirations ● Soft tissue and bony chest wall integrity ● Use of accessory and/or abdominal muscles ● Bilateral breath sounds ● Jugular veins and position of trachea	● Supplemental oxygen ● Bag-valve-mask ventilation ● Needle thoracentesis ● Chest tube ● Nonporous dressing taped on 3 sides
C = Circulation	
● Pulse general rate and quality ● Skin color, temperature, degree of diaphoresis ● External bleeding	● Direct pressure over uncontrolled bleeding sites ● Two large-bore intravenous catheters with warmed lactated Ringer's solution ● Infuse fluid fast with blood tubing ● Blood sample for typing ● Pneumatic antishock garment ● Pericardiocentesis ● ED thoracotomy ● Cardiopulmonary resuscitation and advanced life support measures ● Blood administration ● Surgery
D = Disability	
● Level of consciousness (AVPU) ● Pupils (PERL)	● Perform further investigation ● Hyperventilation

Table 33

SECONDARY ASSESSMENT	
E = Expose Patient	
F = Fahrenheit – Keep Patient Warm	
• Blankets • Warming lights	
G = Get Vital Signs	

• In addition to obtaining a complete set of vital signs, consider:
  ▪ Cardiac monitor and pulse oximeter (SpO$_2$)
  ▪ Urinary catheter if not contraindicated
  ▪ Gastric tube
  ▪ Laboratory studies	

H = History/Head-To-Toe Examination	
History	• MIVT • Patient-generated information • Past medical history
Head and face	• Inspect for wounds, ecchymosis, deformities, drainage from nose and ears, and pupils • Palpate for tenderness, note bony crepitus, deformity
Neck	• Remove the anterior portion of the cervical collar to inspect and palpate the neck. Another team member must hold the patient's head while the collar is being removed and replaced. • Inspect for wounds, ecchymosis, deformities, and distended neck veins • Palpate for tenderness, note bony crepitus, deformity, subcutaneous emphysema, and tracheal position
Chest	• Inspect for breathing rate and depth, wounds, deformities, ecchymosis, use of accessory muscles, paradoxical movement • Auscultate breath and heart sounds • Palpate for tenderness, note bony crepitus, subcutaneous emphysema, and deformity
Abdomen and flanks	• Inspect for wounds, distention, ecchymosis, and scars • Auscultate bowel sounds • Palpate all four quadrants for tenderness, rigidity, guarding, masses, and femoral pulses
Pelvis and perineum	• Inspect for wounds, deformities, ecchymosis, priapism, blood at the urinary meatus or in the perineal area • Palpate the pelvis and anal sphincter tone
Extremities	• Inspect for ecchymosis, movement, wounds, and deformities • Palpate for pulses, skin temperature, sensation, tenderness, deformities, and note bony crepitus

SECONDARY ASSESSMENT	
I = Inspect Posterior Surface	
Posterior surfaces	<ul><li>**Maintain cervical spine stabilization and support injured extremities while the patient is logrolled.**</li><li>Inspect posterior surfaces for wounds, deformities, and ecchymosis</li><li>Palpate posterior surfaces for tenderness, and deformities</li><li>Palpate anal sphincter tone (if not performed previously)</li></ul>

Table 34

PLANNING AND IMPLEMENTATION		
Area	**Diagnostic Studies**	**Interventions**
General		<ul><li>Operative intervention</li><li>Admission or transfer</li><li>Glasgow Coma Scale Score and Revised Trauma Score</li><li>Psychosocial support of patient and family</li><li>Pain medication, as prescribed</li></ul>
Head and face	Radiographic studies, laboratory studies	<ul><li>Position patient</li><li>Medications, as prescribed</li><li>Intracranial pressure monitoring</li></ul>
Neck	Radiographic studies, laboratory studies	<ul><li>Vertebral column immobilization</li><li>Steroids, as prescribed</li></ul>
Chest	Radiographic studies, laboratory studies, ECG, central venous pressure monitoring	<ul><li>Chest tube</li><li>Autotransfusion</li></ul>
Abdomen and flanks	Radiographic studies, laboratory studies, and diagnostic peritoneal lavage	<ul><li>Urinary catheter</li><li>Gastric tube</li><li>Pneumatic antishock garment</li></ul>
Pelvis and perineum	Radiographic studies, laboratory studies	<ul><li>Urinary catheter</li><li>Pneumatic antishock garment</li><li>External pelvic fixator</li></ul>
Extremities	Radiographic studies, laboratory studies	<ul><li>Immobilization</li><li>Elevation, ice</li></ul>
Posterior surfaces	Radiographic studies, laboratory studies	<ul><li>Spinal immobilization</li></ul>

PLANNING AND IMPLEMENTATION		
Area	**Diagnostic Studies**	**Interventions**
Surface trauma		• Irrigation • Wound care • Ice • Care for amputated parts • Tetanus prophylaxis and antibiotics

EVALUATION

Instructors will use a form to evaluate each learner's performance during the Trauma Nursing Process Station. There are specific forms for each case scenario. The * and ** steps indicated on this form are consistent for all case scenarios. Each step counts for one point; performing the double-starred steps in the correct sequence counts for three points.

The single-starred (*) steps are essential skill steps. The single-starred steps must be performed during the skill station demonstration, but their sequence is not critical.

The double-starred (**) steps must be demonstrated during the primary assessment. No points are granted for double-starred steps performed after the primary assessment. If the double-starred steps are accurately demonstrated in order, the learner will receive three points for correct sequence. Failure to perform any of the double-starred steps results in unsuccessful completion of the psychomotor skill station. Learners cannot return to the primary assessment during the secondary assessment and identify double-starred steps.

The following performance information is important for successful completion of the Trauma Nursing Process skill stations:

1. Learners must demonstrate both criteria if two criteria are listed, e.g., auscultates breath sounds **AND** heart tones; inspects **AND** palpates.

2. Learners must demonstrate appropriate assessment techniques, i.e., auscultation and palpation. It is not acceptable for the learner to state, "I would palpate the abdomen" without actually touching the model. The correct method to auscultate breath sounds is dependent upon whether the patient is intubated or not.

369

3. Learners must be specific regarding inspection and palpation, i.e., "I am inspecting and palpating for injuries."

4. Learners must use the appropriate equipment in each station.

5. To assess airway patency in the unconscious patient, the learner should simultaneously manually open the airway using a jaw thrust or chin lift maneuver while assessing for airway patency.

6. For those scenarios that include the patient arriving immobilized on a backboard with a rigid cervical collar, the learner is awarded credit for maintaining spinal immobilization as long as none of the immobilization devices are completely removed.

7. Learners must evaluate the effectiveness of interventions which are expected to have an immediate effect on the patient (e.g., auscultation of breath sounds after intubation).

8. In the primary assessment, observation of skin color is appropriate for assessment of breathing effectiveness and circulation. The learner only has to state the need to observe skin color once to receive credit in both steps.

9. When needle thoracentesis is indicated, the learner will describe the technique (landmarks and equipment).

10. Learners must assess the level of consciousness according to the AVPU mnemonic.

11. Learners must state the need to assess pupils (PERL) but do not need to demonstrate the PERL examination.

12. When learners ask for vital signs, instructors will respond with blood pressure, pulse, respirations, and temperature.

13. To obtain the patient history, learners should obtain any one of the following: any additional information from prehospital providers, patient-generated information, or past medical history if available.

14. Learners need not restate all of the simulated injuries identified during the assessment. Restating the injuries at the end of the assessment is the option of the instructor.

15. If a learner states any "additional appropriate diagnostic studies or interventions" during the primary or secondary assessments, these will count toward the total of five required for performance of the skill step.

TRAUMA NURSING PROCESS SKILL STEPS

The skill steps to complete the Trauma Nursing Process are listed below. In the actual Trauma Nursing Process skill stations, specific case scenarios will be used. However, the following demonstration does not use a case scenario and depicts a more general assessment. In this general demonstration an intervention is identified for each step of the primary assessment (ABCD). In the actual Trauma Nursing Process skill stations, an intervention may not necessarily be required for each step in the primary assessment but will be based on the actual case scenario.

Two Instructors will now demonstrate the skill steps in the Trauma Nursing Process. The skill steps will include a demonstration of the primary and secondary assessment, without a specific case scenario. Actual case scenarios are presented in each of the Trauma Nursing Process teaching and evaluation scenarios.

Instructor Responses	Skill Steps
	** 1. Assesses airway patency, AND if unconscious, manually opens the airway using a jaw thrust or chin lift (at least three of the following)
No vocalization	• Vocalization
No obstruction	• Tongue obstruction
None	• Loose teeth or foreign objects
Blood in the mouth	• Bleeding
No vomitus or secretions	• Vomitus or other secretions
None	• Edema
	2. Maintains spinal stabilization/ immobilization

371

Instructor Responses	Skill Steps
	** 3. Identifies one appropriate airway intervention, e.g., suctions the patient
Airway is patent and clear	4. Assesses effectiveness of airway intervention(s)
	** 5. Assesses breathing effectiveness (at least three of the following)
Present	• Spontaneous breathing
Symmetrical	• Chest rise and fall
Skin color pale	• Skin color
Respirations 10/minute and shallow	• General rate and depth of respirations
No open wounds, chest wall intact	• Soft tissue and bony chest wall integrity
No use of accessory and/or abdominal muscles	• Use of accessory and/or abdominal muscles
Equal and clear bilaterally	• Bilateral breath sounds
No jugular venous distention, no tracheal deviation	• Jugular veins and position of trachea
	** 6. Identifies one appropriate intervention for ineffective breathing, e.g., assist ventilations via bag-valve-mask
Color pale, good rise and fall of chest	7. Assesses effectiveness of breathing intervention(s) • Chest rise and fall • Skin color
Pulse rapid	** 8. Palpates pulse
Skin pale, cool and dry	9. Inspects/palpates skin for color OR temperature OR diaphoresis
Uncontrolled bleeding present from scalp laceration	10. Inspects for external bleeding

Instructor Responses	Skill Steps
	** 11. **Identifies appropriate interventions for ineffective circulation** • Applies direct pressure to areas of uncontrolled external bleeding • States need to cannulate two veins with 14- or 16-gauge intravenous catheters • Initiates infusion of warmed lactated Ringer's solution • Infuses fluid with blood tubing AND at a fast rate • Obtains blood sample for typing
External bleeding controlled	12. Assesses effectiveness of circulatory intervention(s), i.e., control of external bleeding
Unresponsive to painful stimuli	** 13. **Assesses level of consciousness (AVPU)**
PERL	14. Assesses pupils (PERL)
	** 15. **Identifies one appropriate intervention for abnormal neurological findings, e.g., hyperventilation**
	16. Follows the correct sequence of ** steps (three points)
Secondary Assessment	
	17. Removes all clothing
	18. States one measure to prevent heat loss, e.g., places warm blankets on patient
BP 110/70 mmHg Pulse 86 beats/minute Respirations – assist ventilations at 24/min. Temperature 36.8°C (98°F)	19. States need to get a complete set of vital signs
Normal sinus rhythm	20. Places cardiac monitor leads on patient
SpO_2 = 98%	21. Places pulse oximeter probe on patient

373

Instructor Responses	Skill Steps
No contraindications	22. States need to insert urinary catheter
	23. States need to insert gastric tube
Past medical history unknown	24. Describes the pertinent history to be obtained (at least one of the following) • MIVT • Patient-generated information • Past medical history
Demonstrates and describes the head-to-toe assessment by describing appropriate inspection techniques (e.g., lacerations, abrasions, contusions, ecchymosis), demonstrating appropriate palpation techniques, and demonstrating appropriate auscultation techniques. See Table 33, Chapter 15.	
Large laceration to right parietal scalp area	25. Inspects AND palpates head AND face for injuries
"I'll maintain stabilization while you assess the neck" No abnormalities *"I'll replace the collar"*	26. Inspects AND palpates neck for injuries
No abnormalities	27. Inspects AND palpates chest for injuries
Breath sounds equal and clear bilaterally. Normal heart sounds.	28. Auscultates breath AND heart sounds
No abnormalities	29. Inspects the abdomen for injuries
Present	30. Auscultates bowel sounds
No abnormalities	31. Palpates all four quadrants of the abdomen for injuries
No abnormalities	32. Inspects AND palpates the pelvis for injuries
No abnormalities	33. Inspects the perineum for injuries
No abnormalities. Normal neurovascular status in all extremities.	34. Inspects AND palpates all four extremities for neurovascular status and injuries

Instructor Responses	Skill Steps
"We will assist you in logrolling the patient"	35. **Describes method to maintain spinal stabilization when patient is logrolled**
No abnormalities	36. **Inspects AND palpates posterior surfaces for injuries**
	* 37. **Identifies all simulated injuries: Learners do NOT need to restate the injuries they identified during the assessment**
"You have identified certain injuries during the assessment. Now that you have completed the secondary assessment, list five additional diagnostic studies or interventions for this patient." Note to Instructors: If the learner has previously identified any of the appropriate diagnostic studies or interventions listed, include the diagnostic study or intervention into the total of five.	
	* 38. **Identifies appropriate diagnostic studies or interventions (at least five of the following):** • **Cervical spine radiographs** • **Cleanse scalp wound** • **Endotracheal intubation** • **Glasgow Coma Scale Score** • **Head CT** • **Laboratory studies** • **Revised Trauma Score** • **Tetanus immunization**
"What findings need to be re-evaluated?"	
	39. **States need to re-evaluate:** • **Airway effectiveness** • **Breathing effectiveness** • **Circulatory effectiveness** • **Disability** • **Vital signs**

SUMMARY

The Trauma Nursing Process is a standard of care endorsed by the American Nurses Association and the Emergency Nurses Association. The Trauma Nursing Process involves six phases: assessment, nursing diagnosis, outcome identification, planning, implementation, and evaluation. The Trauma Nursing Process skill station is an opportunity for learners to demonstrate their knowledge and understanding of trauma nursing.

PSYCHOMOTOR SKILL STATIONS

OBJECTIVES

In a simulated situation with patients requiring the nursing skills associated with the trauma nursing process, airway and ventilation interventions, spinal immobilization, traction splinting, chest trauma interventions, or helmet removal, the learner will be able to:

1. Identify the priorities of care for the simulated patient.

2. Correctly demonstrate the required nursing skills for the simulated patient.

3. Evaluate the patient's response to the demonstrated nursing skills.

4. The instructor will explain psychomotor skill station evaluation:

   - Double-starred (**) steps must be performed during the primary assessment to successfully complete the station. If they are accurately demonstrated in order, the learner will receive three sequence points.
   - Single-starred (*) steps are critical and must be performed during the station.
   - Criteria for completion: 70% of total points and completion of all * and ** steps.
   - Sample evaluation sheets: lists all * and ** steps and station requirements.
   - Principles: learners must "talk through" the cases and demonstrate skills.
   - Case progression: the instructor will provide patient information in response to the learner's demonstration.

The order of the skill stations is as follows:

TRAUMA NURSING PROCESS STATION #1

I. Introduction

A. Instructor and learner introductions

B. Purpose

Each learner will demonstrate a primary and secondary assessment and initiate appropriate interventions on a simulated patient.

C. Format

1. The Demonstration of the Trauma Nursing Process Station, Chapter 15, previously provided the learner with a general discussion and demonstration of the trauma nursing assessment and interventions.

2. During the Trauma Nursing Process Skill Station #1, the learners in the group will be presented specific case scenarios. Two learners will demonstrate and/or describe a trauma assessment and identify appropriate interventions following Case A; the other two learners will practice Case B.

3. The Instructor will provide additional information as requested by the learner.

D. Evaluation

1. Each learner will be evaluated at one Trauma Nursing Process Station. Do not attempt to memorize the specific scenarios as a new scenario will be used for evaluation.

2. Certain critical steps must be mentioned during the primary assessment. They are marked with an ** on the evaluation form. If these critical steps are accurately demonstrated in order, three sequence points will be included.

3. Additional critical steps are marked with an * on the evaluation form. All of these steps must be demonstrated.

4. At least 70% of the total points must be demonstrated.

5. At the completion of the demonstration, the learner will be asked if there is anything he or she wants to add or revise. Learners may not add or revise any of the ** steps.

II. Principles of the Trauma Nursing Process

A. General principles

1. Assessment, nursing diagnosis, outcome identification, planning, and implementation are the first five steps of the nursing process. Evaluation, the last step, is an ongoing process once the patient arrives in the emergency department.

2. In actual patient care, all personnel who anticipate direct patient contact or contact with the patient's body fluids must wear personal protective equipment. (NOTE: Since TNCC skill stations are simulated situations, the use of personal protective equipment is optional.)

B. Primary assessment

All elements assessed during the primary assessment are of such a critical nature that any major deviations from normal require immediate intervention. Do not proceed until all major life-threatening conditions have been treated. The primary assessment addresses airway (A), breathing (B), circulation (C), and disability or neurologic status (D).

C. Secondary assessment

The secondary assessment is completed after the primary assessment. It includes E through I as described below. The focus of the secondary assessment is to identify ALL injuries in order to determine the priorities for the planning and intervention phases of the nursing process.

A	=	Airway and cervical spine stabilization
B	=	Breathing
C	=	Circulation
D	=	Disability (neurologic status)
E	=	Expose patient
F	=	Fahrenheit – Keep patient warm
G	=	Get vital signs
H	=	History/Head-to-toe examination
I	=	Inspect posterior surfaces

D. Nursing diagnoses, outcome identification, planning, and implementation

The severity of the patient's condition may require simultaneous assessment, diagnosis, and implementation. Appropriate nursing diagnoses are based on assessment findings. Specific patient outcomes are then identified and a plan is developed. The priorities for intervention will depend upon the complexity of the patient's injuries and the availability and qualifications of the emergency department staff and/or trauma nurse. Give priority to those injuries with the greatest potential to compromise airway, breathing, circulation, and/or disability. For the purposes of this station, the learner is NOT expected to identify nursing diagnoses or outcomes.

E. Ongoing evaluation

Evaluate the patient's response to any interventions to determine further interventions. The learner should evaluate the effectiveness of any intervention expected to have an immediate effect on the patient. Any abnormalities identified in the primary assessment and the vital signs must be re-evaluated at the completion of the secondary assessment.

III. Steps in Skill Performance

The learners will be presented a case scenario depicting a trauma victim who is en route or has presented to the emergency department. Two learners will demonstrate Case A, and then two learners will demonstrate Case B. The script and steps in skill performance are listed on page 384 for Case A and on page 389 for Case B.

CASE A: A basic life support ambulance is en route with a 35-year-old unrestrained driver of an automobile which struck a tree. There was extensive vehicular damage requiring lengthy extrication. The patient is alert, blood pressure is 100/70 mmHg, carotid pulse is 120 beats/minute and weak, respirations are rapid and shallow at approximately 30 breaths/minute. Patient has multiple facial contusions and lacerations and a painful, deformed right thigh. The patient is immobilized on a backboard with a rigid cervical collar, the right leg is splinted with a traction splint, and oxygen via nonrebreather mask is being administered. The patient has just arrived in the emergency department. Please proceed with your primary and secondary assessments and appropriate interventions. In the interest of model comfort and safety, assume the model is immobilized on a backboard with a rigid cervical collar.

CASE B: An 18-year-old, assisted by two friends, staggers into triage and states, "I've been shot in the stomach." The patient is brought into the trauma room. Proceed with your primary and secondary assessments and interventions.

IV. Summary

A. Trauma Nursing Process Station #1

1. The Trauma Nursing Process Teaching Station #1 presents the learners with two patient scenarios.

2. During evaluation, the learner must demonstrate all critical steps designated with one and two asterisks (* and **), and 70% of the total number of points. The learner will be evaluated using a new and different scenario. Therefore, concentrate on understanding the principles of the Trauma Nursing Process and not memorizing the specific case scenarios.

B. Critical step review

1. Critical steps as indicated by **

Certain critical steps must be demonstrated/described during the primary assessment. These are designated with ** on the evaluation form. If these steps are accurately demonstrated in order, three sequence points will be included. The total number of possible critical steps (**) in any scenario is eight. However, a scenario may have less steps with **.

a. Assesses airway patency.

b. Identifies one appropriate airway intervention.

c. Assesses breathing effectiveness.

d. Identifies one appropriate intervention for ineffective breathing.

e. Palpates a pulse.

f. Identifies one appropriate intervention for ineffective circulation.

g. Assesses level of consciousness (AVPU).

h. Identifies one appropriate intervention for altered level of consciousness.

2. Critical steps as indicated by *

Additional critical steps demonstrated and/or described during the remainder of the station are designated with a * on the evaluation form. All of these steps must be performed to successfully complete the Trauma Nursing Process station.

a. Identifies all simulated injuries.

b. Identifies at least five appropriate diagnostic studies and/or interventions.

C. Principles and points to remember

1. Correlate the mechanism of injury with potential injuries.

2. Address all life-threatening conditions before the secondary assessment.

3. Maintain cervical spine stabilization during all steps of the nursing process.

4. Caring for a multiple trauma patient requires a team approach and is more efficient when the leader is well identified.

5. Delineate trauma team roles prior to receiving the patient.

6. Assign one team member the responsibility for recording all assessment findings and interventions.

TRAUMA NURSING PROCESS SCENARIO
CASE A

Teaching Scenario Checklist

Prehospital MIVT Report

CASE A: A basic life support ambulance is en route with a 35-year-old unrestrained driver of an automobile which struck a tree. There was extensive vehicular damage requiring lengthy extrication. The patient is alert, blood pressure is 100/70 mmHg, carotid pulse is 120 beats/minute and weak, and respirations are rapid and shallow at approximately 30 breaths/minute. Patient has multiple facial contusions and lacerations and a painful, deformed right thigh. The patient is immobilized on a backboard with a rigid cervical collar, the right leg is splinted with a traction splint and oxygen via nonrebreather mask is being administered. The patient has just arrived in the emergency department. Please proceed with your primary and secondary assessments and appropriate interventions. In the interest of model comfort and safety, assume the model is immobilized on a backboard with a rigid cervical collar.

Instructor Responses	Skill Steps	Demonstrated		
		Yes		No
	1. Assesses airway patency; AND if unconscious, manually opens the airway using a jaw thrust or chin lift (at least three of the following)	** _____		_____
Patient is talking	• Vocalization			
No obstruction	• Tongue obstruction			
No loose teeth or foreign objects	• Loose teeth or foreign objects			
No bleeding	• Bleeding			
No vomitus or secretions	• Vomitus or other secretions			
No edema noted	• Edema			
	2. Maintains spinal immobilization	_____		_____
	3. Assesses breathing effectiveness (at least three of the following)	** _____		_____
Present	• Spontaneous breathing			
Asymmetrical, decreased on left	• Chest rise and fall			
Ashen	• Skin color			
Fast and shallow	• General rate and depth of respirations			
No open wounds, chest wall intact, ecchymotic area on left anterior chest just below the clavicle	• Soft tissue and bony chest wall integrity			
Difficulty breathing, using accessory muscles	• Use of accessory and/or abdominal muscles			

384

Instructor Responses	Skill Steps	Demonstrated		
		Yes		No
No breath sounds on left Jugular venous distention, trachea shifts to right	• Bilateral breath sounds • Jugular veins and position of trachea			
"Air escapes when the needle is inserted"	4. States suspects tension pneumothorax and describes location and equipment for needle thoracentesis	**_____		_____
	5. Reassesses breathing effectiveness (at least three of the following)	_____		_____
Symmetrical	• Chest rise and fall			
Pale	• Skin color			
Slower rate, improved depth	• General rate and depth of respirations			
None	• Use of accessory muscles and/or abdominal muscles			
Equal and clear bilaterally	• Bilateral breath sounds			
No jugular venous distention, trachea midline	• Jugular veins and position of trachea			
Pulse present and fast	6. Palpates pulse	**_____		_____
Pale, cool, slightly diaphoretic	7. Inspects/palpates skin for color OR temperature OR diaphoresis	_____		_____
No uncontrolled external bleeding	8. Inspects for external bleeding	_____		_____
	9. States need to cannulate two veins with 14- or 16-gauge intravenous catheters	**_____		_____
	10. Initiates infusion of warmed lactated Ringer's solution	_____		_____
	11. Infuses fluid with blood tubing AND at a fast rate	_____		_____
	12. Obtains blood sample for typing	_____		_____
Alert	13. Assesses level of consciousness (AVPU)	**_____		_____
PERL	14. Assess pupils (PERL)	_____		_____
	15. Accurately follows the correct sequence of ** steps (three points)	_____		_____
	Secondary Assessment			
	16. Removes all clothing	_____		_____
	17. States one measure to prevent heat loss (blankets, warming lights)	_____		_____
BP = 110/80 mmHg T = 36.8°C (98°F) P = 104 beats/minute R = 24 breaths/minute	18. States need to get a complete set of vital signs	_____		_____

385

Instructor Responses	Skill Steps	Demonstrated		
		Yes		No
ECG = sinus tachycardia without ectopy	19. **Places cardiac monitor leads on patient**	_____		_____
SpO$_2$ = 96%	20. **Places pulse oximeter probe on patient**	_____		_____
No contraindications	21. **States need to insert urinary catheter**	_____		_____
	22. **States need to insert gastric tube**	_____		_____

No new information
 	
Complains of pain in right thigh
 	
Past medical history – unremarkable
	23. **Describes the pertinent history to be obtained (at least one of the following)**
	
	  • **MIVT**
	
	  • **Patient-generated information**
	
	  • **Past medical history**
		_____		_____

Demonstrates and describes the head-to-toe assessment by describing appropriate inspection techniques (e.g., lacerations, abrasions, contusions, ecchymosis), demonstrating appropriate palpation techniques, and demonstrating appropriate auscultation techniques. See Table 33, Chapter 15.				
Multiple facial lacerations and contusions	24. **Inspects AND palpates head AND face for injuries**	_____		_____
"I'll maintain stabilization while you assess the neck" No abnormalities _"I'll replace the collar"_	25. **Inspects AND palpates neck for injuries**	_____		_____
Ecchymotic area on left anterior chest just below the clavicle, otherwise no abnormalities	26. **Inspects AND palpates chest for injuries**	_____		_____
Equal and clear bilaterally. Normal heart sounds.	27. **Auscultates breath AND heart sounds**	_____		_____
Distended abdomen. No obvious injuries.	28. **Inspects the abdomen for injuries**	_____		_____
Decreased bowel sounds	29. **Auscultates bowel sounds**	_____		_____
Painful, rigid, guarding	30. **Palpates all four quadrants of the abdomen for injuries**	_____		_____
No abnormalities	31. **Inspects AND palpates the pelvis for injuries**	_____		_____
No abnormalities	32. **Inspects the perineum for injuries**	_____		_____
Right thigh swollen, deformed and painful. Normal neurovascular status in all extremities. Traction splint is appropriately applied.	33. **Inspects AND palpates all four extremities for neurovascular status and injuries**	_____		_____

Instructor Responses	Skill Steps	Demonstrated		
		Yes		No
	34. **Describes method to maintain spinal stabilization when patient is logrolled**	_____		_____
No abnormalities	35. **Inspects AND palpates posterior surfaces for injuries**	_____		_____
If the learner has not mentioned all of the simulated injuries, ask him or her to identify all simulated injuries	36. **Identifies all simulated injuries** • **Tension pneumothorax** • **Facial lacerations and contusions** • **Abdominal rigidity, guarding, tenderness** • **Swollen, deformed right thigh**	*_____		_____
"You have identified certain injuries during the assessment. Now that you have completed the secondary assessment, list five additional diagnostic studies or interventions for this patient." Note to Instructors: If the learner has previously identified any of the appropriate diagnostic studies or interventions listed, include the diagnostic study or interventions into the total of five.				
	37. **Identifies appropriate diagnostic studies or interventions (at least five of the following)** • **Cervical spine radiographs** • **Chest radiographs** • **Chest tube insertion** • **Clean and dress facial wound** • **Diagnostic peritoneal lavage or abdominal CT** • **ECG** • **Facial radiographs or CT** • **Head CT** • **Glasgow Coma Scale Score** • **Ice to face and/or thigh** • **Laboratory studies** • **Pain control** • **Pelvis radiographs** • **Prepare for admission, surgery, or transfer** • **Psychosocial support** • **Revised Trauma Score** • **Right femur radiographs** • **Tetanus prophylaxis**	*_____		_____

Instructor Responses	Skill Steps	Demonstrated		
		Yes		No
"What findings need to be re-evaluated?"				
	38. States need to re-evaluate breathing effectiveness	_____		_____
	39. States need to re-evaluate circulatory effectiveness, other than vital signs	_____		_____
	40. States need to re-evaluate vital signs	_____		_____
Once the learner has completed his or her Trauma Nursing Process station, ask the learner about his or her performance, and also ask other learners in the group for feedback.				

388

TRAUMA NURSING PROCESS SCENARIO
CASE B

Teaching Scenario Checklist

Prehospital MIVT Report

CASE B: An 18-year-old, assisted by two friends, staggers into triage and states, "I've been shot in the stomach." The patient is brought into the trauma room. Proceed with your primary and secondary assessments and interventions.

Instructor Responses	Skill Steps	Demonstrated		
		Yes		**No**
	1. Assesses airway patency; AND if unconscious, manually opens the airway using a jaw thrust or chin lift (at least three of the following)	** _____		_____
Patient is talking and moaning with pain	• **Vocalization**			
No obstruction	• **Tongue obstruction**			
No loose teeth or foreign objects	• **Loose teeth or foreign objects**			
No bleeding	• **Bleeding**			
No vomitus or secretions	• **Vomitus or other secretions**			
No edema noted	• **Edema**			
	2. Assesses breathing effectiveness (at least three of the following)	** _____		_____
Present, rapid	• **Spontaneous breathing**			
Symmetrical chest rise	• **Chest rise and fall**			
Pale	• **Skin color**			
Shallow and rapid	• **General rate and depth of respirations**			
No open wounds, chest wall intact	• **Soft tissue and bony chest wall integrity**			
None	• **Use of accessory and/or abdominal muscles**			
Equal and clear bilaterally	• **Bilateral breath sounds**			
No jugular venous distention, trachea midline	• **Jugular veins and position of trachea**			
	3. Applies oxygen via nonrebreather mask	** _____		_____
Pulse rapid	**4. Palpates pulse**	** _____		_____
Pale, cool, slightly diaphoretic	**5. Inspects/palpates skin for color OR temperature OR diaphoresis**	_____		_____

Instructor Responses	Skill Steps	Demonstrated		
		Yes		No
No uncontrolled external bleeding. Small amount of oozing from gunshot wound.	6. Inspects for external bleeding	_____		_____
	7. States need to cannulate two veins with 14- or 16-gauge intravenous catheters	** _____		_____
	8. Initiates infusion of warmed lactated Ringer's solution	_____		_____
	9. Infuses fluid with blood tubing AND at a fast rate	_____		_____
	10. Obtains blood sample for typing	_____		_____
Alert but restless	11. Assesses level of consciousness (AVPU)	** _____		_____
PERL	12. Assesses pupils (PERL)	_____		_____
	13. Accurately follows the correct sequence of ** steps (three points)	_____		_____
Secondary Assessment				
	14. Removes all clothing	_____		_____
	15. States one measure to prevent heat loss (blankets, warming lights)	_____		_____
BP = 96/70 mmHg T = 36°C (98°F) P = 120 beats/minute R = 32 breaths/minute	16. States need to get a complete set of vital signs	_____		_____
ECG = sinus tachycardia without ectopy	17. Places cardiac monitor leads on patient	_____		_____
SpO_2 = 98%	18. Places pulse oximeter probe on patient	_____		_____
No contraindications	19. States need to insert urinary catheter	_____		_____
	20. States need to insert gastric tube	_____		_____
Not applicable Patient complains of pain in the abdomen and difficulty breathing. Friends left emergency department. Past medical history – HIV positive	21. Describes the pertinent history to be obtained (at least one of the following) • MIVT • Patient-generated information • Past medical history	_____		_____

Demonstrates and describes the head-to-toe assessment by describing appropriate inspection techniques (e.g., lacerations, abrasions, contusions, ecchymosis), by demonstrating appropriate palpation techniques, and demonstrating appropriate auscultation techniques. See Table 33, Chapter 15.

Instructor Responses	Skill Steps	Demonstrated		
No abnormalities	22. Inspects AND palpates head AND face for injuries	_____		_____

Instructor Responses	Skill Steps	Demonstrated		
		Yes		No
No abnormalities	23. Inspects AND palpates neck for injuries	_____		_____
No abnormalities	24. Inspects AND palpates chest for injuries	_____		_____
Equal and clear bilaterally. Normal heart sounds.	25. Auscultates breath AND heart sounds	_____		_____
Single penetrating injury 3 - 4 inches below the umbilicus	26. Inspects the abdomen for injuries	_____		_____
Absent	27. Auscultates bowel sounds	_____		_____
Rigid and tender	28. Palpates all four quadrants of the abdomen for injuries	_____		_____
No abnormalities	29. Inspects AND palpates the pelvis for injuries	_____		_____
No abnormalities	30. Inspects the perineum for injuries	_____		_____
No abnormalities	31. Inspects AND palpates all four extremities for neurovascular status and injuries	_____		_____
Open wound lateral left flank	32. Inspects AND palpates posterior surfaces for injuries	_____		_____
If the learner has not mentioned all of the simulated injuries, ask him or her to identify all simulated injuries	33. Identifies all simulated injuries • Wound 3 to 4 inches below the umbilicus with pain/rigidity • Wound left flank	*_____		_____

"You have identified certain injuries during the assessment. Now that you have completed the secondary assessment, list five additional diagnostic studies or interventions for this patient."
Note to Instructors: If the learner has previously identified any of the appropriate diagnostic studies or interventions listed, include the diagnostic study or interventions into the total of five.

	Skill Steps	Demonstrated		
	34. Identifies appropriate diagnostic studies or interventions (at least five of the following) • Abdominal radiographs • Antibiotics • Blood administration • Chest radiographs • Control any bleeding • Glasgow Coma Scale Score • Laboratory studies • Prepare for admission, surgery, or transfer • Psychosocial support • Revised Trauma Score • Tetanus prophylaxis	*_____		_____

391

Instructor Responses	Skill Steps	Demonstrated		
		Yes		No
"What findings need to be re-evaluated?"				
	35. States need to re-evaluate breathing effectiveness	_____		_____
	36. States need to re-evaluate circulatory effectiveness, other than vital signs	_____		_____
	37. States need to re-evaluate vital signs	_____		_____
Once the learner has completed his or her Trauma Nursing Process station, ask the learner about his or her performance, and also ask other learners in the group for feedback.				

TRAUMA NURSING PROCESS STATION #2

I. **Introduction**

A. Instructor and learner introductions

B. Purpose

Each learner will demonstrate a primary and secondary assessment and initiate appropriate interventions on a simulated patient.

C. Format

1. The Demonstration of the Trauma Nursing Process Station, Chapter 15, previously provided the learner with a general discussion and demonstration of the trauma nursing assessment and interventions.

2. During the Trauma Nursing Process Skill Station #2, all learners in the group will be presented with specific case scenarios. Two learners will demonstrate and/or describe a trauma assessment and identify appropriate interventions following Case C; the other two learners will practice Case D.

3. The Instructor will provide additional information as requested by the learner.

D. Evaluation

1. Each learner will be evaluated at one Trauma Nursing Process Station. Do not attempt to memorize the specific scenarios as a new scenario will be used for evaluation.

2. Certain critical steps must be mentioned during the primary assessment. They are marked with an ** on the evaluation form. If these critical steps are accurately demonstrated in order, three sequence points will be included.

3. Additional critical steps are marked with an * on the evaluation form. All of these steps must be demonstrated.

4. At least 70% of the total points must be demonstrated.

5. At the completion of the demonstration, the learner will be asked if there is anything he or she wants to add or revise. Learners may not add or revise any of the ** steps.

II. Principles of the Trauma Nursing Process

A. General principles

   1. Assessment, nursing diagnosis, outcome identification, planning, and implementation are the first five steps of the nursing process. Evaluation, the last step, is an ongoing process once the patient arrives in the emergency department.

   2. In actual patient care, all personnel who anticipate direct patient contact or contact with the patient's body fluids must wear personal protective equipment. (NOTE: Since TNCC skill stations are simulated situations, the use of personal protective equipment is optional.)

B. Primary assessment

All elements assessed during the primary assessment are of such a critical nature that any major deviations from normal require immediate intervention. Do not proceed until all major life-threatening conditions have been treated. The primary assessment addresses airway (A), breathing (B), circulation (C), and disability or neurologic status (D).

C. Secondary assessment

The secondary assessment is completed after the primary assessment. It includes E through I as described below. The focus of the secondary assessment is to identify ALL injuries in order to determine the priorities for the planning and intervention phases of the nursing process.

A	=	Airway and cervical spine stabilization
B	=	Breathing
C	=	Circulation
D	=	Disability (neurologic status)
E	=	Expose patient
F	=	Fahrenheit – Keep patient warm
G	=	Get vital signs
H	=	History/Head-to-toe examination
I	=	Inspect posterior surfaces

D. Nursing diagnoses, outcome identification, planning, and implementation

The severity of the patient's condition may require simultaneous assessment, diagnosis, and implementation. Appropriate nursing diagnoses are based on assessment findings. Specific patient outcomes are then identified and a plan is developed. The priorities for intervention will depend upon the complexity of the patient's injuries and the availability and qualifications of the emergency department staff and/or trauma nurse. Give priority to those injuries with the greatest potential to compromise airway, breathing, circulation, and/or disability. For the purposes of this station, the learner is NOT expected to identify nursing diagnoses or outcomes.

E. Ongoing evaluation

Evaluate the patient's response to any interventions to determine further interventions. The learner should evaluate the effectiveness of any intervention expected to have an immediate effect on the patient. Any abnormalities identified in the primary assessment and the vital signs must be re-evaluated at the completion of the secondary assessment.

III. Steps in Skill Performance

The learners will be presented a case scenario depicting a trauma victim who is en route or has presented to the emergency department. Two learners will demonstrate Case C, and then two learners will demonstrate Case D. The script and steps in skill performance are found on page 398 for Case C and on page 402 for Case D.

CASE C: A basic life support ambulance is en route with a 22-year-old assault victim. Bystanders report that the patient was beaten about the face and head with a blunt object. The patient is unconscious and responds only to painful stimuli. The patient has facial contusions, blood in the mouth and a deformed left wrist. The mouth is being suctioned for continued copious bleeding. Blood pressure is 136/80 mmHg, pulse 54 beats/minute, and gurgling respirations at 14 breaths/minute. The patient is immobilized on a backboard with a rigid cervical collar, the left wrist is splinted, and oxygen via nonrebreather mask is being administered. The patient has just arrived in the emergency department. Please proceed with your primary and secondary assessments and interventions. In the interest of model comfort and safety, assume the model is immobilized on a backboard with a rigid cervical collar.

CASE D: An advanced life support ambulance is en route with a 24-year-old patient who fell three stories from a roof. The patient complains of dyspnea and has paradoxical movement of the left chest. The skin color is dusky, the left upper arm is swollen and deformed, and there is a laceration to the forehead. Blood pressure is 110/80 mmHg, peripheral pulse is 110 beats/minute and strong, and respirations are 30 breaths/minute. The patient is responding to verbal stimuli and is restless. The patient is on a backboard with a rigid cervical collar, has two large-bore intravenous catheters with lactated Ringer's solution infusing, and oxygen via nonrebreather mask is being administered. The patient has just arrived in the emergency department. Please proceed with your primary and secondary assessments and appropriate interventions. In the interest of model comfort and safety, assume the model is immobilized on a backboard with a rigid cervical collar.

IV. Summary

A. Trauma Nursing Process Station #2

1. The Trauma Nursing Process Teaching Station #2 presents the learners with two patient scenarios.

2. During evaluation, the learner must demonstrate all critical steps designated with one and two asterisks (* and **), and 70% of the total number of points. The learner will be evaluated using a new and different scenario. Therefore, concentrate on understanding the principles of the Trauma Nursing Process and not memorizing the specific case scenarios.

B. Critical step review

1. Critical steps as indicated by **

Certain critical steps must be demonstrated and/or described during the primary assessment. These are designated with an ** on the evaluation form. If these steps are accurately demonstrated in order, three sequence points will be included. The total number of possible critical steps (**) in any scenario is eight. However, a scenario may have less steps with **.

   a. Assesses airway patency.

   b. Identifies one appropriate airway intervention.

   c. Assesses breathing effectiveness.

   d. Identifies one appropriate intervention for ineffective breathing.

   e. Palpates a pulse.

   f. Identifies one appropriate intervention for ineffective circulation.

   g. Assesses level of consciousness (AVPU).

   h. Identifies one appropriate intervention for altered level of consciousness.

2. Critical steps as indicated by *

Additional critical steps demonstrated and/or described during the remainder of the station are designated with a * on the evaluation form. All of these steps must be performed to successfully complete the Trauma Nursing Process station.

       a.   Identifies all simulated injuries.

       b.   Identifies at least five appropriate diagnostic studies and/or interventions.

C.   Principles and points to remember

   1.   Correlate the mechanism of injury with potential injuries.

   2.   Address all life-threatening conditions before the secondary assessment.

   3.   Maintain cervical spine stabilization during all steps of the nursing process.

   4.   Caring for a multiple trauma patient requires a team approach and is more efficient when the leader is well identified.

   5.   Delineate trauma team roles prior to receiving the patient.

   6.   Assign one team member the responsibility for recording all assessment findings and interventions.

TRAUMA NURSING PROCESS SCENARIO
CASE C

Teaching Scenario Checklist

Prehospital MIVT Report

CASE C: A basic life support ambulance is en route with a 22-year-old assault victim. Bystanders report that the patient was beaten about the face and head with a blunt object. The patient is unconscious and responds only to painful stimuli. The patient has facial contusions, blood in the mouth and a deformed left wrist. The mouth is being suctioned for continued copious bleeding. Blood pressure is 136/80 mmHg, pulse 54 beats/minute, and gurgling respirations at 14 breaths/minute. The patient is immobilized on a backboard with a rigid cervical collar, the left wrist is splinted, an oral airway has been inserted and oxygen via nonrebreather mask is being administered. The patient has just arrived in the emergency department. Please proceed with your primary and secondary assessments and interventions. In the interest of model comfort and safety, assume the model is immobilized on a backboard with a rigid cervical collar.

Instructor Responses	Skill Steps	Demonstrated		
		Yes		No
	1. **Assesses airway patency; AND if unconscious, manually opens the airway using a jaw thrust or chin lift (at least three of the following)**	** ____		____
Oral airway in place	• **Vocalization**			
Gurgling respirations	• **Tongue obstruction**			
No loose teeth or foreign objects	• **Loose teeth or foreign objects**			
Blood present in mouth	• **Bleeding**			
Secretions present	• **Vomitus or other secretions**			
No edema noted	• **Edema**			
	2. **Maintains spinal immobilization**	____		____
	3. **States need to suction patient**	** ____		____
Airway patent	4. **Reassesses airway patency**	____		____
	5. **Assesses breathing effectiveness (at least three of the following)**	** ____		____
Present	• **Spontaneous breathing**			
Symmetrical	• **Chest rise and fall**			
Pale	• **Skin color**			
Nonlabored at 14 breaths/minute	• **General rate and depth of respirations**			

398

Instructor Responses	Skill Steps	Demonstrated		
		Yes		No
No open wounds, chest wall intact	• **Soft tissue and bony chest wall integrity**			
None	• **Use of accessory and/or abdominal muscles**			
Equal and clear bilaterally	• **Bilateral breath sounds**			
No jugular venous distention, trachea midline	• **Jugular veins and position of trachea**			
"Physician now decides to prophylactically intubate patient because of decreased level of consciousness and facial trauma to protect the airway. Tube placement is confirmed and the tube is secured. Patient is placed on a ventilator."				
Pulse present and slow	6. **Palpates pulse**	** _____		_____
Warm, dry, normal color	7. **Inspects/palpates skin for color OR temperature OR diaphoresis**	_____		_____
No uncontrolled external bleeding	8. **Inspects for external bleeding**	_____		_____
	9. **States need to cannulate two veins with 14- or 16-gauge intravenous catheters**	**		_____
	10. **Initiates infusion of warmed lactated Ringer's solution at a slow rate**	_____		_____
	11. **Obtains blood sample for typing**	_____		_____
Withdraws to painful stimuli	12. **Assesses level of consciousness (AVPU)**	** _____		_____
Left dilated and nonreactive; right normal and reactive	13. **Assess pupils (PERL)**	_____		_____
	14. **States need for further investigation during secondary focused assessment OR hyperventilates**	** _____		_____
	15. **Accurately follows the correct sequence of ** steps (three points)**	_____		_____
	Secondary Assessment			
	16. **Removes all clothing**	_____		_____
	17. **States one measure to prevent heat loss (blankets, warming lights)**	_____		_____
BP = 140/76 mmHg T = 36.8°C (98°F) P = 54 beats/minute R = ventilations assisted at 28 breaths/minute	18. **States need to get a complete set of vital signs**	_____		_____
ECG = sinus bradycardia without ectopy	19. **Places cardiac monitor leads on patient**	_____		_____
SpO$_2$ = 100%	20. **Places pulse oximeter probe on patient**	_____		_____
No contraindications	21. **States need to insert urinary catheter**	_____		_____
	22. **States need to insert gastric tube**	_____		_____

Instructor Responses	Skill Steps	Demonstrated		
		Yes		No
No new information Unable to obtain Past medical history unknown	**23. Describes the pertinent history to be obtained (at least one of the following)** • **MIVT** • **Patient-generated information** • **Past medical history**	_____		_____
Demonstrates and describes the head-to-toe assessment by describing appropriate inspection techniques (e.g., lacerations, abrasions, contusions, ecchymosis), demonstrating appropriate palpation techniques, and demonstrating appropriate auscultation techniques. See Table 33, Chapter 15.				
Contusions and ecchymosis to face, edema over left temporal scalp	**24. Inspects AND palpates head AND face for injuries**	_____		_____
"I'll maintain stabilization while you assess the neck" No abnormalities *"I'll replace the collar"*	**25. Inspects AND palpates neck for injuries**	_____		_____
No abnormalities	**26. Inspects AND palpates chest for injuries**	_____		_____
Equal and clear bilaterally. Normal heart sounds.	**27. Auscultates breath AND heart sounds**	_____		_____
No abnormalities	**28. Inspects the abdomen for injuries**	_____		_____
Bowel sounds present	**29. Auscultates bowel sounds**	_____		_____
No abnormalities	**30. Palpates all four quadrants of the abdomen for injuries**	_____		_____
No abnormalities	**31. Inspects AND palpates the pelvis for injuries**	_____		_____
No abnormalities	**32. Inspects the perineum for injuries**	_____		_____
Left wrist swollen and deformed. Normal neurovascular status in all extremities.	**33. Inspects AND palpates all four extremities for neurovascular status and injuries**	_____		_____
	34. Describes method to maintain spinal stabilization when patient is logrolled	_____		_____
No abnormalities	**35. Inspects AND palpates posterior surfaces for injuries**	_____		_____
If the learner has not mentioned all of the simulated injuries, ask him or her to identify all simulated injuries	**36. Identifies all simulated injuries** • **Facial and scalp contusions** • **Possible head injury and/or decreased level of consciousness** • **Deformed left wrist**	*_____		_____

Instructor Responses	Skill Steps	Demonstrated		
		Yes		No
"You identified certain injuries during the assessment. Now that you have completed the secondary assessment, list five additional diagnostic studies or interventions for this patient." Note to Instructors: If the learner has previously identified any of the appropriate diagnostic studies or interventions listed, include the diagnostic study or interventions into the total of five.				
	37. **Identifies appropriate diagnostic studies or interventions (at least five of the following)** • **Arterial blood gas** • **Cervical spine radiographs** • **Chest radiographs** • **Elevate and ice left wrist** • **Facial radiographs** • **Glasgow Coma Scale Score** • **Head CT** • **Ice to face** • **Laboratory studies** • **Left wrist radiographs** • **Prepare for admission, surgery, or transfer** • **Revised Trauma Score** • **Tetanus prophylaxis**	*_____		_____
"What findings need to be re-evaluated?"				
	38. **States need to re-evaluate airway**	_____		_____
	39. **States need to re-evaluate breathing**	_____		_____
	40. **States need to re-evaluate level of consciousness and pupils**	_____		_____
	41. **States need to re-evaluate vital signs**	_____		_____
Once the learner has completed his or her Trauma Nursing Process station, ask the learner about his or her performance, and also ask other learners in the group for feedback.				

TRAUMA NURSING PROCESS SCENARIO
CASE D

Teaching Scenario Checklist

Prehospital MIVT Report

CASE D: An advanced life support ambulance is en route with a 24-year-old patient who fell three stories from a roof. The patient complains of dyspnea and has paradoxical movement of the left chest. The skin color is dusky, the left upper arm is swollen and deformed, and there is a laceration to the forehead. Blood pressure is 110/80 mmHg, peripheral pulse is 110 beats/minute and strong, respirations are 30 breaths/minute. The patient is responding to verbal stimuli and is restless. The patient is on a backboard with a rigid cervical collar, has two large-bore intravenous catheters with lactated Ringer's solution infusing, and oxygen via nonrebreather mask is being administered. The patient has just arrived in the emergency department. Please proceed with your primary and secondary assessments and appropriate interventions. In the interest of model comfort and safety, assume the model is immobilized on a backboard with a rigid cervical collar.

Instructor Responses	Skill Steps	Demonstrated		
		Yes		No
	1. **Assesses airway patency; AND if unconscious, manually opens the airway using a jaw thrust or chin lift (at least three of the following)**	** _____		_____
Patient is talking	• **Vocalization**			
No obstruction	• **Tongue obstruction**			
No loose teeth or foreign objects	• **Loose teeth or foreign objects**			
No bleeding	• **Bleeding**			
No vomitus or secretions	• **Vomitus or other secretions**			
No edema noted	• **Edema**			
	2. **Maintains spinal immobilization**	_____		_____
	3. **Assesses breathing effectiveness (at least three of the following)**	** _____		_____
Present	• **Spontaneous breathing**			
Asymmetrical with para-doxical movement on left	• **Chest rise and fall**			
Dusky, ashen	• **Skin color**			
Rapid and shallow	• **General rate and depth of respirations**			
Paradoxical movement and ecchymosis left anterolateral chest	• **Soft tissue and bony chest wall integrity**			
Labored respirations with sternocleidomastoid re-tractions	• **Use of accessory and/or abdominal muscles**			

402

Instructor Responses	Skill Steps	Demonstrated		
		Yes		No
Present bilaterally but shallow No jugular venous distention, trachea midline	• **Bilateral breath sounds** • **Jugular veins and position of trachea**			
"There is difficulty in assisting the patient's respirations. Physician decides to sedate and intubate patient. Intubation has just been accomplished. What is your next step?"	4. **States need for assisted ventilation via bag-valve-mask**	** _____		_____
No gurgling over epigastrium, chest rises and falls, breath sounds equal bilaterally, ventilation continued	5. **Assess endotracheal tube placement by auscultating over the epigastrium while observing chest for rise and fall; AND then auscultates lungs**	_____		_____
Pulse present and rapid	6. **Palpates pulse**	** _____		_____
Pale, cool, dry	7. **Inspects/palpates skin for color OR temperature OR diaphoresis**	_____		_____
No uncontrolled external bleeding; oozing from forehead laceration	8. **Inspects for external bleeding**	_____		_____
Intravenous lines patent	9. **Assesses patency of prehospital intravenous lines**	_____		_____
	10. **Obtains blood sample for typing**	_____		_____
Unresponsive due to effects of sedation	11. **Assesses level of consciousness (AVPU)**	** _____		_____
PERL	12. **Assesses pupils (PERL)**	_____		_____
	13. **Accurately follows the correct sequence of ** steps (three points)**	_____		_____
	Secondary Assessment			
	14. **Removes all clothing**	_____		_____
	15. **States one measure to prevent heat loss (blankets, warming lights)**	_____		_____
BP = 124/80 mmHg T = 36.6°C (97.8°F) P = 104 beats/minute R = ventilator, rate of 14 breaths/minute	16. **States need to get a complete set of vital signs**	_____		_____
ECG = sinus tachycardia without ectopy	17. **Places cardiac monitor leads on patient**	_____		_____
SpO$_2$ = 97%	18. **Places pulse oximeter probe on patient**	_____		_____
No contraindications	19. **States need to insert urinary catheter**	_____		_____
	20. **States need to insert gastric tube**	_____		_____

Instructor Responses	Skill Steps	Demonstrated		
		Yes		No
No new information Dyspnea, pain in the left chest, increased with breathing. Complaints of pain in left arm. Past medical history – not available due to sedation	21. **Describes the pertinent history to be obtained (at least one of the following)** • **MIVT** • **Patient-generated information** • **Past medical history**	————		————
Demonstrates and describes the head-to-toe assessment by describing appropriate inspection techniques (e.g., lacerations, abrasions, contusions, ecchymosis), demonstrating appropriate palpation techniques, and demonstrating appropriate auscultation techniques. See Table 33, Chapter 15.				
4 cm laceration to forehead	22. **Inspects AND palpates head AND face for injuries**	————		————
"I'll maintain stabilization while you assess the neck" No abnormalities *"I'll replace the collar"*	23. **Inspects AND palpates neck for injuries**	————		————
Ecchymosis and crepitus left chest, decreased paradoxical chest movement. Unable to assess tenderness due to effects of sedation.	24. **Inspects AND palpates chest for injuries**	————		————
Breath sounds while on the ventilator are equal and clear bilaterally. Normal heart sounds.	25. **Auscultates breath AND heart sounds**	————		————
No abnormalities	26. **Inspects the abdomen for injuries**	————		————
Bowel sounds present	27. **Auscultates bowel sounds**	————		————
No abnormalities	28. **Palpates all four quadrants of the abdomen for injuries**	————		————
No abnormalities	29. **Inspects AND palpates the pelvis for injuries**	————		————
No abnormalities	30. **Inspects the perineum for injuries**	————		————
Left upper arm swollen, deformed and the vascular status is normal. The vascular status in all other extremities is normal. Unable to test neurological status due to sedation.	31. **Inspects AND palpates all four extremities for neurovascular status and injuries**	————		————
	32. **Describes method to maintain spinal stabilization when patient is logrolled**	————		————
No abnormalities	33. **Inspects AND palpates posterior surfaces for injuries**	————		————

404

Instructor Responses	Skill Steps	Demonstrated		
		Yes		**No**
If the learner has not mentioned all of the simulated injuries, ask him or her to identify all simulated injuries	**34. Identifies all simulated injuries** • **4 cm forehead laceration** • **Left flail chest** • **Left humerus deformity**	*_____		_____
"You have identified certain injuries during the assessment. Now that you have completed the secondary assessment, list five additional diagnostic studies or interventions for this patient." Note to Instructors: If the learner has previously identified any of the appropriate diagnostic studies or interventions listed, include the diagnostic study or interventions into the total of five.				
	35. Identifies appropriate diagnostic studies or interventions (at least five of thc following) • **Abdominal CT** • **Arterial blood gas** • **Cervical spine radiographs** • **Chest radiographs** • **Clean and dress facial wound** • **Diagnostic peritoneal lavage** • **ECG** • **Glasgow Coma Scale Score** • **Head CT** • **Humerus radiographs** • **Laboratory studies** • **Pelvis radiographs** • **Prepare for admission, surgery, or transfer** • **Psychosocial support** • **Revised Trauma Score** • **Skull radiographs** • **Splint arm and apply ice** • **Tetanus prophylaxis**	*_____		_____
"What findings need to be re-evaluated?"				
	36. States need to re-evaluate breathing effectiveness	_____		_____
	37. States need to re-evaluate vital signs	_____		_____
	38. States need to re-evaluate level of consciousness	_____		_____
Once the learner has completed his or her Trauma Nursing Process station, ask the learner about his or her performance, and also ask other learners in the group for feedback.				

AIRWAY AND VENTILATION INTERVENTIONS
SKILL STATION

I. **Introduction**

A. Instructor and learner introductions

B. Purpose

Each learner will demonstrate an assessment of airway patency, identify the appropriate interventions to obtain and maintain a patent airway, and demonstrate and describe interventions to ensure effective ventilation.

C. Format

1. The Instructor will discuss and demonstrate:

a. Jaw thrust and chin lift maneuver.

b. Oropharyngeal suctioning.

c. Insertion of oropharyngeal or nasopharyngeal airways.

d. Oxygen delivery methods.

e. Bag-mask-valve ventilation.

f. Assessment of endotracheal tube placement.

g. Pulse oximetry, end-tidal CO_2 monitoring, and surgical airways: These sections are optional components.

2. The learners will practice:

a. Jaw thrust and chin lift maneuver.

b. Insertion of an oropharyngeal airway.

c. Bag-valve-mask ventilation.

d. Assessment of endotracheal tube placement.

Note: Learners should practice each skill as it is demonstrated and prior to practicing the case scenario.

The learner will be presented a case scenario and asked to demonstrate and describe airway and ventilation assessments with appropriate interventions. The Instructor will provide additional information as requested by the learner.

D. Evaluation

1. Each learner will be evaluated in the Airway and Ventilation Interventions Skill Station. Evaluation will not include cricothyroidotomy or transtracheal jet insufflation.

2. All critical steps must be demonstrated. These steps are marked with double asterisks (**) on the evaluation form.

3. At least 70% of the total points must be demonstrated.

4. At the completion of the demonstration, the learner will be asked if there is anything he or she wants to add or revise.

II. Principles of Airway and Ventilation

A. General principles

1. The first priority in nursing care of the trauma patient is the establishment of a patent airway.

2. Airway management for the trauma patient must be achieved without hyperextension of the neck. Hyperextension of the cervical spine may cause additional damage in the presence of cervical spine trauma.

3. In actual patient care, all personnel who anticipate direct patient contact or contact with the patient's body fluids must wear personal protective equipment. (NOTE: Since TNCC skill stations are simulated situations, the use of personal protective equipment is optional.)

B. Maneuvers to open and clear the airway

1. Assess airway patency in the conscious patient. In the unconscious patient, manually open the airway using a jaw thrust or chin lift and assess airway patency.

   a. Vocalization

   b. Tongue obstruction

   c. Loose teeth or foreign objects

   d. Bleeding

e.   Vomitus or other secretions

f.   Edema

2. Lifting the patient's mandible lifts the tongue and opens the airway. To position the mandible without hyperextending the cervical spinc, use a jaw thrust or chin lift maneuver.

  a.   Jaw thrust maneuver – Stand at the patient's head and lift the mandible forward (see Figure 39).

Figure 39
Jaw Thrust Maneuver

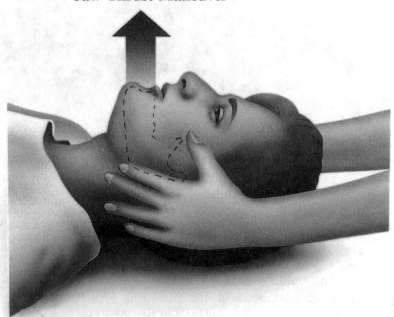

  b.   Reassess airway patency.

  OR

  c.   Chin lift maneuver – Stand at the side of the patient and place one hand on the victim's forehead to stabilize the head and neck. Grasp the mandible between the thumb and index finger with the other hand and lift the mandible (see Figure 40).

  d.   Reassess airway patency.

Figure 40
Chin Lift Maneuver

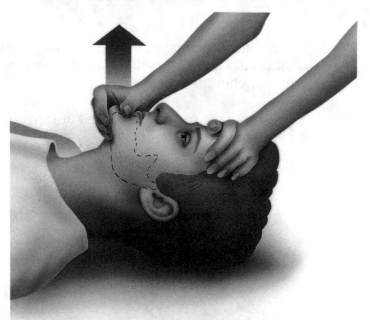

3. Suction to clear the airway of blood, mucus, foreign objects, vomitus or other materials.

C. Airway adjuncts

1. Once a patent airway has been established, an airway adjunct may be required to maintain the airway in an open position.

2. A nasopharyngeal airway can be used in conscious or unconscious patients, but not in patients with facial trauma or a basilar skull fracture.

    a. Use the largest size that will fit in the patient's nostril. Select the correct length of nasopharyngeal airway by measuring from the tip of the nose to the earlobe.[1]

    b. Lubricate the airway with a water-soluble lubricant prior to insertion.

    c. Insert the nasopharyngeal airway with the bevel facing the nasal septum. Direct the airway posteriorly and slightly rotate it towards the ear until the flange rests against the nostril. Avoid inserting the airway into a nostril obstructed by septal deviation, polyps, etc.

    d. Reassess airway patency.

3. An oropharyngeal airway can be used in unconscious patients.

    a. Select the correct sized airway by measuring the airway device from the corner of the mouth to the tip of the earlobe.

b. Insert the airway with the distal tip of the oropharyngeal airway turned towards the roof of the mouth. As the airway device passes across the back of the tongue, gently rotate the airway 180 degrees.

OR

c. Use a tongue blade to hold the tongue against the floor of the mouth and insert the airway following the curvature of the mouth. The flange should rest against the patient's lips.

d. Reassess airway patency.

D. Assess breathing effectiveness

1. Spontaneous breathing

2. Chest rise and fall

3. Skin color

4. General rate and depth of respirations

5. Soft tissue and bony chest wall integrity

6. Use of accessory and/or abdominal muscles

7. Bilateral breath sounds

8. Jugular veins and position of trachea

E. Oxygen delivery methods

1. A tight fitting nonrebreather mask delivers the highest concentration of oxygen to a spontaneously breathing nonintubated patient.

2. A patient with inadequate or absent respirations will require manual ventilation before definitive airway control. See Table 35 for additional information regarding oxygen delivery devices.

Table 35

	OXYGEN DELIVERY DEVICES		
Device	**Oxygen Concentration Delivered**	**Liter Flow (liters/min)**	**Comments**
Nasal cannula	24 to 44%	1 to 6	Difficult to tolerate flow rates greater than 6 liters
Simple face mask	40 to 60%	8 to 10	Flow meter must be set greater than 8 liters to avoid CO_2 accumulation
Nonrebreather mask	60 to 90%	12 to 15	Prevents accumulation of CO_2
Bag-valve-mask with oxygen reservoir	60 to 100%	15	Delivers highest concentration of O_2

F. Bag-valve-mask ventilation

1. A bag-valve-mask must have an oxygen reservoir system and be connected to an oxygen source.

2. Effective bag-valve-mask ventilation requires a tight seal of the face mask, in conjunction with adequate compression of the bag. Achieving this seal may require two people.

   a. Bag-valve-mask ventilation via one person technique: Stand at the patient's head and place the narrow end of the mask over the patient's nose. Hold the mask firmly with the thumb over the patient's nose; grasp and lift the mandible with the fingers. Compress the bag with the other hand. Individuals with small hands may be able to generate a larger tidal volume by compressing the bag against their bodies.

   b. Bag-valve-mask ventilation via two person technique: One person stands at the patient's head and places the thumbs on each side of mask; he or she then grasps and lifts the mandible with the fingers of both hands. The second person stands to the patient's side and compresses the bag.

3. Assess for effective ventilation by inspecting for chest rise and fall and skin color.

G. Endotracheal tube placement

1. The proper placement of the endotracheal tube can be confirmed by the following:

   a. Absence of gurgling over the epigastrium, symmetrical chest rise and fall, and presence of bilateral, equal breath sounds. Endotracheal tube placement is assessed immediately by auscultating over the epigastrium

412

while observing for rise and fall of the chest wall. If stomach gurgling occurs and chest wall expansion is not evident, inadvertent esophageal intubation should be assumed and no further breaths delivered.[2] If the chest rises and falls symmetrically and gastric insufflation is not heard, auscultate the lungs at the second intercostal space, midclavicular line and at the fifth intercostal space anterior axillary line bilaterally.

b. Equal breath sounds indicate proper endotracheal tube placement. Inflate the cuff, secure the tube, and continue ventilations.

c. Unilaterally absent or decreased breath sounds may indicate improper tube placement or a pneumothorax.

d. To rule out improper tube placement, slightly withdraw the tube and reassess breath sounds.

e. Absence of breath sounds indicates esophageal placement; immediately remove the tube and hyperventilate the patient.

2. Additional indicators of correct tube placement include:

a. Direct visualization of the endotracheal tube passing through the cords.

b. Normal oxygen saturation. (SpO_2 is slow to respond to incorrect tube placement)

c. Normal end-tidal CO_2 measurement.

End-tidal CO_2 devices are adjuncts, but not substitutes, for determining correct placement of an endotracheal tube. In emergency settings, monitoring carbon dioxide levels to assure proper endotracheal tube placement usually refers to monitoring end-tidal carbon dioxide ($PetCO_2$) in a patient who has been endotracheally intubated. Once the endotracheal tube has been inserted, a disposable end-tidal CO_2 detector can be placed on the end of the tube. The color of the detector changes based on the concentration of carbon dioxide.

- Purple – during inspiration when CO_2 is very low

- Yellow – during expiration when CO_2 is high

- Beige – intermediate concentrations of CO_2

If the device is purple during expiration, the tube is most likely misplaced in the esophagus. Patients who have consumed carbonated beverages may have false (yellow) readings as there is enough carbon dioxide in gastric air. Other end-tidal CO_2 sensing devices are available. These devices use a disposable (or reusable if properly cleaned) sensor attached to a portable recording machine. More sophisticated capnometers and capnographs that continuously monitor carbon dioxide concentrations during each breath are used in operating rooms and intensive care units to monitor the patient's respiratory, metabolic, and ventilation to perfusion ratios.[3]

    d.   Chest radiograph confirmation.

3.   Inflate the cuff, if not already inflated, and secure endotracheal tube.

H.   Pulse Oximetry

Pulse oximetry is an available method to monitor a patient's oxygen saturation or the percentage of hemoglobin saturated with oxygen (SpO_2). Pulse oximeters do not measure oxygen tension (PO_2) or alveolar ventilation. However, the oxyhemoglobin dissociation curve demonstrates that when the PO_2 is 60 mmHg (8 KPa) the oxygen saturation is approximately 90%, and when the PO_2 is 40 mmHg (5.3 KPa), the oxygen saturation is approximately 75%. Normally, 98% of hemoglobin is saturated with oxygen. At the higher range of oxygen saturation, i.e., 94 to 98%, the oxyhemoglobin dissociation curve is relatively flat. Therefore, a small change in oxygen saturation could correlate with significant changes in oxygen tension. The usefulness of pulse oximetry is related to detection of "unsuspected hypoxemia."[4]

The pulse oximeter probe attached to the patient (usually to a finger) contains light-emitting diodes (LEDs), a photo diode, and a microprocessor that interprets the amount of light in the sensor during a pulse beat. The oxygen saturation is calculated by the oximeter based on the differential absorption of light by the patient's oxyhemoglobin. The probe attached to the patient is connected by a cord to a machine that digitally displays the SpO_2 and the pulse (which is also audible).

Pulse oximetry has certain limitations related to conditions that may not generate an adequate signal, e.g., vasoconstriction, hypothermia, malplacement of the probe, or low tissue perfusion. Additionally, certain circumstances may be interpreted by the oximeter as pulsations, e.g., flickering fluorescent lights, hand tremors, or positive pressure ventilation.[4-6] Methemoglobin (oxidation of the iron molecule in the blood from the ferrous to the ferric state caused by injury or toxic substances) and carboxyhemoglobin (hemoglobin combined with carbon monoxide) cannot be distinguished from oxyhemoglobin. If any dyshemoglobin is suspected, monitor blood gases, pH, and oxygen saturation from arterial blood samples.

Advantages of pulse oximetry:

1.   Noninvasive and painless.

2.   Portable, lightweight, and compact.

3. Less costly as compared to arterial blood gases.

4. Adjunct for monitoring the need for intubation, or deterioration or improvement of a patient's respiratory status.

5. Can be attached to a finger, earlobe, toe, corner of the mouth, or other available body part.

I.   Surgical airway access

1. In the rare event that endotracheal intubation cannot be performed, surgical cricothyroidotomy may be considered. This procedure is indicated when intubation is necessary but not possible or is contraindicated, i.e., massive facial trauma, fractured larynx or severe oropharyngeal hemorrhage which obstructs the glottic opening. This procedure is not recommended in children under age 12.[7]

   Surgical cricothyoidotomy is accomplished by making an incision into the cricothyroid membrane (see Figure 41) and inserting an endotracheal or tracheostomy tube into the trachea.

2. When intubation or surgical, cricothyroidotomy are contraindicated or not possible, needle cricothyroidotomy is performed to establish a temporary airway. A large-bore (12- or 14-gauge) over-the-needle intravenous catheter is inserted through the cricothyroid membrane (see Figures 42 and 43).

Figure 41
Anterior Cervical Anatomy of the Larynx and Trachea

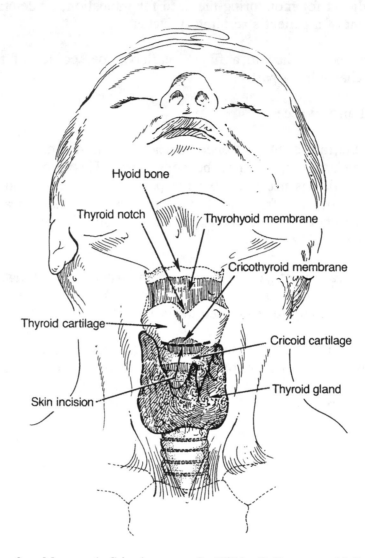

(Reprinted with permission from Moncure A. Cricothyrotomy. In: Wilkins E. *Emergency Medicine Scientific Foundations and Current Practice*. Baltimore, Md: Williams & Wilkins; 1989:997.)

Figure 42
Needle Cricothyroidotomy

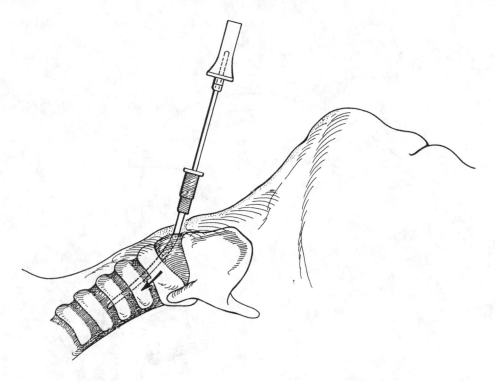

(Reprinted with permission from McCabe C. Needle cricothyrotomy. In: Wilkins E. *Emergency Medicine Scientific Foundations and Current Practice*. Baltimore, Md: Williams & Wilkins; 1989:999.)

3. There are several ventilation methods which may be used. Transtracheal jet insufflation provides a temporary means of providing oxygen and ventilation to the patient with an airway obstruction until a definitive airway is established. The transtracheal jet insufflation technique consists of inserting a large-bore plastic over-the-needle catheter (12- or 14-gauge), through the cricothyroid membrane. The needle is inserted at a 45-degree angle into the trachea, below the oropharyngeal obstruction. Using a plastic "Y" connecting device inserted into the over-the-needle catheter, oxygen is delivered at a high pressure (30 - 60 psi) in an intermittent fashion (one insufflation every five seconds).[1,5,7] Since inadequate exhalation results in the patient gradually retaining carbon dioxide, transtracheal jet insufflation should be used for a limited time (not to exceed 45 minutes), especially in the patient with alterations in consciousness. Observe the patient for any signs of complications associated with high pressure ventilation (e.g., tension pneumothorax).[7]

J. Learners should practice skills as desired.

Figure 43
Intravenous Catheter in Position

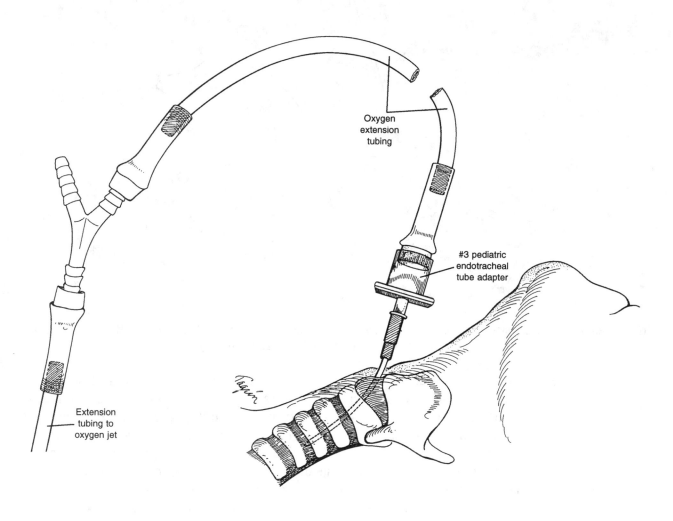

Oxygen
extension
tubing

#3 pediatric
endotracheal
tube adapter

Extension
tubing to
oxygen jet

(Reprinted with permission from McCabe C. Needle cricothyrotomy. In: Wilkins E. *Emergency Medicine Scientific Foundations and Current Practice.* Baltimore, Md: Williams & Wilkins; 1989:1000.)

418

III. Steps in Skill Performance

The learners will be presented with a case scenario and asked to demonstrate and/or describe airway and ventilation assessments and appropriate interventions.

TEACHING CASE: "A trauma patient arrives in the emergency department unresponsive but breathing. Cervical spine immobilization is being maintained. Please proceed with your assessment and appropriate interventions."

1. Assesses airway patency; AND if unconscious, manually opens the airway using a jaw thrust or chin lift maneuver (at least three of the following):**

   - Vocalization

   - Tongue obstruction

   - Loose teeth or foreign objects

   - Bleeding

   - Vomitus or other secretions

   - Edema

2. Suctions the airway.**

3. Reassesses airway patency.

4. Inserts an oral or nasal airway.

   - Determines the correct size.

   - Demonstrates proper insertion technique.

5. Reassesses airway patency.

6. Assesses breathing effectiveness (at least three of the following):**

   - Spontaneous breathing

   - Rise and fall of the chest wall

   - Skin color

   - General rate and depth of respirations

   - Soft tissue and bony chest wall integrity

- Use of accessory and/or abdominal muscles

- Bilateral breath sounds

- Jugular veins and position of trachea

7. Demonstrates bag-valve-mask ventilation.**

8. Assesses effectiveness of bag-valve-mask ventilation.

    - Chest rise and fall

    - Skin color

9. Auscultates over the epigastrium while observing for rise and fall of the chest, with bag-valve ventilations continued.

10. Removes endotracheal tube and hyperventilates the patient via bag-valve-mask.**

11. Auscultates over the epigastrium while observing for rise and fall of the chest, with bag-valve ventilations continued.

12. Auscultates breath sounds.

13. Inflates the endotracheal tube cuff.

14. States need to secure endotracheal tube and continue ventilation.

IV. **Summary**

A. The Airway and Ventilation Interventions Skill Station presents learners with information regarding the assessment of and interventions for airway and ventilation. The learner will be evaluated on the ability to apply this information to a case scenario. The learner must demonstrate all ** steps and 70% of the total points.

B. Critical step review

Critical steps as indicated by **

There are five critical steps that must be demonstrated and/or described. These are designated with double asterisks (**) on the evaluation form.

1. Assesses airway patency; **AND** if unconscious, manually opens the airway using a jaw thrust or chin lift maneuver.

2. Suctions the airway.

3. Assesses breathing effectiveness.

4. Demonstrates bag-valve-mask ventilation.

5. Removes endotracheal tube and hyperventilates the patient via bag-valve-mask.

C. Principles and points to remember

1. The first priority in trauma care is the establishment of a patent airway.

2. Avoid nasal airways in patients with severe head and/or facial trauma.

3. Do not use oropharyngeal airways in a patient with a gag reflex.

4. To confirm endotracheal placement auscultate over the epigastrium while observing for rise and fall of the chest wall. If the chest rises and falls symmetrically and gastric insufflation is not heard, auscultate the lungs at the second intercostal space, midclavicular line and at the fifth intercostal space anterior axillary line bilaterally.

5. Breath sounds that are consistently louder on one side despite efforts at repositioning the endotracheal tube may signal a pneumothorax or hemothorax.

6. Ventilate the patient between all intubation attempts.

REFERENCES

1. Heckman JD. Ventilation equipment and oxygen therapy. In: Heckman JD, ed. *Emergency Care and Transportation of the Sick and Injured.* 5th ed. Park Ridge, Ill: American Academy of Orthopaedic Surgeons; 1992:166-185.

2. Emergency Cardiac Care Committee and Subcommittees, American Heart Association. Guidelines for cardiopulmonary resuscitation and emergency cardiac care. *JAMA.* 1992;268:16:2202.

3. Bongard FS, Sue DY. Critical care monitoring. In: Bongard FS, Sue DY, eds. *Current Critical Care Diagnosis and Treatment.* Norwalk, Conn: Appleton & Lange; 1994:170-190.

4. Severinghaus JW, Kelleher JF. Recent development in pulse oximetry. *Anesthesiology.* 1992;76:1018-1038.

5. Dailey RH. Respiratory adjuncts: diagnostic. In: Dailey RH, Simon B, Young GP, Stewart RD, eds. *The Airway: Emergency Management.* St. Louis, Mo: Mosby-Year Book; 1992:210-215.

6. Padolina RM, Siler JN. Monitoring for trauma anesthesia. In: Grande CM, ed. *Textbook of Trauma Anesthesia and Critical Care.* St. Louis, Mo: Mosby-Year Book; 1993:432-444.

7. American College of Surgeons Committee on Trauma. *Advanced Trauma Life Support® Course for Physicians (Student Manual).* 5th ed. Chicago, Ill: Author; 1993.

AIRWAY AND VENTILATION

Evaluation Form

TEACHING CASE: A trauma patient arrives in the emergency department unresponsive but breathing. Cervical spine stabilization is being maintained. Please proceed with your assessment and appropriate interventions.

Instructor Responses	Skill Steps	Demonstrated		
		Yes		No
	1. Assesses airway patency; AND if unconscious, manually opens the airway using a jaw thrust or chin lift (at least three of the following)	** _____		_____
Does not vocalize	• Vocalization			
No obstruction. Bleeding is noted from a laceration.	• Tongue obstruction			
No loose teeth or foreign objects, bleeding is noted	• Loose teeth or foreign objects			
Blood is present in the oropharynx	• Bleeding			
Secretions are present in the oropharynx	• Vomitus or other secretions			
No edema noted	• Edema			
	2. Suctions the airway	** _____		_____
"I have suctioned the airway."				
Patient remains unresponsive. There is no further blood or secretions in the oropharynx.	3. Reassesses airway patency	_____		_____
	4. Inserts an oral or nasal airway	_____		_____
	• Determines the correct size			
	• Demonstrates proper insertion technique			
Airway is patent	5. Reassesses airway patency	_____		_____
	6. Assesses breathing effectiveness (at least three of the following)	** _____		_____
Present, shallow, and labored	• Spontaneous breathing			
Symmetrical, but shallow	• Rise and fall of the chest wall			
Dusky	• Skin color			
Slow, rate 8 breaths/minute and shallow	• General rate and depth of respirations			
No open wounds, chest wall intact	• Soft tissue and bony chest wall integrity			

Instructor Responses	Skill Steps	Demonstrated	
		Yes	No
Accessory muscle use present Markedly diminished bilaterally No jugular venous distention, trachea midline	• **Use of accessory and/or abdominal muscles** • **Bilateral breath sounds** • **Jugular veins and position of trachea**		
	7. **Demonstrates bag-valve-mask ventilation**	** ⎯⎯	⎯⎯
	8. **Assesses effectiveness of bag-valve-mask ventilation** • **Chest rise and fall** • **Skin color**	⎯⎯	⎯⎯
"There is good rise and fall of the chest with assisted ventilations. Skin is pale. The physician elects to intubate the patient due to the decreased level of consciousness. Intubation has just been accomplished. What is your next step?"			
No rise and fall of chest, gurgling sounds are heard over the epigastrium with assisted ventilation	9. **Auscultates over the epigastrium while observing for rise and fall of the chest wall, with bag-valve ventilations continued.**	⎯⎯	⎯⎯
	10. **Removes endotracheal tube and hyper-ventilates the patient via bag-valve-mask**	** ⎯⎯	⎯⎯
"The intubation is repeated."			
No gurgling sounds over the epigastrium, bilateral rise and fall of the chest is observed with assisted ventilation.	11. **Auscultates over the epigastrium while observing for rise and fall of the chest, with bag-valve ventilations continued.**	⎯⎯	⎯⎯
Breath sounds are equal and clear bilaterally	12. **Auscultates breath sounds**	⎯⎯	⎯⎯
	13. **Inflates the endotracheal tube cuff**	⎯⎯	⎯⎯
	14. **States need to secure endotracheal tube and continue ventilation**	⎯⎯	⎯⎯

SPINAL IMMOBILIZATION SKILL STATION

I. **Introduction**

A. Instructor and learner introductions

B. Purpose

Each learner will demonstrate the appropriate method for spinal immobilization with the patient strapped in a supine position on a backboard with a cervical collar.

C. Format

1. The Instructor will discuss and demonstrate:

a. Principles of spinal immobilization.

b. Importance of the leader in directing the procedure and instructing three assistants.

b. Application of a rigid cervical collar.

d. Logrolling using three assistants.

e. Securing the patient to the backboard.

2. The learners will practice:

a. Application of a rigid collar.

b. Logrolling using three assistants.

c. Securing the patient to the backboard.

3. Each learner rotates through the leader position. Learners should rotate as the patient on teaching day unless contraindicated or they have a strong preference not to be the patient.

D. Evaluation

1. Each learner will be evaluated while performing the leader role.

2. All critical steps (*) must be demonstrated.

3. At least 70% of the total points must be demonstrated.

4. At the completion of the learners demonstration, the learner will be asked if there is anything he or she wants to add or revise.

II. Principles of Spinal Immobilization

A. General principles

1. The leader is responsible for **VERBALLY** directing the procedure and instructing assistants.

2. The leader is responsible for stabilizing the patient's cervical spine during logrolling.

3. Three assistants are required to perform this skill utilizing the team approach.

4. All unresponsive trauma patients must be immobilized.

5. Thoroughly evaluate all patients by radiographs and physical exam prior to removal of any spinal immobilization devices.

6. Keep the vertebral column aligned and immobilized.

7. Cervical collars alone do not immobilize the cervical spine. The head and torso must also be immobilized to prevent flexion, extension, rotation, and lateral movements.

8. In actual patient care, all personnel who anticipate direct patient contact or contact with the patient's body fluids must wear gown, gloves, masks, and eye protection. (NOTE: Since TNCC skill stations are simulated situations, the use of personal protective equipment is optional.)

B. Indications:

1. Any patient whose mechanism of injury, symptoms, or physical findings suggest a spinal injury.

2. The following are associated with potential spinal injury:

a. Mechanism of injury:

1) Motor vehicle crash

2) Falls

3) Diving injury

426

4) Near-drowning

5) Direct force applied to spine or head

6) Missile and other penetrating trauma to spine

7) Ejection from vehicle

8) Spontaneous structural failure from pre-existing bone disease

b. Symptoms:

1) Neck pain and tenderness: posterior or anterior

2) Occipital headache

3) Back pain

4) Paresthesia

5) Paralysis/weakness

c. Physical findings:

1) Head injury: laceration, contusion, hematoma, fracture

2) Alteration in level of consciousness

3) Edema and tenderness over spine

4) Muscle spasm of neck/back/shoulders

5) Penetrating wounds of neck or vertebral column

6) Impaled object in neck or vertebral column

7) Respiratory compromise

8) Loss of urinary and/or sphincter tone

9) Bradycardia and hypotension

C.   Contraindications:

    1.   Patients with a compromised airway (e.g., facial trauma) who sit up and lean forward, or stand and lean over, must not be forced to immediately lie down. Prepare for immediate and definitive control of their airways.

    2.   Insufficient number of assistants.

III.   Steps in Skill Performance

A.   Leader takes position at head of patient and positions hands on each side of head, with thumbs along mandible and fingers behind the head on the occipital ridge. Maintain gentle but firm stabilization of the neck throughout the entire procedure. The leader briefly explains to the patient what to expect and not to move head or neck.

B.   Leader asks patient to wiggle his or her toes and fingers, **OR** gently lift an arm and a leg, and determines if sensation is present.

C.   While maintaining firm control of patient's head (see #1), the leader assigns the assistants to locations beside the patient's body.

    1.   Assistant 1 – near the patient's head and upper body.

    2.   Assistant 2 – beside Assistant 1, near the patient's hips and legs.

    3.   Assistant 3 – opposite side of patient.

D.   Leader directs Assistant 1 to remove the jewelry (earrings, necklace).

E.   Leader directs Assistant 1 to apply and secure an appropriate-sized rigid cervical collar. A properly fitted collar will fit between the point of the chin and the suprasternal notch, resting on the clavicles and supporting the lower jaw. The Stifneck collar is one type of rigid collar. To properly size and apply a Stifneck collar:

    1.   Determine the appropriate size by measuring from the patient's chin to the shoulder. Place your fingers on top of the shoulder where the collar will rest and measure the distance to the point of the chin (not the angle of the jaw). Compare this distance on the collar by placing the same number of fingers below the black fastener. The correct size collar is equal to the measurement between the black fastener and the edge of the rigid plastic at the bottom of the collar (not the foam portion of the collar).

    2.   Assemble the collar by moving the chin piece up and snapping the black fastener into the hole on the side of the collar.

    3.   Preform the collar.

4. Slide the back portion of the collar under the patient's neck until the velcro can be seen on the patient's other side.

5. Slide the collar up the sternum until the chin piece fits snugly under the chin.

6. Secure and fasten the velcro.

F. Leader directs Assistant 2 to straighten patient's arms at patient's side and to straighten legs.

G. On the count of three, the leader directs Assistants 1 and 2 to roll the patient as a unit towards them onto the patient's side. Leader monitors the alignment (nose with umbilicus) continually rather than watching backboard placement.

H. Leader directs Assistant 3 to position backboard on its side up against the patient's back.

I. On the count of three, the leader directs Assistants 1 and 2 to gently roll the patient as a unit onto the backboard as Assistant 3 guides the board.

J. Leader maintains stabilization of head until the straps are correctly placed. Leader directs assistants to place straps to encircle the patient and backboard at the shoulders, hips, and proximal to the knees.

K. Leader directs Assistants to place head support devices (i.e., towel rolls, or rigid foam blocks) on either side of head. Secures the head to the backboard with tape to prevent movement of head. Tape is NOT placed across chin.

L. Leader continually maintains manual stabilization of the head and neck until the head is immobilized. Once the head is immobilized, leader may remove hands from patient's head.

M. Leader reassesses motor and sensory function.

IV. **Summary**

A. The Spinal Immobilization skill station allows learners to practice the technique of manual stabilization of a patient's neck while directing assistants to complete spinal immobilization. The learner must demonstrate all * steps and 70% of the total points.

B. Critical step review

Critical steps are indicated by an asterisk (*).

There are four critical steps that must be demonstrated and/or described. These steps are designated with an * on the evaluation form.

1. Demonstrates control by stabilizing patient's head with hands and informs patient not to move neck or turn head.

2. On the count of three, directs logrolling of patient up onto side.

3. On the count of three, directs logrolling of patient down onto backboard.

4. Continually maintains manual stabilization of head and neck until head support devices are properly secured.

C. Principles and points to remember

1. An unresponsive trauma patient is assumed to have a spinal injury until definitive evaluation is completed.

2. Absence of fracture on a lateral cervical spine radiograph does not necessarily rule out cervical spine injury.

3. If a patient is transported to the emergency department on a scoop-type stretcher, first place a long backboard on the emergency department stretcher. The patient on the scoop-type stretcher can then be placed on top of the backboard.

4. A patient with suspected spinal injury or in a high-risk category for spinal injury who is not on a backboard, needs to be first evaluated for life-threatening injuries.

5. Avoid logrolling the patient onto the side with a suspected extremity injury.

6. Position the pregnant trauma patient on a backboard, tilted 15 to 20 degrees to the left.

SPINAL IMMOBILIZATION

Evaluation Form

Skill Steps	Demonstrated	Not Demonstrated
1. Stabilizes patient's head **AND** informs patient not to move neck or turn head	*	
2. Determines motor **AND** sensory function		
3. Assigns assistants to appropriate areas of patient's body		
4. Directs Assistant 1 to remove jewelry		
5. Directs Assistant 1 to apply and secure appropriate-sized rigid cervical collar		
6. Directs Assistant 2 to place patient's arms at sides and to straighten legs		
7. Directs logrolling of patient onto side (on count of 3)	*	
8. Directs Assistant 3 to position backboard		
9. Directs logrolling of patient down onto the backboard	*	
10. Describes correct placement of backboard straps		
11. Directs correct placement of head support devices and tape		
12. Continually maintains manual stabilization of head/neck until head support	*	
13. Reassesses motor **AND** sensory function		

SKILL PERFORMANCE RESULTS

Course Participant _____

Evaluator _____

Total Possible Demonstrated Points   =   13

   Learner Demonstrated Points   = ___

Demonstrated all ** Steps   ☐ Yes   ☐ No

Evaluator Recommendation (Check One)

☐   Station successfully completed
   - At least 9 out of 13 points
   - All * critical steps demonstrated

☐   Incomplete, needs minimal instruction before re-evaluation

☐   Incomplete, needs considerable instruction before re-evaluation

Potential Instructor   ☐ Yes   ☐ No

CHEST TRAUMA
INTERVENTIONS SKILL STATION

I. Introduction

A. Instructor and learner introductions

B. Purpose

The Instructor will demonstrate and describe the indications, contraindications, and management of patients with needle thoracentesis and chest drainage systems. Each learner will be given the opportunity to practice based on personal learning needs.

C. Format

1. The Instructor will discuss and demonstrate:

a. Needle thoracentesis.

b. Nurse's role in chest tube insertion.

c. Management of chest drainage systems using patient situations.

d. Autotransfusion: This section of the station is an optional component.

2. The learners will practice any of the above skills based on personal learning needs.

D. Teaching station only.

II. Principles of Chest Trauma Interventions

A. General principles

1. A needle thoracentesis may be required to rapidly correct a tension pneumothorax.

2. A chest tube thoracostomy is required to evacuate air or blood from the pleural cavity.

3. Autotransfusion is a procedure to transfuse patients with their own shed blood.

4. Preparation and maintenance of chest drainage systems is a nursing responsibility. Trauma nurses must be familiar with the specific chest drainage units and autotransfusion systems used at their facilities.

5. In actual patient care, all personnel who anticipate direct patient contact or contact with the patient's body fluids must wear personal protective equipment. (NOTE: Since TNCC skill stations are simulated situations, the use of personal protective equipment is optional.)

B. Needle thoracentesis

1. Indications: A tension pneumothorax. Signs and symptoms include respiratory distress, hypotension, hypoxia, unilaterally decreased or absent breath sounds, jugular venous distention, and tracheal shift. Cardiac arrest may result if a tension pneumothorax is not promptly decompressed.

2. Precautions:

   a. In the absence of a tension pneumothorax, a needle thoracentesis may create a pneumothorax or injure the lung.[1]

   b. Diaphragmatic rupture with herniation of abdominal contents into the thoracic cavity may mimic a pneumothorax. Needle thoracentesis is not indicated and, if performed, may result in intestinal content contamination of the pleural cavity.[2]

3. Steps in skill performance

   a. Identify the insertion site

   The insertion site is the second intercostal space, midclavicular line. Insert the needle on the same side as the decreased/absent breath sounds, and on the opposite side of the tracheal shift.

   b. Insert the needle

   Insert a 14-gauge over-the-needle catheter, 3 to 6 cm in length, over the top of the third rib into the pleural space until air escapes. Air should exit under pressure. Remove the needle and leave the catheter in place until replaced by a chest tube.

   c. Prepare for chest tube insertion since needle thoracentesis is a temporary measure.

C. Chest tube insertion and chest drainage systems

1. Indications: Open or closed pneumothorax or hemothorax. Signs and symptoms of pneumothorax include respiratory distress, decreased or absent breath sounds, and hyperresonance on the injured side. Hemothorax has similar signs and symptoms except percussion produces dullness. Chest tubes may also be inserted in patients with "substantial chest injury" who require positive pressure ventilation or those who require transfer to another facility.[3]

434

2. Contraindications: The only contraindication is the need for an immediate open thoracotomy.

3. Chest drainage systems: If air or blood accumulates in the pleural cavity, negative pressure is lost and the lung collapses. The therapeutic goal of drainage devices is restoration of negative pressure. There are two types of chest drainage systems:

   a. In underwater systems, the water in the water seal chamber has a one-way valve allowing blood or air to escape while preventing backflow.

   b. The waterless drainage systems have a mechanical valve in place of water, to allow blood and/or air drainage. The one-way valve prevents backflow.

4. Steps in skill performance

   a. Preparing the patient

      1) Administer analgesic medications as prescribed.

      2) Document patient's respiratory status, including breath sounds, prior to the procedure.

   b. Inserting the chest tube

      1) Assemble the chest drainage unit, per manufacturer's directions, by placing sterile water in the water seal chamber (if necessary) and in the suction chamber (if necessary).

      2) Ensure the patient has at least one large-bore intravenous catheter infusing a crystalloid solution.

      3) Assist with chest tube insertion by positioning the patient supine, with the head of the bed elevated 45° (if possible) and the arm over the head. Clean the insertion site, fourth or fifth intercostal space, anterior or midaxillary line.

   c. Securing the chest tube

      1) After the chest tube is inserted, connect the chest tube to the drainage tubing.

      2) Attach suction chamber tubing to wall suction. In water systems, regulate the wall suction to maintain a gentle continuous bubbling action.

3) Tape all tubing connections between the patient and underwater seal or chest drainage unit to prevent inadvertent disconnection.

d. Applying a dressing. Apply a petroleum-impregnated, occlusive dressing (dressing may vary by institutional protocol), around the chest tube insertion site and cover with 4 x 4 gauze dressings. Apply tincture of benzoin and secure the tube with heavy tape.

e. Documenting correct tube placement. Obtain a chest radiograph to document correct tube placement

f. Managing a chest drainage system

1) Maintain the chest drainage unit below the level of the chest to facilitate the flow of drainage and prevent reflux into the chest cavity. With water seal chest drainage units, keep the unit upright to prevent the loss of the water seal.

2) The tubing should be gently coiled without dependent loops or kinks.

3) Assess and document fluctuation, output, color of drainage, and air leak (FOCA).

4) Consider notifying the physician if initial chest drainage output is > 1,500 ml or a there is continued blood loss > 200 ml/hour.

g. Assessing for an air leak

1) The water level in the water seal chamber should gently rise and fall with each breath. Assess for an air leak by looking for bubbling in the water seal chamber. Constant bubbling in the water seal chamber indicates an air leak either in the lung or in the chest drainage unit or tubing.

2) An air leak is an expected finding with an unexpanded lung.

3) Leaks may originate from[5]:

- The chest tube drainage system.

- A continued air leak in the lung.

- Injury to the esophagus or bronchus.

- A malpositioned chest tube.

436

4) If an air leak is suspected, assess that all connections are tight. Turn off suction and reassess after one minute.

5) To assess the location of the leak, intermittently occlude the chest tube or drainage tubing beginning at the dressing site, progressing to the chest drainage unit, if needed. If the bubbling in the water seal chamber immediately stops when the chest tube is occluded at the dressing site, the air leak is inside the patient's chest or under the dressing. Reinforce the occlusive dressing and notify the physician.[4]

6) If the bubbling does not stop when the chest tube is occluded at the dressing site, continue to intermittently occlude down the tubing at various positions until the bubbling stops. When the bubbling stops, the air leak is between the occlusion and the patient's chest.

7) If the bubbling does not stop with occlusion, replace the chest drainage unit.

h. Assessing tube patency

If a clot is suspected, as when fresh bleeding suddenly stops or slows, gently manipulate the tube by squeezing the drainage tubing in a proximal to distal direction. Do not squeeze the tube enough to collapse it as it may increase the negative pressure.[6,7] The need to dislodge a suspected clot is the only indication for squeezing the drainage tubing.[6,7]

i. Clamping chest tube

During patient transport, clamping of chest tubes is not necessary. Clamping a chest tube before the patient's lung is fully re-expanded may lead to the development of a tension pneumothorax.[4]

j. Using a one-way valve

A one-way valve is used primarily during transport to ensure one-way drainage in the event the chest drainage unit is damaged or placed above the level of the chest. The one-way valve may also be used temporarily until a chest drainage unit is obtained. In addition, it is sometimes used instead of a chest drainage unit for a small, spontaneous pneumothorax (see Figure 44).[4]

Figure 44
One-Way Valve

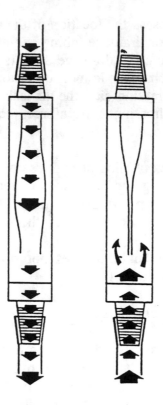

(Reprinted with permission from Besson A, Saegesser F. Pleural drainage. In: Besson A, Saegesser F, eds. *Color Atlas of Chest Trauma and Associated Injuries. Volume One.* Oradell, NJ: Medical Economics Books; 1983:224.)

D. Chest drainage system problems to discuss

Problems	Interventions
• Patient returns from radiology. • Drainage unit is between patient's legs. • Patient is dyspneic.	• Lower chest drainage unit. • Assess patient's respiratory distress and auscultate breath sounds. • Ensure correct water levels are present in the water-seal and suction chambers.
• Patient pulls out chest tube.	• Apply a petroleum-impregnated dressing; tape the dressing on three sides. • Auscultate breath sounds and assess for the development of a pneumothorax. • Notify the physician.
• Substantial increase in bloody drainage.	• Notify physician. • Prepare for operative intervention as indicated.
• Sudden decrease or no drainage in collection chamber.	• Assess tubing for kinks. • Assess for obstruction by clots.
• No bubbling in water-seal chamber	• Consider the lung has re-expanded.
• Drainage unit was tipped over. • Water in suction control chamber is below desired level.	• Add water to the suction chamber.
• While patient is transferred from one bed to another, chest tube disconnects from chest drainage unit.	• Change the drainage unit. • Consider temporary use of a Heimlich valve.
• Patient develops sudden onset of dyspnea.	• Assess for the development of a tension pneumothorax. • Assess integrity of system.

E. Autotransfusion

1. Indications: To transfuse patients with their own shed blood. In the emergency department, autotransfusion is usually limited to blood drained from a hemothorax. In significant chest trauma, autotransfusion should be anticipated and the collection device prepared before chest tube insertion, if possible.

2. Precautions/contraindications:

   a) Blood contaminated with bowel contents or infection at the site of blood retrieval. Blood salvaged from a bacteria-contaminated cavity is considered in dire emergencies or when no alternative source of blood is available.[8,9]

   b) Blood potentially contaminated with malignant cells.[8,9]

   c) Injuries from four to six hours old.[5]

   d) Autotransfusion greater than 50% of patient's estimated blood loss.[5]

   e) Carefully consider autotransfusion in patients with hepatic or renal dysfunction.

3. Steps in skill performance

   a. Assemble the chest drainage unit and autotransfusion device per manufacturer's directions.

   b. Instill anticoagulant, if prescribed.

      Citrate phosphate dextrose (CPD) is the most common anticoagulant. The recommended amount is 1 ml of CPD for every 7 to 10 ml of blood collected. CPD prevents clot formation; however, it does not dissolve clots. Since the amount of blood cannot be measured prior to collection, it is best to instill 60 to 70 ml of CPD into the autotransfusion collection chamber. When one unit of blood (approximately 500 ml) has been collected, it may be transfused. If not, an additional 60 to 70 ml of CPD may be instilled in preparation for additional blood collection.[5]

   c. Prepare to return the collected blood per manufacturer's directions. Avoid infusion of the collected blood under high pressure infusion to prevent hemolysis.

E. Learners practice skills as desired.

III. Summary

A. The Chest Trauma Interventions station reviews information and skills pertinent to the management of patients with thoracic trauma.

B. Critical step review

   1. Identifies correct insertion site for needle thoracentesis.

2. Correctly places sterile water into the water seal drainage chamber if necessary.

3. Applies an appropriate dressing to the chest tube insertion site.

4. Positions the chest drainage unit and tubing below the level of the patient.

5. Describes indications and contraindications for clamping of chest tubes.

C. Principles and points to remember

1. Clamping a chest tube is contraindicated as it may precipitate the development of a tension pneumothorax.

2. Obtain chest radiographs following chest tube insertion to document tube placement and verify lung re-expansion.

3. Avoid squeezing the chest tube to the point of collapse as it may cause lung injury.

D. Skill station steps summary

1. Needle thoracentesis

   a. Identifies the insertion site.

   b. Describes insertion of the needle.

   c. States needle thoracentesis is a temporary measure and chest tube placement should be anticipated.

2. Chest tube insertion and chest drainage units

   a. Assembles the chest drainage unit.

   b. Assists with the chest tube insertion.

   c. Connects chest drainage unit to chest tube.

   d. Connects chest drainage unit to suction.

   e. Describes appropriate dressing for insertion site.

   f. Describes assessment for air leak.

   g. Describes indications/contraindications for squeezing chest tubes.

   h. Describes indications/contraindications for clamping chest tubes.

441

  i. Describes indications and use of a one-way valve.

3. Autotransfusion

  a. Identifies indications for autotransfusion.

  b. Identifies contraindications to autotransfusion.

  c. Prepares the autotransfusion unit for blood collection.

  d. Describes use of anticoagulant.

  e. Prepares autotransfusion unit to reinfuse blood.

REFERENCES

1. American College of Surgeons Committee on Trauma. Chest trauma management. In: *Advanced Trauma Life Support® Course for Physicians (Student manual)*. 5th ed. Chicago, Ill: Author; 1993:135-140.

2. Taylor LD. Needle thoracostomy. In: Proehl JA, ed. *Adult Emergency Nursing Procedures*. Boston, Mass: Jones and Bartlett; 1993:129-131.

3. American College of Surgeons Committee on Trauma. Thoracic trauma. In: *Advanced Trauma Life Support Course® for Physicians (Students Manual)*. 5th ed. Chicago, Ill: Author; 1993:111-125.

4. Gray MD. Management of chest drainage systems. In: Proehl JA, ed. *Adult Emergency Nursing Procedures*. Boston, Mass: Jones and Bartlett; 1993:136-137.

5. Bickell W, Pepe PE, Mattox KL. Complications of resuscitation. In: Mattox KL, ed. *Complications of Trauma*. New York, NY: Churchill Livingstone; 1994:101-138.

6. Erickson RS. Mastering the ins and outs of chest drainage: part 2. *Nursing*. 1989;19:46-49.

7. Duncan C, Erickson R. Pressures associated with chest tube stripping. *Heart Lung*. 1982;11:166-171.

8. American Medical Association Council on Scientific Affairs. Autologous blood transfusions. *JAMA*. 1986;256:2378-2380.

9. American Association of Blood Banks. *Guidelines for Blood Salvage and Reinfusion in Surgery and Trauma*. Bethesda, Md: Author; 1993:1-9.

CHEST DRAINAGE SYSTEM MANUFACTURERS

To receive specific product information, the manufacturers of chest drainage systems can be contacted directly at the addresses listed below.

Thora-Klex®

> Davol, Inc.
> P.O. Box 8500
> Cranston, RI 02920
> Phone: (800) 556-6275

Pleur-evac®

> Deknatel, Inc.
> P.O.Box 2980
> Fall River, MA 02722-8600
> Phone: (800) 843-8600

Atrium®

> Atrium Medical Corporation
> 17 Clinton Drive
> Hollis, NH 03049
> Phone: (800) 528-7486

Thora-Seal®

> Sherwood Medical
> 1815 Olive Street
> St. Louis, MO 63103
> Phone: (800) 428-4400

TRACTION SPLINT SKILL STATION

I. Introduction

A. Instructor and learner introductions

B. Purpose

Each learner will demonstrate the application of a traction splint on the leg.

C. Format

1. The Instructor will discuss and demonstrate the principles of traction splinting and application of a traction splint.

2. Learners will practice application of a specific traction splint utilized in their geographical area.

D. Teaching station only.

II. Principles of Traction Splinting

A. General principles

1. Life-threatening injuries must be assessed and treated first.

2. Fractures of the femur may result in:

   a. Spasms of the large muscles of the thigh.

   b. Significant deformity of the extremity with shortening of the affected limb.

   c. Significant blood, 500 to 1,000 ml, can be lost and may result in hypovolemic shock. The application of a traction splint can help to decrease blood loss by stabilizing the injury and alleviate pain by decreasing muscle spasm.

3. Countertraction is applied to produce enough opposing force to stabilize the leg and prevent further injury, not to realign ends of fractured bones.[1] Traction devices hold the fracture immobile by securing the device proximally in the groin area, attaching an ankle hitch, and then applying traction. Once traction has been applied to an extremity, do not release traction until definitive care has begun.

4. An assistant is required to perform this skill.

5. Consider pain control measures prior to application of the splint, after excluding other injuries and based upon hemodynamic status.

6. Assess distal neurovascular status before and after splinting. If neurovascular function is present before, but not after splinting, remove the splinting device and resplint.

7. Do not attempt to reposition protruding bone ends. If the bone ends retract under the skin while traction is being applied, do not apply any further traction. If a wound is present, it should be covered with a dry, sterile dressing.

8. A backboard supports the hip and facilitates moving a patient with a traction splint.

9. If the patient arrives with a traction splint, assure neurovascular function distal to the injury is intact, and leave the splint in place until radiographic studies and care are completed.

10. Radiographs can be taken with the splint in place.

11. In actual patient care, all personnel who anticipate direct patient contact or contact with the patient's body fluids must wear personal protective equipment. (NOTE: Since TNCC skill stations are simulated situations, the use of personal protective equipment is optional.)

B. Indications: A traction splint is indicated to align and stabilize a fracture of the femur or proximal tibia.[2]

C. Contraindications: Traction splints are not indicated for any other extremity fractures.

III. **Steps in Skill Performance**

A. Hare® traction splint

A Hare® traction splint consists of a metal frame with padded ischial bar, ratchet device, and a heel stand. Additional parts include an ankle hitch and elasticized velcro straps. A Hare® traction splint works by applying a padded device to the back of the pelvis or ischium. The leg is attached to the end of the splint by an ankle hitching device and countertraction is applied.[2]

1. Leader explains procedure to patient and assistant.

2. Assistant removes shoes and clothing from the leg.

3. Leader palpates pedal pulses in the injured extremity and asks patient to wiggle his or her toes, and determines if sensation is present.

4. Assistant measures and extends splint to proper length, locks it into position, and opens velcro straps. The splint is measured with the ring at the ischial tuberosity and the ratchet device extended eight to 12 inches beyond the foot.

5. Assistant places ankle hitch under the foot and crosses straps over the top of the foot.

6. Assistant applies traction; holds the dorsum of foot with one hand and the ankle and heel with the other hand.

7. Assistant gently applies traction and lifts leg just high enough so leader can slide splint under leg. Leader places top of padded bar against ischial tuberosity and pads groin as needed.

8. Assistant lowers the leg onto the splint.

9. Assistant maintains traction with hands while leader fastens ischial strap around leg.

10. Leader moves to foot and attaches ankle hitch to ratchet and turns ratchet until enough traction is applied to maintain limb alignment and relieve pain.

11. Leader asks patient for feedback regarding comfort of traction.

12. Leader fastens two velcro straps below the knee and two straps above the knee. Avoids the fracture site. The leader lowers heel stand into place to elevate the limb.

13. Leader reassesses neurovascular function.

B. Sager® splint

The Sager® splint is a splint placed along the medial aspect of the leg with a groin cushion fitting snugly against the groin and ischial tuberosity. The Sager® splint is light, compact, and consists of a metal bar with a padded arch support for the groin and an attached pulley and cable apparatus for the application of countertraction. Additional parts include an ankle strap, 6-inch wide elastic straps and a long narrow strap.[2]

1. Leader explains the procedure to patient and assistant.

2. Assistant removes shoes and clothing from the leg.

3. Assistant palpates pedal pulses in the injured extremity. Assistant asks patient to wiggle toes and determines if sensation is present.

4. Assistant applies traction by holding the dorsum of the foot with one hand and the heel and ankle with the other hand.

5. Leader prepares traction splint for application.

    a. Leader adjusts groin strap so the buckle will be over lateral thigh when fastened.

    b. Leader adjusts splint shaft to four inches past the heel, using the uninjured leg as a guide. The wheel of the pulley should be aligned with the heel.

    c. Leader prepares ankle strap to fit around lower leg just above the ankle. If the strap will not fit snugly, additional padding may be necessary.

6. The leader positions the splint in the patient's groin with the padded bar resting in the groin; avoid the external genitalia.

7. The leader secures the thigh strap.

8. The leader connects the ankle harness to the splint and applies the ankle harness around the injured leg just above the ankle. The loop of the ankle harness is shortened by pulling on the strap threaded through the buckle.

9. The leader extends the splint until the desired amount of traction registers on the pulley wheel markings. The appropriate amount of traction is based upon an approximation of the patient's body weight. (10% patient's body weight equated to pounds of tension, but no greater than 22 to 25 pounds).

10. Leader asks patient for feedback regarding comfort of traction.

11. Leader fastens 6-inch wide straps:

    a. Longest strap around the thigh.

    b. Second longest strap around the knee.

    c. Shortest strap around the ankle encompassing ankle harness and pole.

12. Leader fastens long narrow strap under ankles in a figure eight fashion to secure the splint.

13. Leader reassesses neurovascular function.

Alternate methods of Sager® splint application include placing the splint to the outside of leg if perineal injury or pelvic fracture is present and application of bilateral Sager® splints.

C. Thomas half-ring® splint

The Thomas half-ring® splint is a padded device applied to the back of the pelvis or ischium. The leg is attached to the end of the splint by an ankle hitching device and countertraction is applied.[2] The Thomas half-ring® splint consists of a metal frame with a padded ischial half-ring. Additional equipment needed are a minimum of 6 cravats and padding material.[2]

1. Leader explains procedure to patient and assistant.

2. Assistant removes shoes and clothing from the leg.

3. Assistant prepares metal frame by attaching four cravats to act as a sling.

4. Assistant palpates pedal pulses in the injured extremity. Assistant asks patient to wiggle his or her toes and determine if sensation is present.

5. Assistant applies traction by holding the dorsum of the foot with one hand and the heel and ankle with other hand.

6. Leader positions splint under the patient's leg with the padded half-ring facing down and the shorter side of the splint on the inside of the leg. The ring is fitted snugly under the hip against the ischial tuberosity.

7. Leader ties two support cravats above the knee and two below the knee.

8. Leader attaches top ring strap over the thigh and padding.

9. Leader applies padding to foot and ankle.

10. Leader applies traction hitch around foot and ankle and attaches it to the end of splint. Increase traction by forming a windlass action using a stick or tongue depressors.

11. Assistant gently transfers pull of traction from hands to traction pull of splint.

12. Leader asks patient for feedback regarding comfort of traction.

13. Leader reassesses neurovascular function.

D. Donway® splint

The Donway® splint is a variation of the Thomas half-ring® splint and can be applied by one person. Traction is applied through the use of a pneumatic pump.[2]

1. Leader explains procedure to patient and assistant (if used).

2. Leader supports the leg and maintains traction while an assistant removes shoes and clothing from the leg.

3. Assistant palpates pedal pulses in the injured extremity. Assistant asks patient to wiggle his or her toes and determines if sensation is present.

4. Assistant places the ischial ring under the knee, adjusts around the thigh, and fastens the buckle.

5. Assistant depresses the air release valve to ensure no excess pressure is retained in the system.

6. Assistant unlocks the collets, raises the footplate into the upright position, and then places the splint over the leg.

7. Assistant adjusts the sidearms of the splint to the proper length, attaches the ischial ring pegs, and locks the splint by turning the side arms.

8. Assistant applies ankle strap around the foot and ankle.

   a. Places the patient's heel in the padded portion of the strap with the foot against the footplate.

   b. Adjusts the lower velcro attachment to ensure the padded support member is positioned high on the ankle.

   c. Criss-crosses the top straps tightly over the instep starting with the longest strap.

   d. Tightens and secures the straps around the footplate.

9. Assistant applies pneumatic pressure with the pump up to the desired level of traction (the operating range of the splint is 10 to 40 pounds of traction). Tightens the strap to secure the ring in the ischial load-bearing position.

10. Leader releases manual traction and reassesses neurovascular function.

11. Leader aligns the opened leg supports with the calf and thigh. Feeds the leading tapered edge under the leg, over the top of the frame of the opposite side arm, and back under the leg. Adjusts the tension to provide the required support and secures with the button fastener.

12. Leader raises the heel stand.

13. Leader turns the collets until hand tight and applies a further quarter turn to lock the position of the side arms. Releases the pneumatic pressure device by depressing the air release valve until the gauge reads zero.

IV. Summary

A. The Traction Splint skill station reviews the principles and skills associated with application of a traction splint.

B. Critical step review

    1. Assesses neurovascular function distal to the injury before and after splinting.

    2. Demonstrates correct splint application.

C. Principles and points to remember

    1. Position patient on a backboard.

    2. Keep splint in place until definitive care is implemented if neurovascular status is intact.

    3. Keep splint in place during transport.

    4. Note the effectiveness of the interventions including pain control and stability of neurovascular function.

D. Skill station steps summary

    1. Identifies life-threatening problems first.

    2. Assesses neurovascular function distal to injury before splinting.

    3. Splints extremity correctly.

    4. Maintains traction once initiated until entire splint is applied.

    5. Reassesses neurovascular function distal to injury after splinting.

    6. Repositions extremity and/or splint in the presence of neurovascular compromise (cyanosis, no pulse, loss of sensation).

REFERENCES

1. Grant H, Murray R, Bergeron JD. Injuries II: The lower extremities. *Emergency Care.* 5th ed. Englewood Cliffs, NJ: Brady; 1990:267-293.

2. American College of Emergency Physicians. Using traction splints. *Basic Trauma Life Support: Advanced Prehospital Care.* 2nd ed. Englewood Cliffs, NJ: Brady; 1988:298-302.

HELMET REMOVAL SKILL STATION

I.   **Introduction**

A.   Instructor and learner introductions

B.   Purpose

Each learner will demonstrate the correct method to remove a supine patient's helmet while stabilizing the patient's head and cervical spine.

C.   Format

1.   The Instructor will discuss and demonstrate the principles of helmet removal and the correct method to remove a helmet while stabilizing the patient's neck.

2.   Each learner will practice the removal of a helmet while stabilizing the patient's neck. Learners should rotate as the patient unless contraindicated or they have a strong preference not to be the patient.

D.   Teaching station only.

II. **Principles of Helmet Removal**

A.   General principles

1.   An unresponsive trauma patient should be assumed to have potential cervical spine injuries.

2.   During helmet removal, the leader has the responsibility to:

a.   Verbally direct the assistant.

b.   Ensure the patient's cervical spine is continually stabilized throughout the skill performance.

c.   Emphasize teamwork.

3.   An assistant is required to perform this skill.

4.   If the helmet has a full face shield, lift the shield to talk to the patient.

5.   If the helmet has detachable pieces, remove the pieces prior to helmet removal.

6. Avoid pressure on the soft tissues of the neck.

7. Avoid manual traction or pulling on the head and neck.

8. Jewelry may make it difficult to remove the helmet.

9. Place a pad between the head and stretcher to maintain the head in a neutral position.

10. In actual patient care, all personnel who anticipate direct patient contact or contact with the patient's body fluids must wear gown, gloves, masks, and eye protection. (NOTE: Since TNCC skill stations are simulated situations, the use of personal protective equipment is optional.)

B. Indications: Any patient who has sustained trauma and who is wearing protective head gear or some type of helmet.

C. Contraindications:

1. Presence of injuries prohibiting manual stabilization of the head/neck (e.g., impaled objects).

2. Lack of an assistant to help remove the helmet (relative contraindication).

III. Steps in Skill Performance

A. Leader takes a position at the head of the patient, places hands on each side of helmet with the thumbs on the victim's mandible, AND instructs the patient not to move.

B. Leader briefly explains procedure to patient.

C. Leader asks patient to wiggle his or her toes and fingers and gently lift an arm or leg. Determines if sensation is present.

D. Leader maintains stabilization of helmet and mandible and then instructs assistant to remove the chin strap and other removable parts of the helmet (face shield, ear pads, mouth guards, etc.).

E. Leader instructs assistant to take a position at the side of the patient. Assistant cups the patient's mandible with thumb and index finger of one hand and places the other hand on the occipital ridge.

F. Leader asks assistant to state when ready. Leader then transfers stabilization responsibility to the assistant.

G. Leader, still at the head, spreads sides of helmet and gently removes it. If a void exists, leader places a small pad between occiput and stretcher.

H. Leader resumes cervical stabilization by placing hands on either side of neck, both thumbs on mandible, and fingers of both hands on occipital ridge. When leader is ready, assistant transfers stabilization responsibility to the leader.

I. Leader reassesses motor and sensory functions.

J. Leader states that spinal immobilization will now be performed.

IV. **Summary**

A. The Helmet Removal skill station demonstrates the skills associated with the removal of a helmet.

B. Critical step review

Maintains cervical stabilization and alignment throughout the procedure.

C. Principles and points to remember

1. An unresponsive trauma patient is assumed to have a cervical spine injury.

2. Perform a limited assessment of motor and sensory functions before helmet removal to establish a baseline, and after helmet removal to determine any changes.

D. Skill station steps summary

1. Assumes control, informs patient, and directs assistant.

2. Assesses motor and sensory function.

3. Maintains stabilization and vertebral alignment.

4. Reassesses motor and sensory function.

NURSING DIAGNOSES
NORTH AMERICAN NURSING DIAGNOSIS ASSOCIATION
AS OF THE
ELEVENTH NATIONAL CONFERENCE[1]

The following is the current (1994) taxonomy of nursing diagnoses developed by the North American Nursing Diagnosis Association. The taxonomy includes nine response patterns: exchanging, communication, relating, valuing, choosing, moving, perceiving, knowing, and feeling.[1] NANDA no longer uses the term "high risk" but does classify diagnoses as actual or risk.[1] Those diagnoses labeled with an * are new diagnoses added to the taxonomy in 1994.

EXCHANGING

Altered Nutrition
- More than body requirements
- Less than body requirements
- Potential for more than body requirements

Altered Physical Regulation
- Risk for infection
- Risk for altered body temperature
  - Hypothermia
  - Hyperthermia
  - Ineffective thermoregulation
- Dysreflexia

Altered Elimination
- Constipation
  - Perceived
  - Colonic
- Diarrhea
- Bowel incontinence
- Altered urinary elimination
  - Incontinence
    - Stress
    - Reflex
    - Urge
    - Functional
    - Total
  - Retention

Altered Circulation
- Tissue perfusion
  - Renal
  - Cerebral
  - Cardiopulmonary
  - Gastrointestinal
  - Peripheral
- Fluid volume
  - Excess
  - Deficit
    - ◆ Risk for fluid volume deficit
- Decreased cardiac output

Altered Oxygenation
- Impaired gas exchange
- Ineffective airway clearance
- Ineffective breathing pattern
  - Inability to sustain spontaneous ventilation
  - Dysfunctional ventilation weaning response

Altered Physical Integrity
- Risk for injury
  - Risk for suffocation
  - Risk for poisoning
  - Risk for trauma
  - Risk for aspiration
  - Risk for disuse syndrome
- Altered protection
  - Impaired tissue integrity
    - ◆ Oral mucous membranes
    - ◆ Risk for impaired skin integrity
- Decreased adaptive capacity: intracranial*
- Energy field disturbance*

COMMUNICATION

Altered Communication
- Verbal
  - Impaired

RELATING

Altered Socialization
- Impaired social interaction
- Social isolation
- Risk for loneliness*

Altered Role
- Altered role performance
  - Parenting
    - ♦ Risk for altered parent/infant/child attachment*
  - Sexual
    - ♦ Dysfunction
- Altered family processes
  - Caregiver role strain
  - Risk for caregiver role strain
    - ♦ Altered family process: alcoholism*
- Altered role conflict
  - Parental role conflict

Altered Sexuality Patterns

VALUING

- Altered spiritual state
  - Spiritual distress (distress of the human spirit)
  - Potential for enhanced spiritual well-being*

CHOOSING

Altered Coping
- Individual coping
  - Ineffective
    - ♦ Impaired adjustment
    - ♦ Defensive coping
    - ♦ Ineffective denial
- Family coping
  - Ineffective
    - ♦ Disabled
    - ♦ Compromised
  - Potential for growth
  - Potential for enhanced community coping*
  - Ineffective community coping*
- Management of therapeutic regimen*
  - Ineffective (individuals)*
    - ♦ Noncompliance*
  - Ineffective (families)*
  - Ineffective (community)*

Altered Judgment
- Individual
  - Decisional conflict

Health Seeking Behaviors

MOVING

Altered Activity
- Physical mobility
  - Impaired
    - Risk for peripheral neurovascular dysfunction
    - Risk for perioperative positioning injury*
  - Activity intolerance
    - Fatigue
  - Risk for activity intolerance

Altered Rest
- Sleep pattern disturbance

Altered Recreation
- Diversional activity
  - Deficit

Altered Activities of Daily Living
- Home maintenance management
  - Impaired
- Altered health maintenance
- Feeding self-care deficit
  - Impaired swallowing
  - Ineffective breastfeeding
  - Ineffective infant feeding pattern
- Bathing/hygiene self-care deficit
- Dressing/grooming self-care deficit
- Toileting self-care deficit

Altered Growth and Development
Relocation Stress Syndrome
*Risk for Disorganized Infant Behavior**
*Disorganized Infant Behavior**
*Potential for Enhanced Organized Infant Behavior**

PERCEIVING

Altered Self-Concept
- Body image disturbance
- Self-esteem disturbance
  - Chronic low self-esteem
  - Situational low self-esteem
- Personal identity disturbance

Altered Sensory/Perception
- Visual
- Auditory
- Kinesthetic
- Gustatory
- Tactile
- Olfactory
  - Unilateral Neglect

Altered Meaningfulness
- Hopelessness
- Powerlessness

KNOWING

Altered Knowing
- Knowledge deficit (specify)
- Impaired environmental interpretation syndrome*
- Acute confusion*
- Chronic confusion*

Altered thought processes
- Impaired memory*

FEELING

Altered Comfort
- Pain
  - Chronic

Altered Emotional Integrity
- Grieving
  - Dysfunctional
  - Anticipatory
- Risk for violence: self-directed or directed at others
- Risk for self-mutilation
- Posttrauma response
  - Rape-trauma syndrome
    - Compound reaction
    - Silent reaction

Altered Emotional Stress
- Anxiety
- Fear

DEFINITIONS[2]

Actual	Existing at the present moment; existing in reality.
Acute	Severe but of short duration.
Chronic	Lasting a long time; recurring; habitual; constant.
Decreased	Smaller; lessened; diminished; lesser in size, amount, or degree.
Deficient	Inadequate in amount, quality, or degree; not sufficient; incomplete.
Depleted	Emptied wholly or partially; exhausted of.
Disturbed	Agitated; interrupted; interfered with.
Dysfunctional	Abnormal; impaired or incompletely functioning.
Excessive	Characterized by an amount or quantity that is greater than is necessary, desirable, or usable.
Impaired	Made worse, weakened; damaged, reduced; deteriorated.
Increased	Greater in size, amount, or degree; larger, enlarged.
Ineffective	Not producing the desired effect; not capable of performing satisfactorily.
Intermittent	Stopping and starting again at intervals; periodic; cyclic.

NANDA defines an **actual nursing diagnosis** as: "describes human responses to health conditions/life processes that exist in an individual, family or community. It is supported by defining characteristics (manifestations/signs and symptoms) that cluster in patterns of related cues or inferences."[2]

A **risk nursing diagnosis** is defined as: "describes human responses to health conditions/life processes which may develop in a vulnerable individual, family or community. It is supported by risk factors that contribute to increased vulnerability."[2]

REFERENCES

1. North American Nursing Diagnosis Association. *Nursing Diagnoses: Definitions and Classification, 1995-1996.* Philadelphia, Pa: Author; 1994.

2. Carroll-Johnson RM, Paquette M, eds. *Classification of Nursing Diagnoses Proceedings of the Tenth Conference.* Philadelphia, Pa: JB Lippincott Co; 1994.

EPIDEMIOLOGY OF TRAUMA

OBJECTIVES

Upon completion of this appendix, the learner should be able to:

1. Define the terms trauma, epidemiology, injury control, and prevention.
2. Identify five characteristics associated with trauma.
3. Describe the injury model, including three phases (preinjury, injury, and postinjury), and the three factors (human, vehicle, and environment).
4. Compare and contrast three approaches to injury prevention and control.

INTRODUCTION

Trauma epidemiology, from the Greek word to visit (epidemion), is the study of the distribution of trauma in populations, the determinants of injury, and the associated causes and risk factors.[1] Trauma or injury is defined as the damage to human tissues and organs resulting from the transfer of energy from the environment. Injuries are therefore caused by some form of energy that is beyond the body's resilience to tolerate.[1,2]

The term "accident" is obsolete in injury epidemiology since the term has a tendency to mean "without intent" as well as implies focus on the behavior of the injured victim. For example, the phrase motor vehicle accident had been substituted by the phrase motor vehicle crash or collision (MVC) and injuries are now classified as intentional or unintentional. The study of injuries not only quantifies the incidence of injury events and the mechanisms associated with the transfer of energy, but also describes the scope of the problem in order to formulate meaningful public health policies and injury control programs.

UNITED STATES

Incidence and Severity of Trauma

The incidence of trauma refers to the actual number of persons who sustain an injury from various causes. Total numbers are more meaningful when computed as a rate which adjusts for the population. For example, to calculate the death rate from trauma for persons between the ages of 15 and 24 years, the number of injury deaths in that age group are divided by the total population of persons in the same age group. Mortality figures for trauma over recent years reflect the stability of trauma as the third leading cause of death for all ages combined in the United States, and the first leading cause of death for those persons between the ages of one and

44[3-9] (see Table 36). The death rates due to trauma over a seven-year period (1985 to 1991) have decreased for motor vehicle crashes and trauma overall, but have recently increased for suicide and homicide. The overall death rate due to all trauma events is 57.2 deaths/100,000 population in the United States.[9]

Table 36

FIVE LEADING CAUSES OF DEATH IN THE UNITED STATES – 1992[9]		
Cause	**Number of Deaths**	**Rate***
• Diseases of the heart	717,706	281.4
• Malignant neoplasms	520,578	204.1
• Accidents and adverse effects; suicides; and homicides/legal interventions	145,655	57.2
• Cerebrovascular diseases	143,769	56.4
• Chronic obstructive pulmonary disease	91,938	36.0
* Rate per 100,000 population		

From death certificates, the US Government calculates figures related to the cause of the injury death but does not provide figures related to the body system injured. Mortality data are published annually, available usually during the month of September each year, and address those deaths occurring in the US two years previous to the publication date. For example, mortality data for deaths occurring in 1994 will not be published until 1996. The government still uses the term "Accidents and Their Adverse Effects" to represent the aggregate number of injury deaths and uses separate categories for suicides and homicides/legal intervention. During 1992, there were 145,655 deaths due to trauma with 28% (40,982) due to motor vehicle crashes, 21% (30,484) due to suicide, 17.5% (25,488) due to homicides and legal intervention, and 33.5% (48,701) due to all other trauma events and their adverse effects (see Table 37).

Table 37

CAUSES OF INJURY DEATHS IN THE UNITED STATES – 1992[9]		
Cause	**Number**	**%**
• Motor vehicle crashes	40,982	28%
• Suicide	30,484	21%
• Homicide/legal intervention	25,488	17.5%
• All other events	48,701	33.5%
Total	**145,655**	**100%**

Deaths from injury are better documented than nonfatal injuries. It is known that of the 30.8 million patients (excluding newborns) discharged from short-stay hospitals in the United States, 2.7 million were due to injuries and/or poisonings.[10] The 10 leading causes of unintentional injuries are motor vehicle crashes, falls, poisonings, fires and burns, drowning, aspiration (nonfood), aspiration (food), firearm-related, machinery-related, and aircraft-related.[11] Intentional injury deaths are considered those deaths related to suicide and homicide.

Human Characteristics

The Subcommittee on Epidemiology of the American Trauma Society has guidelines for trauma systems to monitor the epidemiology of trauma. They suggest that demographic data elements such as age, gender, and ethnicity be collected to link particular populations with specific mechanisms of injury for injury prevention planning.

Age

Injuries resulted in the death of more persons between the ages of 25 and 34 years than in any other age group (see Table 38). Those persons between the ages of 15 and 24 years were the group with the second largest number of injury deaths. Although the incidence of trauma is greatest in these two age groups, the death rate (number of deaths/age group divided by the total number in age group) is greatest for those over the age of 85 years. Those persons between the ages of 75 and 84 have the second highest ranking death rate from trauma but represent the age group ranked sixth in terms of incidence.[9]

The leading cause of death for every age from six to 33 years is motor vehicle crashes.[12] Of the 22 million people in the United States who are 70 years of age or older, 14.7 million are licensed drivers (representing 8.6% of all drivers). This older age group represents 12% of all traffic fatalities and 18% of all pedestrian fatalities.[12]

Table 38

INJURY DEATHS AND DEATH RATES BY AGE IN THE UNITED STATES											
Rates per 100,000 population in each age group											
Age Groups	<1	1-4	5-14	15-24	25-34	35-44	45-54	55-64	65-74	75-84	>84
Accidents (All except suicide & homicide)	961	2,665	3,660	15,278	14,774	11,752	7,137	6,556	8,137	10,142	8,165
Death rate	24.0	17.5	10.2	42.0	34.5	29.9	27.7	31.2	44.5	98.3	258.4
Suicide			266	4,751	6,514	5,767	3,983	3,241	3,084	2,426	758
Homicide	380	428	519	8,159	7,801	4,571	2,112	1,156	738	438	130
Other	48	41	50	323	635	672	275	176	122	101	41
TOTAL	1,389	3,134	4,495	28,511	29,724	22,762	13,507	11,129	12,081	13,108	9,094

Gender

The death rate (deaths/100,000 population) from injuries for males is 84.0 compared to 31.4 for females.[9] There are differences in the ratio of male to female injury death rates depending on the cause of the injury. The overall death rate for injuries is two times more for males than females. The ratio of males to females, for example, for falls from ladders/scaffolds is as high as 29:1; for motorcyclist death it is 11:1; for suicide from firearms it is 6:1; and, for suicide by poisoning it is 1:1.[11] Exposure to the injury-producing event, the amount of risk involved, occupation, and cultural norms have been considered reasons for the gender differences.

Race

The causes of deaths from injuries vary by race. The overall injury death for whites was 54.0, for blacks 84.9, and for all others 73.4 (death rates are per 100,000 population of each group).[9] The suicide rate for whites was twice that for blacks and the homicide rate for blacks was almost seven times greater than for whites. The Native American has a death rate from motor vehicle crashes that is twice that for whites and almost four times that for Asians. Injury-related death from motor vehicles is ranked first for whites, Native Americans, Hispanics, and Asians while homicide is ranked first for blacks, second for Native Americans and Hispanics, and third for whites and Asians.[11]

Alcohol

The relationship of alcohol to fatal motor vehicle crashes is well studied. The estimate of fatal motor vehicle crashes related to alcohol dropped from 56.8% in 1982 to 45.1% in 1992.[12,13] In nearly half of all motor vehicle collisions resulting in a fatality, the driver of the motor vehicle or, in some circumstances, the pedestrian who was struck had been drinking alcohol. The National Highway Traffic Administration (NHSTA) publishes *The Fatal Accident Reporting System* (FARS) annually. This report is a wealth of information related to all fatal motor vehicle-related crashes. According to NHSTA, a fatal alcohol-related crash is considered one in which either the driver or pedestrian (if it is a pedestrian-related motor vehicle crash) has a blood alcohol concentration (BAC) of 0.01% or greater.

In most states it is considered illegal to drive when the BAC is 0.10% or greater. Some states have dropped the BAC level to 0.08% as the illegal level to drive. Of the 39,235 persons fatally injured in motor vehicle traffic crashes in one year, 36% were involved in a crash where the driver or pedestrian was considered intoxicated (BAC $\geq 0.10\%$). The incidence of drivers involved in fatal crashes was three times greater during night hours than during the day. The male to female ratio for driving while intoxicated and being involved in a fatal traffic crash was 2:1. Motorcycle drivers involved in fatal crashes had the highest incidence of driving with an illegal blood alcohol concentration of 0.10% or greater (35.6%), followed by drivers of light trucks (25.5%) and then drivers of passenger cars (21.7%).[12]

Violence

The presence of violence in American society has led to the injury and death of thousands; it is estimated that assaultive violence results in 19,000 to 23,000 deaths/year in the United States.[14] Assaultive violence includes both nonfatal and fatal interpersonal violence where physical force or other means is used by one person with the intent of causing harm, injury, or death to another.[14]

The statistics from firearm mortality are the most telling of the escalation of violence in America. In 1990, 17.6% of deaths of persons between the ages of one and 34 were due to firearm injury.[15] The firearm death rate for teenagers (15 to 19 years old) rose at the alarming rate of 77% from 1985 to 1990. The rate for those aged 10 to 14 increased 18%. Among black males between 10 to 14 years of age, the death rate from firearms more than doubled (46.5/100,000 to 119.9) from 1985 to 1990. The overall homicide death rate from firearms increased from 3.0/100,000 to 6.9/100,000; the homicide death rate from firearms for black teen-aged males tripled in 1990.

Abuse is a specific form of violence. It is estimated that 1.8 million women per year are victims of physical abuse inflicted by their partners.[16] The Pregnancy Risk Monitoring System in four states (Alaska, Maine, Oklahoma, and West Virginia) demonstrated that from 3.4% to 6.9% of pregnant women were assaulted.[17] The following characteristics of the victims were identified:

- Less than 12 years of education

- Race other than white

- Nineteen years old or less

- Unmarried

- Living in crowded conditions

- Delayed or no prenatal care

- Unintended pregnancy

The dramatic increase in violence in America has raised the awareness of public officials. Violence and prevention are being viewed as a public health problem which should be approached in similar fashion to the government's successful campaign against smoking. With this strategy the risks and predetermining factors, such as gang culture, the lack of male role models, drug culture, and the consequences of hate and rage, would be investigated.[18]

THE INJURY EVENT

An epidemiologic model to account for the factors and phases associated with the injury event was developed by William Haddon, the first director of the National Highway Traffic Safety Institute (NHTSA).[19] The intent of the model is to construct injury prevention strategies and programs that can alter the injury occurrence, depending on where the injury-producing factors are emphasized for a particular injury event. The model is divided into the three phases of preinjury, injury, and postinjury. The three factors are those related to the human who sustained the injury, the vehicle or agent of the energy transfer, and the environmental characteristics surrounding the injury event.[1]

Examples of factors are seen in Table 39. The clinical role of trauma nurses usually does not become activated until cell #9, after the event has occurred. With more emphasis on nurses becoming involved in injury control, many nurses have roles other than clinical practice. For example, nurses are involved in educational programs in the community to teach responsible driving behaviors to young teen-age drivers.

Table 39

THE HADDON INJURY MATRIX			
Phases	**Human**	**Vehicle**	**Environment**
Preinjury	1 Alcohol or drug use	4 Window visibility	7 Break-away poles
Injury	2 Pre-existing medical conditions which compound injury	5 Old shatter type windshield	8 Car fire postcrash
Postinjury	3 Cerebral ischemia	6 Weight of vehicle on occupant	9 Nursing response

INJURY PREVENTION/CONTROL

Injury prevention focuses on reducing the incidence of injury events. Injury control is a broader concept to include not only reducing the incidence but also reducing the severity.[1] The Centers for Disease Control and Prevention (CDC) has officially designated the National Center for Injury Prevention and Control a "center" within the CDC. The Center identified five areas of injury control where funds may be awarded: injury epidemiology, prevention, biomechanics, acute care, and rehabilitation.[20] Most injury control strategies can be classified as one of the following[21]:

- Engineering and technologic interventions, e.g., high-mounted rear brake lights

- Legislative and enforcement interventions, e.g., seat belt laws

- Education and behavioral interventions, e.g., school-based injury prevention programs

Altering the engineering and technologic aspects of injury-producing products and objects is the most effective strategy to reduce injuries. Regulating peoples' behavior through laws and regulations is the second most effective. Educational programs are the least effective.

For more information on injury prevention, the National Center for Injury Prevention & Control of the Centers for Disease Control can be contacted in Atlanta, Georgia (404-448-4365). There are also six Injury Control Research Centers in the United States: University of Alabama Injury Prevention Center, Harvard University Injury Prevention Center, University of California at San Francisco Injury Prevention Center, Harborview Injury Prevention Center, University of North Carolina Injury Prevention Center, and The Johns Hopkins School of Public Health Injury Prevention Center.

Vehicular Occupant Protection

Some familiarity with occupant protection technology will contribute to understanding the patterns of injury. Vehicle crashworthiness, friendly interiors, and restraint systems are the three main occupant protection concepts.[22] Examples of friendly interiors are cars equipped with energy-absorbing steering systems or high penetration-resistant windshields.

Restraint systems used in modern cars are safety belt restraints, car seats for infants and children, and inflatable restraints, i.e., air bags. The rapid inflation of the air bag (which uses a pyrotechnic technique to fill the bag with nitrogen) and occasional debris from the air bag pose some risk to the occupant. The air bag is a passive restraint system, meaning the occupant does not have to engage the system for it to be effective. It provides protection that does not rely on the occupant's behavior. Air bags do not replace safety belts. Since the air bag immediately deflates and is not activated during side impacts, seat belt restraints should be worn to protect the occupant from vehicular ejection. In general, air bags have prevented serious and fatal injuries; the injuries that may result from air bag inflation are limited to minor abrasions and ocular irritation.[23] The use of lap and shoulder safety belts reduces the risk of fatal injury to front seat passengers by 45% and reduces the risk of moderate to critical injury by 50%.[12]

There are many varieties of car seats for infants and children. Some car manufacturers are constructing back seats which can be converted into car seats for children. The use of different styles of infant and child car seats is based on the weight and age of the occupant. Rear-facing child car seats should not be used in front passenger seats that are equipped with air bags.[24]

All 50 states and the District of Columbia have some form of child restraint law.[12] It is estimated that there is a 69% reduction in fatalities to infants less than one year of age and a 47% reduction in fatalities to toddlers between the ages of one and four because of the use of child safety seats.

TRAUMA IN THE 1990s

The incidence of trauma and the specific statistics related to the various causes of injury are published frequently as the events change over time. For example, it is well known that over 30% of all deaths due to trauma in the US are related to motor vehicle crashes. However, because the actual number of these deaths is decreasing from year to year and the number of firearm-related deaths is increasing, the state-by-state picture varies.

The only state where there were more firearm deaths than motor-vehicle deaths for 17 of the years between 1968 and 1991 was Alaska. The District of Columbia for all of these 24 years had more firearm-related deaths. But as violence has escalated in the 1990s, five states in 1990 (Alaska, Louisiana, Maryland, New York, and Texas) and seven states in 1991 (California, Louisiana, Maryland, Nevada, New York, Texas, and Virginia) had more deaths due to firearms than motor vehicles.[25]

Researchers in Los Angeles County recently studied the incidence and causes of occupational deaths. They found that homicide was the leading cause of such deaths, accounting for almost half of all on-the-job deaths.[26] Homicide is also the number one cause of occupational deaths in New York City.

New reports from New Mexico and other states also demonstrate the epidemiologic changes in the leading causes of trauma. In New Mexico, it has been reported that the most frequent mechanism of head or neck injury is a gunshot, not motor vehicle crashes.[27] Although injury has been the leading cause of death for adult males, AIDS deaths are increasing in this age/gender group. In California, Florida, Massachusetts, New Jersey, and New York the number one cause of death for males between the ages of 25 and 44 is not trauma but AIDS.[28]

Statewide trauma registries, along with information generated from the federal government, provide useful data for all health professionals interested in preventing and controlling the incidence and prevalence of injuries.

AUSTRALIA

Incidence

In Australia, mortality figures over recent years indicate that trauma is the fourth leading cause of death for all ages (73 deaths per 100,000) behind cancer, ischemic heart disease and cerebrovascular deaths.[29] There were 23,127 injury deaths in Australia between 1990 and 1992.[30]

The leading causes of fatal injury were motor vehicle crashes which accounted for 31% of both male and female injury deaths, and suicide, which accounted for 31% of male injury deaths and 18% of female injury deaths.[31]

By 1991 suicide deaths continued to increase in number, overtaking deaths from motor vehicle crashes.[29] Other injury-related deaths are caused by incidents involving trains, boats, and aircraft. A significant number of deaths and injuries result from industrial accidents, sporting, and leisure activities.

The Australian Bureaus of Statistics classifies trauma deaths as accidents, poisonings, or violence. The accident category includes motor vehicle crashes, accidental falls, and all other accidents (see Table 40).

Table 40

CAUSES OF INJURY DEATHS FOR AUSTRALIA IN 1990[32]		
Cause	Number	%
Motor vehicle crashes	2,489	36.2
Suicide	2,161	25.7
Homicide	385	4.1
All other events	2,900	34
Total	7,935	100

Human Characteristics

Age

Deaths from the external causes of accidents, poisonings, and violence are a major cause of premature death, representing 6.8% of deaths of people of all ages and 19% of deaths in the 15 to 64 year age group. Injuries accounted for 50.1% of deaths in persons between the ages of one and 44 years.[29] The age group with the highest injury deaths is 15 to 24 years of age (see Table 41). Those between 25 and 44 years form the second largest group of injury deaths.

Table 41

DEATHS AT AGES 15 TO 24 YEARS MAIN CAUSES 1989 TO 1991[33]			
Cause of Death	1989	1990	1991
All causes	2,270	2,189	2,078
Malignant neoplasms	150	143	149
Accidents, poisoning and violence	1,703	1,596	1,533
Motor vehicle traffic accidents	931	785	696
Suicide	380	439	462

Gender

Males account for 70.3% of deaths from accidents, poisonings, and violence. They account for 78.5% of suicide deaths, 71.1% of motor vehicle crash deaths, and 44.8% of accidental fall deaths. Approximately 95% of nontraffic, work-related deaths involve males.[34] Exposure to the injury-producing event, amount of risk involved, occupation, and cultural norms are possible reasons for the gender differences (see Table 42).

Table 42

RaRA Category	Unintentional	Rate	Suicide	Rate	Interpersonal Violence	Rate
DISTRIBUTION OF INJURY DEATHS BY AREA, INTENT AND SEX: TOTAL NUMBERS OF DEATHS, AUSTRALIA, 1990-1992[30]						
Males						
Capital city	5,171	33.5	3,207	20.8	373	2.4
Other major urban	814	37.4	519	23.8	43	2.0
Rural major	1,177	42.4	639	23.0	69	2.4
Rural other	1,764	53.5	798	24.2	68	2.1
Remote major	182	60.4	67	22.2	21	7.0
Remote other	462	86.2	162	30.2	59	11.0
All areas	**9,570**	**39.0**	**5,392**	**22.0**	**633**	**2.6**
Females						
Capital city	2,686	16.9	982	6.2	248	1.5
Other major urban	423	19.0	133	6.0	38	1.7
Rural major	670	23.4	134	4.7	38	1.3
Rural other	720	22.6	134	4.2	39	1.2
Remote major	58	20.3	11	3.9	15	5.3
Remote other	152	32.1	18	3.8	34	7.2
All areas	**4,709**	**18.9**	**1,412**	**5.7**	**412**	**1.6**

Race

Aboriginal people have the highest death rate in Australia. The Aboriginal male has a 3.5 times greater death rate from accidents, poisoning, or violence than nonAboriginal males. Injury-related deaths were responsible for 20% of the excess mortality. The Aboriginal female death rate is 3.8 times greater than the nonAborigincal death rate. The injury-related deaths were responsible for 13% of the excess mortality in Aboriginal females.[34] The increased death rates among Aboriginal people may be due to many factors, including the fact that many people travel in open vehicles, such as trucks, which do not have safety restraints.

Alcohol

The use and especially the abuse of alcohol has been linked to accidents, injuries, and death. Therefore, it is expected that a reduction in alcohol use will lead to a reduction in injury and death. This area of prevention has continued to receive attention throughout the 1980s and 1990s with some authorities attributing the decline in motor vehicle deaths to random breath testing (RBT), particularly in NSW. Others report a decline due to adverse economic conditions. A report in New South Wales claims that RBT produced an average annual savings of 274 lives.[29]

Violence

The homicide rate of just over 4% is relatively small compared to that of other countries. While this figure is small, it should be noted that the amount of severe injury from personal violence and terrorism is rising.[35] The incidence of violent acts such as rape, physical assault, child abuse, and violence against women is increasing in our society despite awareness, help and prevention programs. There were 1,860 firearm deaths during the three-year period from 1990 to 1992, with 84% of these due to suicide, 14% due to interpersonal violence, and 5% due to unintentional personal injury.[30]

At present, laws restricting the ownership of guns and, especially, handguns, may play a signif-icant role in limiting the amount of gun-related violence in Australia. The Sporting Shooters Association of Australia estimates there are up to four million firearms in Australia.[36]

The incidence of violence is increasing throughout the world. Table 43 illustrates the number of persons killed by handguns in various countries. Firearms are involved in 28% of the 1.8 million violent crimes in the US.[38] The US Bureau of Alcohol, Tobacco and Firearms estimates that, of the 220 million firearms owned by US citizens, 72 million are handguns.[37] Although the actual number of homicide deaths in the US is over 19,000, the rate of homicide deaths is greater in other countries. Handguns are less easily obtainable in other Western countries due to tighter restrictions on gun ownership.

Table 43

INTERNATIONAL HANDGUN AND HOMICIDE DEATHS (ONE YEAR)		
Country	Number Killed by Handguns[39]	Total Male Homicide Rate*[14]	Total Homicide Number
Puerto Rico	–	30.6	579
Paraguay	–	13.6	182
USA	10,728	12.7	19,628
Northern Ireland	–	6.6	58
Israel	58	2.9	91
Australia	–	2.5	314
New Zealand	–	2.5	66
Canada	52	2.7	537
Sweden	21	1.7	104
Switzerland	34	1.2	93
West Germany	42	1.2	726
Japan	48	1.0	1,017
Great Britian	8	0.8	344
*Rate is per 100,000 population			

Suicide

In Australia, suicide accounted for 5,392 male deaths and 1,412 female deaths between 1990 and 1992. The crude rate of male deaths attributed to suicide has been fairly steady in the most recent years after a sharp increase in the mid-1980s to a peak in 1987. The rate for females has slightly declined since 1987. The pattern for females is different, generally rising with age. A long-term decline in female suicide rates in the mid-adult years continued in 1990. Continuing the pattern that emerged for males during the early 1980s, suicide rates were high for all age groups from 15 years, though a little lower for middle-aged men than for younger or older men.

In 1991 the suicide rate for males increased and has now become the leading cause of injury-related deaths in males 15 to 24 years.[29] Reasons for this rise have been attributed to the socioeconomic situation of widespread unemployment for youth and also the lessening of the social stigma that was once attached to suicide.

Prevention

The number of deaths and injuries in Australia from motor vehicle crashes has shown a steady decrease over the past 20 years. Between 1960 and the late 1970s, the annual fatality rate fluctuated around 25 deaths per 100,000, but has since declined by 5% per year to 13.6 deaths per 100,000 in 1990.[31] There was a 6% decline from 1980 to 1990 in the number of deaths per million vehicle kilometers travelled. This death rate was 1.6 deaths per million vehicle kilometers travelled in 1990. In 1991 the incidence of highway fatalities further declined an additional 9.4%, resulting in 2,112 fatalities.[31] Bicyclist fatalities dropped 27.5%, which may have been due to greater publicity or widespread adoption of protective headgear.[29] In 1991 the number of road fatalities was 22.8%, below the average for 1986.[31] The reason for this decrease is largely due to continuous and aggressive prevention programs in each state. These programs include mandatory seatbelt legislation and drink-driving laws.[29] Drink-driving laws, specifying the blood alcohol level considered not to impede driving judgment and response (0.05 to 0.08% varying with each state), were introduced in the early 1980s. Following introduction of these laws, a further decrease in deaths associated with drinking and motor vehicle crashes was noted. Other areas of prevention relate to highway regulations and vehicular design. Enforcement of traffic regulations, with more sophisticated entrapment procedures, such as speed cameras, slant radar and red light cameras, have contributed to a decrease in road fatalities.[29]

REFERENCES

1. Robertson L. *Injury Epidemiology*. New York, NY: Oxford University Press; 1993.

2. Robertson L. *Injuries: Causes, Control Strategies, and Public Policy*. Lexington, Mass: Lexington Books; 1983.

3. Advance report of final mortality statistics, 1986. *Monthly Vital Statistics Report*. National Center for Health Statistics, Hyattsville, Md: 1988;37:1-55.

4. Advance report of final mortality statistics, 1987. *Monthly Vital Statistics Report*. National Center for Health Statistics, Hyattsville, Md: 1989;38:1-48.

5. Advance report of final mortality statistics, 1988. *Monthly Vital Statistics Report*. National Center for Health Statistics, Hyattsville, Md: 1990;39:1-48.

6. Advance report of final mortality statistics, 1989. *Monthly Vital Statistics Report*. National Center for Health Statistics, Hyattsville, Md: 1991;40:1-52.

7. Advance report of final mortality statistics, 1990. Monthly Vital Statistics Report. National Center for Health Statistics, Hyattsville, Md: 1992;41:1-52.

8. Advance report of final mortality statistics, 1991. *Monthly Vital Statistics Report*. National Center for Health Statistics, Hyattsville, Md: 1993;42:1-64.

9. Advance report of final mortality statistics, 1992. *Monthly Vital Statistics Report*. National Center for Health Statistics, Hyattsville, Md: 1994;43:1-76.

10. 1990 summary: national hospital discharge survey. *Vital and Health Statistics*. National Center for Health Statistics, Hyattsville, Md: 1992;210:1-12.

11. Baker SP, O'Neill B, Ginsburg MJ, Guohua LM. *The Injury Fact Book*. 2nd ed. New York, NY: Oxford University Press; 1992.

12. National Highway Traffic Safety Administration. *Traffic Safety Facts 1992*. US Department of Transportation, National Center for Statistics and Analysis: Washington, DC; 1993; DOT HS 808 022.

13. National Highway Traffic Safety Administration. *Traffic Safety Facts 1993*. US Department of Transportation, National Center for Statistics and Analysis: Washington, DC; 1994; DOT HS 808 169.

14. Rosenberg ML, Fenley MA. *Violence in America: A Public Health Approach*. New York, NY: Oxford University Press; 1991.

15. Fingerhut LA. Firearm mortality among children, youth, and young adults 1-34 years of age, trends and current status: United States 1985-90. *Advance Data from Vital and Health Statistics*. Hyattsville, Md: National Center for Health Statistics; 1993;231:1-20.

16. Strauss MA, Gelles RJ. How violent are American families? In: Strauss MA, Gelles RJ, eds. *Physical Violence in American Families: Risk Factors and Adaptations to Violence in 8,145 Families*. New Brunswick, NJ: Transaction Publishers; 1990:95-112.

17. Physical violence during the 12 months preceding childbirth-Alaska, Maine, Oklahoma, and West Virginia, 1990-1991. *MMWR*. Atlanta, Ga: Centers for Disease Control; 132-137.

18. Prothrow-Stith D. *Deadly Consequences: How Violence is Destroying Our Teenage Population and a Plan to Begin Solving the Problem*. New York, NY: Harper Perennial; 1991.

19. Haddon W Jr. A logical framework for categorizing highway phenomena and activity. *J Trauma*. 1972;12:197-207.

20. Committee to Review the Status and Progress of the Injury Control Program at the Centers for Disease Control. *Injury Control*. Washington, DC: The National Academy Press; 1988.

21. The National Committee for Injury Prevention and Control. *Injury Prevention Meeting the Challenge*. New York, NY: Oxford University Press; 1989.

22. Viano DC. Cause and control of automotive trauma. *Bulletin of the New York Academy of Medicine*. 1988;64:376-421.

23. Insurance Institute for Highway Safety. *Special Issue: Air Bags in Perspective*. Washington, DC; 1993.

24. American Public Health Association. *The Nation's Health*. Washington, DC; July 1993:6.

25. Death resulting from firearm-and motor-vehicle related injuries, United States, 1968-1991. *MMWR*. Atlanta, Ga: Centers for Disease Control; 1994;43:1-42.

26. American Public Health Association. Homicide replaces accident as top killer on the job in LA county. *The Nation's Health*. Dec. 1993:14.

27. Nelson DE, Sacks JJ, Parrish RG, Sosin DM, McFeeley P, Smith SM. Sensitivity of multiple-cause mortality data for surveillance of deaths associated with head or neck injuries. *MMWR*. Atlanta, Ga: Centers for Disease Control; 1994;42(SS-5):29-35.

28. The bad news. *Time*. June 1993:28. Article.

29. Grant C, Lapsley HM. *The Australian Health Care System 1992*. Sydney, Australia: University of New South Wales; 1993.

30. Moller J. The spatial distribution of injury deaths in Australia: urban, rural and remote areas. *Australian Injury Prevention Bulletin*. Bedford Park, South Australia: Australian Institute of Health and Welfare; 1994;8:1-8.

31. *Third Biennial Report of the Australian Institute of Health and Welfare. Australia's Health.* Canberra, Australia: Australian Government Publishing Service; 1992.

32. *National Injury Surveillance Unit.* Sydney, Australia; 1991.

33. Australian Bureau of Statistics. *Causes of Death.* 1991.

34. Glover J, Woollacott T. *A Social Health Atlas of Australia.* Adelaide, Australia: South Australian Health Commission; 1992.

35. National Health and Medical Research Council. *Discussion Paper on the Management of Severe Injuries.* Canberra, Australia: Australian Government Publishing Service; 1988.

36. Harford S. *Sydney Morning Herald.* February 5 1994:29. Newspaper article.

37. Eastern Association for the Surgery of Trauma. Violence in America: a public health crisis, the role of firearms. *J Trauma.* 1995;38:163-168.

38. Zimring SE. Firearms, violence and public policy. *Scientific American.* 1991:48.

39. Southward J. *Sun Herald.* January 30 1994:35. Newspaper article.

APPENDIX THREE

UNIVERSAL PRECAUTIONS

Universal precautions is an infection control method. All body fluids and blood are considered infectious for human immunodeficiency virus, hepatitis B virus, and other bloodborne pathogens. The Bloodborne Pathogens Standard developed by the Occupational Health and Safety Administration (OSHA) and endorsed by the Centers for Disease Control (CDC) became effective March 6, 1992. This standard requires the following:

1. Employers shall establish a written Exposure Control Plan designed to eliminate or minimize employee exposure.[1] This plan must identify workers who are at risk of occupational exposure to blood and other potentially infectious materials, and specify means to protect and train the workers.

2. Employees shall follow universal precautions to prevent contact with blood or other potentially infectious materials.[1] All body fluids shall be considered potentially infectious materials.

3. Engineering and work practice controls shall be used to eliminate or minimize employee exposure.[1] These controls include use of puncture-resistant containers for used needles; enforcement of work practices such as handwashing to reduce contamination; and appropriate use of personal protective equipment including gowns, gloves, eye protection, masks, and face shields.[2]

4. Personal protective equipment (PPE) shall be available to employees at no cost. The equipment shall be available in appropriate sizes and must be readily accessible. All personal protective equipment shall be removed prior to leaving the work area and placed in an appropriately designated area or container for storage, washing, or decontamination.[1]

    a. Gloves shall be worn whenever the employee may have hand contact with blood, other potentially infectious materials, mucous membranes, and nonintact skin. Gloves shall be worn during vascular access procedures and when handling or touching contaminated items or surfaces.[1]

    b. Masks in combination with eye protection devices shall be worn whenever splashes, spray, splatter, or droplets of blood or other potentially infectious materials may occur.[1]

    c. Gowns, aprons, and other protective clothing shall be worn in situations where exposure may occur.[1]

    d. Surgical caps and/or shoe covers shall be worn whenever gross contamination can be reasonably anticipated.[1]

5. Written housekeeping procedures shall be developed addressing decontamination procedures, written schedules for cleaning, discarding of contaminated needles and other sharp instruments, handling of regulated wastes, and handling of contaminated laundry.[2]

6. Employers shall make available the hepatitis B vaccine and vaccination series to all employees who have occupational exposure. They must also provide postexposure evaluation and follow-up to all employees who have had an exposure incident. The vaccine must be offered at no cost to the employee.[1] If the employee initially declines the vaccine and then decides to accept the vaccine at a later date, the employer must make the vaccine available.

   Following an exposure, the employer shall provide the employee with medical evaluation and follow-up. A record must be established and maintained with the employer following an occupational exposure.[1]

7. Employers shall provide employees with an annual training program offered during the employee's working hours and at no cost to the employee.[1]

In addition to the Bloodborne Pathogens Standard, OSHA has released the Enforcement Policy and Procedure for Occupational Exposure to Tuberculosis. This document sets forth requirements that[3]:

- Health care workers shall receive purified protein derivative (PPD) skin testing at least yearly and more often depending on the circumstances of the workplace.

- Specialized isolation rooms for the patient who is suspected or known to have TB must be developed.

- Certain types of face masks shall be worn while caring for the possibly infectious TB patient.

Members of the trauma team should be familiar with the requirements of the above standards and understand their implications for practice.[4] Universal precautions are indicated for all patients whenever there is a potential for exposure to blood or body fluids. The use of personal protective equipment and adherence to universal precautions will help prevent the transmission of infectious agents. Reminder: Patients may have an allergy to the latex used in gloves.

REFERENCES

1. Department of Labor. Occupational exposure to bloodborne pathogens: final rule. *Federal Register.* 1991;56:63861-64186.

2. Trauma Nursing Coalition. Preventing transmission of infectious agents in blood and body fluids. *Resource Document for Nursing Care of the Trauma Patient.* Denver, Co: Author; 1992:89-90.

3. Occupational Safety and Health Administration. *Enforcement Policy and Procedure for Occupational Exposure to Tuberculosis.* October 8, 1993:1-9.

4. Curry J. Identifying the patient with tuberculosis and protecting the emergency department staff. *JEN.* 1994;20:293-304.

PHARMACOLOGIC ADJUNCTS FOR ENDOTRACHEAL INTUBATION

INTRODUCTION

Numerous papers were published in the 1980s dealing with the use of drugs to facilitate emergency endotracheal intubation.[1-4] Some reports are limited to the use of neuromuscular blocking agents,[5-6] while others address the full protocol of rapid sequence induction.[2]

The phrase "rapid sequence induction" (RSI) is an established phrase that refers to the use of certain drugs, techniques, and a sequence of steps to induce anesthesia. Anesthesia is a three-stage process, distinguished by varying degrees of analgesia and decreased levels of consciousness. Induction is a term that relates to the first two stages of anesthesia. In stage 1 the patient is conscious but analgesic; in stage 2 the patient is unconscious but skeletal muscles are not relaxed. Stage 3 has four planes in which the patient is unconscious with varying degrees of skeletal muscle relaxation. Most surgical operations are done in the second or third plane of stage 3.[7]

RSI was introduced in the field of obstetrics in 1946.[8] BA Sellick[9] introduced the Sellick maneuver or cricoid pressure into the RSI protocol in 1961. The protocol was refined for the combat arena in 1976.[10] The "I" of RSI refers to induction; however, the field of emergency medicine has frequently substituted the word "intubation" for induction.[1,8]

RSI was classically used for patients who required endotracheal intubation for general anesthesia purposes but who had full stomachs increasing the threat of aspiration during intubation. Also, in the classic use of RSI, patients are not ventilated with positive pressure during the induction since such pressure could precipitate regurgitation.[11]

Protocols for the Use of Drugs to Facilitate Intubation

The use of drugs to facilitate endotracheal intubation in patients who are traumatized, awake, and in need of definitive airway control is not without risk. It is suggested that a multidisciplinary team representing trauma surgery, anesthesiology, and nursing develop institution-specific protocols. There are many different drugs in multiple drug categories that have the potential to be included. Physician preference and experience with these agents will influence the drugs selected for the protocol.

Having predetermined protocols that address the use of drugs to facilitate endotracheal intubation assist the health care team in identifying the indications, precautions, sequence of administration, and pharmacodynamics of various drugs. The purpose of RSI in the emergency department is usually not to induce anesthesia for surgery but to medicate an awake patient to facilitate the insertion of an endotracheal tube.

It is recommended that the trauma nurse be familiar with the particular drugs in the predetermined protocol. Before drugs are administered, determine the following:

- Age and estimated weight of the patient

- Type of injuries (certain drugs are contraindicated in patients with head injuries who have the potential for increased intracranial pressure)

- Allergies, e.g., barbiturates

- Patient's hemodynamic stability (in the military arena hemodynamic instability is an absolute contraindication to RSI by forward surgical teams [FST][12])

- Level of consciousness prior to intubation

- Immediate availability of skilled intubationist

- Immediate availability of ventilation equipment

- Immediate availability of a nurse to monitor the patient during and after the use of medications that will alter the patient's level of consciousness and/or use of skeletal muscles

MEDICATIONS

The following drug groups include certain medications that may be considered to paralyze, sedate, or induce anesthesia:

- Neuromuscular blocking agents (skeletal relaxants)

- Sedatives

- Hypnotics

- Narcotic and nonnarcotic analgesics

- Induction anesthetics

Neuromuscular Blocking Agents (NBA)

NBAs peripherally induce skeletal muscle relaxation by interfering with the cholinergic (acetylcholine) transmission in the neuromuscular junction. They are classified as either nondepolarizing or depolarizing. The nondepolarizing agents compete with acetylcholine for the receptor site to block acetylcholine's function of depolarizing the postsynaptic membrane and, therefore, prevent contraction of the muscle.[13] The common nondepolarizing agents are tubocurarine, atracurium (Tacrium), pancuronium (Pavulon), and vecuronium (Norcuron). Vecuronium has fewer side effects, e.g., mild hypertension, tachycardia,[13] than pancuronium.

486

Vecuronium is therefore preferred over pancuronium for patients with a questionable hemodynamic status. Since these agents produce hypertension and tachycardia, the patient's myocardial oxygen consumption and ventricular ejection fraction may be compromised.[14]

Depolarizing agents depolarize the postsynaptic membrane and then continue to occupy the receptor site, delaying repolarization and further depolarization. The only depolarizing agent used clinically is succinylcholine (Anectine). When administered it causes an initial muscle contraction (fasciculations), followed by flaccid paralysis. Anectine may cause hyperkalemia in trauma patients, especially those with chronic renal failure.

NBAs must be used with caution or avoided in normotensive trauma patients who have either eye or head injuries or who have pre-existing cardiovascular disease such as hypertension. The use of succinylcholine in children may precipitate bradycardia.[14] The onset of skeletal muscle relaxation varies depending on the drug administered (see Table 44).

Table 44[15]

NEUROMUSCULAR BLOCKING AGENTS			
Drug	ED$_{90}$ Dose*	Maximum Effect In Minutes	Total Duration In Minutes +
Atracurium	0.19 mg/kg	6.7	32
Vecuronium	0.05 mg/kg	4.5	24.9
Pancuronium	0.06 mg/kg	4.9	73.2
Tubocurarine	0.34 mg/kg	9.9	96.4
Succinylcholine	0.51 mg/kg#	1	2 to 4
* Effective dose to cause 90% loss of muscle twitch + From time of injection to 90% recovery # Effective dose to cause 95% loss of muscle twitch			

Sedatives and Hypnotics

Sedatives by definition are "chemical substances that reduce nervousness, excitability, or irritability by producing a calming or soothing effect." Whereas, hypnotics "are used to induce sleep." The major difference between a sedative and a hypnotic is the degree of CNS depression induced.[16] Benzodiazepines do not have a general CNS depressant effect, but different benzodiazepines have different locations and mechanisms of action. As muscle relaxants, they block synaptic reflexes decreasing muscle activity.[16] Diazepam (Valium) and midazolam (Versed) are two benzodiazepines. Versed has antianxiety, sedative, hypnotic, and amnesic effects. If used with a narcotic or if given too rapidly it may produce severe respiratory depression; a drug warning has been issued for the use of Versed intravenously.

487

Opioid Analgesics

Fentanyl (Sublimaze) and alfentanil (Alfenta) are two opioid analgesics that affect the mu opioid receptors. These agents also produce unconsciousness in higher doses and are used as anesthesia induction agents. If the trauma patient is hemodynamically stable, both fentanyl (4 to 5 μg/kg) and alfentanil (10 μg/kg) have been cited as possible drugs to use to reduce the side effects of hypertension and tachycardia from some of the skeletal muscle relaxants used in an RSI protocol.[14]

Induction Anesthetics

Thiopental (Pentothal) and etomidate are two induction anesthetics. Etomidate is classified as a nonbarbiturate short-acting hypnotic. Etomidate (0.3 mg/kg) is useful for injured children since it "maintains cardiovascular stability without increasing ICP."[17] The use of drugs to facilitate intubation in children requires careful planning of an RSI protocol. The International Trauma Anesthesia and Critical Care Society states "a rapid-sequence technique with cricoid pressure is the preferred method of performing endotracheal intubation in the traumatized uncooperative child in whom the airway appears normal."[17] Etomidate is contraindicated in pregnant patients[18] and is considered a substitute for thiopental in some RSI protocols.[1,18]

Thiopental is an ultrashort-acting barbiturate and a CNS depressant. It is frequently used in combination with other drugs for anesthesia purposes. Thiopental has been suggested as an RSI agent to intubate head trauma patients.[1] However, the hemodynamic stability of the head injured patient is important in deciding the dose of thiopental. Because it can depress cardiovascular function, a lower dose is suggested in patients who have some hemodynamic compromise. It is not recommended for hypotensive patients.[1]

Cricoid Pressure

The Sellick maneuver or cricoid pressure, is performed by a trauma team member using a thumb and forefinger to compress the patient's cricoid cartilage while exerting downward pressure onto C-6, occluding the esophagus. This maneuver is frequently part of an RSI protocol since intubating a patient who has a potentially full stomach may precipitate aspiration. However, cricoid pressure must not be released until the endotracheal tube is inserted properly.

Precautions

The International Trauma Anesthesia and Critical Care Society indicates caution in the following statement: "Obviously the use of any sedative or potent analgesic is contraindicated in a hypotensive patient, but such agents are appropriate in the majority of trauma victims once fluid resuscitation has been undertaken."[18] The decision whether to perform an endotracheal intubation in an awake patient using a sedative and opioid (e.g., 0.05 mg/kg of Valium or 0.03 mg/kg of Versed in combination with Fentanyl at a dose of 1.5 μg/kg), is not the same procedure as RSI. If there is a need to medicate the patient before endotracheal intubation is attempted, the decision must be made to use one or two drugs which will not render the patient unconscious or to use the RSI approach. Indications vary for performing RSI versus an awake intubation (see Table 45).

Table 45

POSSIBLE INDICATIONS FOR AWAKE INTUBATION AND RAPID SEQUENCE INDUCTION TECHNIQUES IN THE TRAUMA PATIENT WITH FULL STOMACH	
Awake Intubation	**Rapid Sequence Induction**
• Obstructed or compromised airway	• Uncooperative patient
• Anatomical variations of the face, neck and upper airway with the potential of causing difficult intubation	• Head injury
• Suspected difficulty of bag-valve-mask ventilation and intubation	• Ischemic heart disease
• Neck injuries that are not evaluated adequately	• Reactive airway disease
• Active upper airway bleeding	• Asthma
• Cardiac tamponade	• Suspected major vessel injury without active bleeding
• Shock	

(Reprinted with permission from Capan, LV. Airway management. In: Capan LV, Miller SM, Turndorf H, eds. *Trauma Anesthesia and Intensive Care*. Philadelphia, Pa: JB Lippincott; 1991:48.)

In the event that the endotracheal intubation using RSI fails, LV Capan[14] suggests two approaches depending on whether the patient can or cannot be bag-valve-mask ventilated:

• Ventilate using a bag-valve-mask while maintaining cricoid pressure. Then attempt to intubate under direct laryngoscopy with a different laryngoscope blade.

• If bag-valve-mask ventilation cannot be done, reduce cricoid pressure and attempt to ventilate. If the ventilation cannot be done, perform a surgical cricothyroidotomy and provide positive pressure ventilation OR perform a needle cricothyroidotomy and jet ventilate the patient. Attempt to perform an awake intubation.

Nursing Implications

Nursing knowledge of the procedures, assessment, intervention, and evaluation includes:

• Determining the patient's hemodynamic status

• Providing psychosocial support prior to administration of the medication and during the procedure

• Documenting the exact time, route, and dose of each agent used

• Assessing patient responses to each drug

- Determining and documenting the time analgesia, sedation, or skeletal muscle relaxation is achieved

- Providing the immediate availability of resuscitation equipment

SUMMARY

The use of drugs to facilitate performing an endotracheal intubation in the emergency department requires critical thinking skills on the part of the trauma team. The indication should be well identified. The selection of agents used will be influenced by: the physician prescribing the drugs; the hemodynamic stability of the patient; type of injuries; pre-existing medical conditions and allergies; degrees of sedation, hypnosis, analgesia, muscle relaxation, and induction required; patient's level of consciousness; availability of personnel and equipment to provide immediate definitive airway control; and institution-specific protocols.

REFERENCES

1. Walls RM. Rapid-sequence intubation in head trauma. *Ann Emerg Med.* 1993;70:1008-1013.

2. Talucci RC, Shaikh KA, Schwab CW. Rapid sequence induction with oral endotracheal intubation in the multiply injured patient. *Am Surg.* 1988;54:185-187.

3. Yamato LG, Gregory KY, Britten AG. Rapid sequence anesthesia induction for emergency intubation. *Pediatr Emerg Care.* 1990;6:201-213.

4. Glaser RB. Sedation and rapid induction anesthesia for emergency intubation. In: Callaham ML, ed. *Current Therapy in Emergency Medicine.* Toronto, Canada: BC Decker; 1987:21-26.

5. Syverud SA, Borron SW, Storer DL. Prehospital use of neuromuscular blocking agents in a helicopter ambulance program. *Ann Emerg Med.* 1988;17:236-242.

6. Degarmo BH, Dronen S. Pharmacology and clinical use of neuromuscular blocking agents. *Ann Emerg Med.* 1983;12:48-55.

7. McKenry LM, Salerno E. Anesthetics. *Mosby's Pharmacology in Nursing.* 19th ed. St. Louis, Mo: Mosby-Year Book; 1995:279-303.

8. Simon B. Pharmacologic aids in airway management. In: Dailey RH, Simon B, Young GP, Stewart RD, eds. *The Airway: Emergency Management.* St. Louis, Mo: Mosby-Year Book; 1992:145-170.

9. Sellick BA. Cricoid pressure to control regurgitation of stomach contents during induction of anesthesia. *Lancet.* 1961;2:404-406.

10. Cromartie RS. Rapid anesthesia induction in combat casualties with full stomachs. *Anesth Analg.* 1976;55:816.

11. Dornette WHL, McAlary BG, Grande CM. Medicolegal issues in trauma anesthesia. In: Grande CM, ed. *Textbook of Trauma Anesthesia and Critical Care.* St. Louis, Mo: Mosby-Year Book; 1993:1205-1223.

12. Lichtmann MW. Military and battlefield anesthesia. In: Grande CM, ed. *Textbook of Trauma Anesthesia and Critical Care.* St. Louis, Mo: Mosby-Year Book; 1993:1297-1324.

13. Malseed RT, Goldstein FJ, Balkon N. Skeletal muscle relaxants. *Pharmacology Drug Therapy and Nursing Considerations.* 4th ed. Philadelphia, Pa: JB Lippincott; 1995:143-155.

14. Capan LV. Airway management. In: Capan LV, Miller SM, Turndorf H, eds. *Trauma Anesthesia and Intensive Care.* Philadelphia, Pa: JB Lippincott; 1991:43-81.

15. Booij LHDJ. Muscle relaxants. In: Grande CM, ed. *Textbook of Trauma Anesthesia and Critical Care*. St. Louis, Mo: Mosby-Year Book; 1993:479-484.

16. McKenry LM, Salerno E. Antianxiety, sedative, and hypnotic drugs. *Mosby's Pharmacology in Nursing*. 19th ed. St. Louis, Mo: Mosby-Year Book; 1995:304-333.

17. Harris MM, Berry FA. Pediatric trauma patients. In: Grande CM, ed. *Textbook of Trauma Anesthesia and Critical Care*. St. Louis, Mo: Mosby-Year Book; 1993:619-627.

18. Cicala RS, Grande CM, Stene JK, Behringer. Emergency and elective airway management for trauma patients. In: Grande CM, ed. *Textbook of Trauma Anesthesia and Critical Care*. St. Louis, Mo: Mosby-Year Book; 1993:344-360.

PAIN ASSESSMENT AND CONTROL

OBJECTIVES

Upon completion of this appendix, the learner should be able to:

1. Identify three sources of pain in the multiply injured patient.
2. Discuss the effects of pain on the multiply injured patient.
3. Identify the pathophysiology of pain.
4. Discuss the nursing management of pain in the injured patient.
5. Describe the effects of selected medications used to manage pain in the injured patient.
6. Discuss additional nursing interventions to help manage pain in the injured patient.

INTRODUCTION

Pain is an unpleasant sensory and emotional experience arising from actual or potential tissue damage.[1] Pain has serious physiologic consequences, yet it continues to be inadequately managed in the injured patient.[2-6] There are several reasons why pain management may not be considered a priority in the injured patient. These include the health care team's lack of knowledge about pain management, fear on the part of the health care team and the patient about the patient becoming addicted to pain medication, concern about side effects such as respiratory depression and hypotension, and the high priority given to stabilizing the patient's vital functions.

SOURCES

The sources of pain for the injured patient include:

- Injuries

- Procedures

  - Intravenous cannulation

  - Chest tube insertion and removal

  - Intubation

  - Wound care

- Fracture reduction

- Laceration repair

- Sexual assault examination

● Environment

- Light

- Noise

♦ Cardiac monitors
♦ Intravenous monitors
♦ Pulse oximeter

● Extrication

- Tools

- Breaking windows

● Transport noise

- Ground ambulance

- Rotor or fixed wing

● Diagnostic procedures

- CT scan

- MRI

- Ultrasonography

- Endoscopy

PHYSIOLOGY

Pain Receptors

The body has five types of sensory receptors: mechanoreceptors, thermoreceptors, electromagnetic receptors, chemoreceptors, and nociceptors.[7] Nociceptors are free nerve endings distributed throughout the skin, dural extensions, dental pulp, and in some internal organs. They are sensitive to physical or chemical tissue damage. Both physiologic and psychologic events interact to cause pain in the injured patient. Mechanical, thermal, or chemical forces are potential painful

494

stimuli. When tissue is initially damaged, endogenous substances are released. Substances such as bradykinin, histamine, and prostaglandins influence the sensation of pain experienced by persons with tissue injury.[7]

Sources of Pain

The many causes of pain are related to painful stimuli in various portions of the body. The source of the pain is either from the skin or subcutaneous tissue (cutaneous); muscles, joints, tendons, or blood vessels (deep somatic); organs (visceral or splanchnic); or from functional or psychogenic sources whereby the pain is present but the source is unknown.

Intrinsic Analgesic System

The body also has its own intrinsic analgesic system. The endogenous analgesia center (EAC) is located in the midbrain. The EAC apparently is able to receive messages from the spinothalamic tracts and connects to the limbic system where emotional responses to pain are processed. Through complex connections of the EAC fibers to the medulla and the dorsal horn of the spinal cord, it is postulated that excitation of the neurons of the medulla inhibits the transmission of pain.[8] Two additional opioid chemicals, endorphins and enkephalins located in the brain, produce morphine-like analgesia. Serotonin is also an endogenous chemical that may play a role in reducing chronic pain. There is evidence that drugs which block serotonin uptake (e.g., antidepressants) produce some analgesia.[8]

Pain Transmission

The transmission of pain from the nociceptors to the spinal cord, thalamus, and parietal cortex of the brain occurs via two types of afferent peripheral nerve fibers. A-delta fibers are considered fast pain fibers since transmission velocity is 5 to 30 m/second. These are myelinated fibers that respond to mechanical and temperature stimuli to produce a pain that is sharp, stabbing, or acute, e.g., pinprick. C fibers have a transmission velocity of 0.5 to 2.0 m/second and, therefore, are referred to as slow pain fibers that respond to mechanical stimuli, temperature, and chemicals released from damaged tissues. The type of pain transmitted via C fibers is described as a burning, throbbing, aching, or chronic pain.

The spinal cord, thalamus, limbic system, and the cerebral cortex have roles in the pain experience. The anterolateral sensory nerve fiber tracts and their three spinothalamic tracts transmit pain from the spinal cord. The thalamus is the area where the pain sensation is realized. The refinement of the pain is the function of the cerebral cortex.

Physiologic and Psychologic Responses to Pain

Physiologically, pain activates the sympathetic portion of the autonomic nervous system leading to:

- Increase in heart rate and force of cardiac contraction

- Peripheral vasoconstriction and pallor

- Tachypnea

- Muscle tension leading to guarding or splinting as a reflex to protect painful structures

- Loss of parasympathetic tone with anorexia, nausea, and vomiting

- Release of adrenal gland catecholamines resulting in an increase in blood pressure, cardiac afterload, and myocardial oxygen consumption

Psychologically, the response to pain is related to past experiences, age, gender, culture, threshold, tolerance, and environmental circumstances surrounding the painful experience.

NURSING CARE OF THE INJURED PATIENT WITH PAIN

Assessment

The Agency for Health Care Policy and Research of the US Department of Health and Human Services, published the clinical practice guidelines *Acute Pain Management: Operative or Medical Procedures and Trauma*.[9] This document contains pain assessment tools and guidelines for pain control. The report states: *"The single most reliable indicator of the existence and intensity of acute pain and any resultant affective discomfort or distress is the patient's self-report."*[9] This statement reinforces the concept that pain is an individual perception and experience that is best described in terms of its presence and relief by that individual.

History

- What is the source of pain?

- Where is the pain located?

- When did the pain start?

- What has been done to manage the pain?

- Has the patient ever had similar pain before?

Physical Assessment

INSPECTION

- Observe general response to pain which may include

  - Tachypnea

  - Shallow respirations[9]

- Nausea and vomiting

- Diaphoresis

- Muscular guarding, e.g., abdominal muscles

- Protective behavior, e.g., requests not to be touched

- Pinched facial expressions

- Clenched fist or teeth

- Moaning

- Crying

- Facial mask of pain

- Assess level of pain using a pain intensity scale such as[9]:

  - 0 – No pain

  - 1 – Mild pain

  - 2 – Moderate

  - 3 – Severe

  - 4 – Very severe

  - 5 – Worst possible pain

PALPATION

- Skin temperature

- Area of pain

- Pulses

POSSIBLE NURSING DIAGNOSIS AND EXPECTED OUTCOMES	
Nursing Diagnosis	**Expected Outcome**
Pain related to: • Tissue injury	The patient will experience relief of pain as evidenced by: • Diminishing or absent level of pain through patient's self-report using an objective measurement tool • Absence of physiologic indicators of pain that include: tachycardia, tachypnea, pallor, diaphoretic skin, increasing blood pressure • Absence of nonverbal cues of pain: crying, grimacing, inability to assume position of comfort • Ability to cooperate with care as appropriate

Planning and Implementation

Various methods may be used to manage pain. These include analgesics, conscious sedation, cutaneous stimulation, therapeutic touch, and provision of comfort measures.

Desirable properties of medications used in the emergency management of pain include minimal side effects, easy and painless administration, amnesic effect, short-term duration of action, few contraindications, and sedative as well as analgesic effects.

• Monitor the patient following pain medication administration for:

   ■ Respiratory depression

   ■ Hypotension

   ■ Altered mental status

   ■ Allergic reaction

   ■ Nausea and vomiting

• Facilitate conscious sedation, as prescribed

   ■ Conscious sedation is defined as a medically controlled state of altered consciousness that allows patients to maintain their protective reflexes, maintain an adequate airway, and respond appropriately to physical or verbal stimulation.[10]

   ■ Medications used for conscious sedation may provide analgesia, amnesia, altered pain perception, muscle relaxation, and euphoria. Even though these drugs have positive effects, they also have potential side effects (see Table 46).

   ■ The most common medications used for conscious sedation in the adult patient include opioid analgesics and benzodiazepines. Recently, research has demonstrated that conscious sedation may be more effective if agents are employed that not only alter the patient's response to pain, but also block the physiological changes that may occur as the result of injury. Ketorolac, a nonsteroidal anti-inflammatory agent, is often used with an opioid and/or benzodiazepine to manage pain from injury (see Table 47).

Table 46

SIDE EFFECTS OF CONSCIOUS SEDATION
• Respiratory depression
• Hypotension
• Bradycardia
• Muscle rigidity
• Nausea and vomiting
• Hallucinations from medications
• Agitation

Table 47

DRUGS USED FOR CONSCIOUS SEDATION		
Drug	**Route**	**Side Effects**
Opioids		
Morphine	IV, IM, SC	• Respiratory depression • Hypotension • Muscular rigidity • Miosis • Urinary retention • Nausea and vomiting
Fentanyl	IV, IM	• Respiratory depression • Muscular rigidity (especially the chest wall) • Facial puritis • Hypotension
Benzodiazepines		
Midazolam (Versed)	IV, PO	• Respiratory depression • Hypotension • Agitation • Nausea and vomiting • Hiccough
Diazepam (Valium)	IV, PO	• Respiratory depression • Headaches
Lorazepam (Ativan)	IV, IM, PO	• Respiratory depression
Nonsteroidal Anti-Inflammatory Agents		
Ketorolac (Toradol)	IM	• Nausea and vomiting • Dizziness • Nephrotoxicity

- Consider alternative pain management

  - Epidural and intrathecal methods may be used to provide analgesia for selected injuries.[11]

  - Other alternative pain management methods include:

    - Therapeutic touch
    - Accupressure
    - Positioning
    - Application of heat or cold
    - Distraction
    - Relaxation
    - Guided imagery
    - General comfort measures

- Remove or adjust pain-producing objects or equipment, e.g., shattered glass

- Assure immediate availability of:

  - Oxygen source with flow meter, tubing and mask

  - Resuscitation bag with an appropriately-sized mask

  - Suction regulator and rigid tonsil suction

  - Naloxone (Narcan) if narcotics are administered

  - Flumazenil (Mazicon) if benzodiazepines are administered

Evaluation and Ongoing Assessment

Monitor:

- Depth and rate of respiration

- Blood pressure

- Pulse

- Level of consciousness

- Signs of allergic reaction

- Gastrointestinal disturbances, e.g., nausea and vomiting

- Oxygen saturation

- Electrocardiogram

SUMMARY

Pain is an unpleasant sensory and emotional experience arising from actual or potential tissue damage. Causes of pain include:

- Tissue damage due to injuries

- Therapeutic and diagnostic procedures

- Environmental stimuli

If conscious, have the patient describe the location, intensity, or type of the pain. The methods used to control pain include the use of analgesics, conscious sedation, and nonpharmacologic relaxation and comfort measures.

REFERENCES

1. International Association for the Study of Pain. Pain terms: a list with definitions and notes on usage. *Pain*. 1979;6:249.

2. Friedland L, Kulick R. Emergency department use of analgesics in pediatric trauma victims with fractures. *Ann Emerg Med*. 1994;23:203-207.

3. Kaiser K. Assessment and management of pain in the critically ill trauma patient. *Crit Care Nurs*. 1992;15:14-34.

4. Puntillo K. The physiology of pain and its consequences in critically ill patients. In: Puntillo K, ed. *Pain in the Critically Ill*. Gaithersburg, Md: Aspen Publications; 1991:30.

5. Selbst M, Clark M. Analgesic use in the emergency department. *Ann Emerg Med*. 1990;19:1010-1013.

6. Stewart R. Analgesia in the field. *Prehospital and Disaster Medicine*. 1989;4:31-34.

7. Guyton AC. Somatic sensations, pain, headache, and thermal sensations. *Textbook of Medical Physiology*. 8th ed. Philadelphia, Pa: WB Saunders Co; 1991:520-531.

8. Curtis SM, Curtis RL. Somatosensory function and pain. In: Porth CM, ed. *Pathophysiology Concepts of Altered Health States*. 4th ed. Philadelphia, Pa: JB Lippincott Co; 1994:973-1006.

9. Acute Pain Management Guideline Panel. *Acute Pain Management: Operative or Medical Procedures and Trauma*. Clinical Practice Guideline. AHCPR Pub. No: 92-0032. Rockville, MD: Agency for Health Care Policy and Research, Public Health Service, US Department of Health and Human Services; February 1992.

10. Schlag K. *Conscious Sedation: Standards and Procedures*. Dublin, Ca: Contemporary Forums; 1994.

11. Dyble K. Epidural and intrathecal methods of analgesia in the critically ill. In: Puntillo K, ed. *Pain in the Critically Ill*. Gaithersburg, Md: Aspen Publications; 1991:95-114.

TETANUS PROPHYLAXIS

TETANUS AND PRIMARY VACCINATION

Tetanus is a serious, often fatal disease caused by the bacillus, *Clostridium tetani*. The disease leads to convulsions, muscle spasms, stiffness of the jaw, coma, and death. The bacilli are found in the intestines of animals and humans. The spores can be found in soil and dust and are spread by animal and human feces. The bacillus organism enters the human host through an open wound, particularly those caused by nails, splinters, insect bites, or gunshots.

Immunization with tetanus toxoid, improved wound management, and tetanus prophylaxis after injury have reduced the number of cases of tetanus in the United States. Since 1947, tetanus has been a reportable disease. During 1947, there were 560 cases and, in 1987, the incidence dropped to only 48 cases.[1] Sixty-eight percent of all patients with tetanus are 50 years of age or older; there are no reported cases of neonatal tetanus, and the case-fatality rate is 21%.[1] Of those patients who contracted tetanus following an acute injury in 1987 and 1988, 58% did not receive any medical care for the injury. Of those patients who did receive medical care and did contract tetanus, 81% were not given the appropriate tetanus prophylaxis as recommended by the CDC's Advisory Committee on Immunization Practices.

Table 48 outlines the routine vaccination schedule for those children less than seven years of age. Table 49 describes the vaccination schedule for those seven years of age and older.[1]

Table 48

ROUTINE DIPHTHERIA, TETANUS, AND PERTUSSIS (DPT) VACCINATION FOR CHILDREN LESS THAN 7 YEARS OF AGE			
Dose	**Age**	**Age/Interval**	**Product***
Primary 1	2 months	6 weeks old or older	DPT
Primary 2	4 months	4 to 8 weeks after 1st dose	DPT
Primary 3	6 months	4 to 8 weeks after 2nd dose	DPT
Primary 4	15 months	6 to 12 months after 3rd dose	DPT
Booster	4 to 6 years (not necessary if fourth primary dose administered after fourth birthday)		DPT
Additional Boosters	Every 10 years after last dose		Td
* Use DT if pertussis vaccine is contraindicated. If the child is 1 year old or older at the time that primary dose three is due, a third dose 6 to 12 months after the second completes primary vaccination with DT.			

Table 49

ROUTINE DIPHTHERIA, TETANUS, AND PERTUSSIS (DPT) VACCINATION FOR THOSE 7 YEARS OF AGE OR OLDER		
Dose	**Age/Interval**	**Product**
Primary 1	Fist Dose	Td
Primary 2	4 to 8 weeks after 1st dose	Td
Primary 3	6 to 12 months after 2nd dose	Td
Booster	Every 10 years after last dose	Td

TETANUS PROPHYLAXIS AFTER TRAUMA

Determination of the need for tetanus prophylaxis following trauma depends on:

- Condition of the wound

- Patient's past vaccination history

First determine whether the patient has ever received primary vaccination. Any person with military experience since 1941 "can be considered to have received at least one dose."[1] Table 50 describes the guidelines for tetanus prophylaxis.[1] The two drugs used for tetanus prophylaxis are tetanus-diptheria toxoid (Td) and tetanus immune globulin (TIG).

Table 50

TETANUS PROPHYLAXIS IN WOUND MANAGEMENT				
Vaccination History	**Clean/Minor Wounds**		**All Others***	
	Td+	**TIG**	**Td+**	**TIG**
Unknown or <three	Yes	No	Yes	Yes
Three or more§	No¶	No	No+	No
* Such as, but not limited to, wounds contaminated with dirt, feccs, soil, and saliva; puncture wounds; avulsions; and wounds resulting from missiles, crushing forces, burns, and frostbite.				
+ For children <7 years old; DPT (DT, if pertussis vaccine is contraindicated) is preferred to tetanus toxoid alone. For persons 7 years of age or older, Td is preferred to tetanus toxoid.				
§ If only three doses of fluid toxoid have been received, then a fourth dose of toxoid, preferably an absorbed toxoid, should be given.				
¶ Yes, if >10 years since last dose.				
+ Yes, if >5 years since last dose. More frequent boosters are not needed and can accentuate side effects.				

REFERENCES

1. US Department of Health and Human Services. Public Health Service, Centers for Disease Control, National Center for Prevention Services, Division of Immunization. Diphtheria, tetanus, and pertussis: recommendations for vaccine use and other preventive measures. *MMWR*. 1991:40(RR-10).

INJURY SEVERITY INDICES

INTRODUCTION

Injury severity indices identify patient risk by converting a number of patient variables into a numerical format. They are utilized to quantify the magnitude of injury, determine priorities of care in the prehospital setting, and identify patients with needs that may require the resources available at a designated trauma center. Additionally, they quantify injuries for the purpose of comparing patients with varying case mixes for research and trauma quality improvement activities. Injury severity indices developed for triage purposes are usually based on physiologic indicators or a combination of physiologic status, anatomic site of injury, and mechanism of injury.

REVISED TRAUMA SCORE

The Revised Trauma Score is the most utilized physiologic severity index in the prehospital setting for identifying severely injured patients.[1] The precursors of the Revised Trauma Score are the Triage Index[2] and the Trauma Score.[3] The Revised Trauma Score consists of three components: the Glasgow Coma Scale, respiratory rate, and systolic blood pressure. Each component is assigned a rank value of 0 to 4. The sum of the three coded values can range from 0 to 12 (see Table 51).

GLASGOW COMA SCALE

The Glasgow Coma Scale was developed in 1974 by Teasdale and Jennett as a tool for examination of the patient with impaired consciousness.[4] The scale is based on eye opening ability, best verbal response, and best motor response to stimuli. Each is graded to indicate the degree of dysfunction. The greater the degree of impaired consciousness, the lower the score. The score ranges from 3 to 15 (see Table 52).

Table 51

REVISED TRAUMA SCORE	
Area of Measurement	**Coded Value**
Systolic Blood Pressure (mmHg)	
>89	4
76-89	3
50-75	2
1-49	1
0	0
Respiratory Rate **(spontaneous inspirations/minute)***	
10-29	4
>29	3
6-9	2
1-5	1
0	0
*patient-initiated, not artificial ventilations	
Glasgow Coma Scale Score	
13-15	4
9-12	3
6-8	2
4-5	1
3	0
Total Possible Points	**0-12**

Table 52

GLASGOW COMA SCALE	
Areas of Response	**Points**
Eye Opening	
Eyes open spontaneously	4
Eyes open in response to voice	3
Eyes open in response to pain	2
No eye opening response	1
Best Verbal Response	
Oriented (e.g., to person, place, time)	5
Confused, speaks but is disoriented	4
Inappropriate, but comprehensible words	3
Incomprehensible sounds but no words are spoken	2
None	1
Best Motor Response	
Obeys command to move	6
Localizes painful stimulus	5
Withdraws from painful stimulus	4
Flexion, abnormal decorticate posturing	3
Extension, abnormal decerebrate posturing	2
No movement or posturing	1
Total Possible Points	**3-15**
Major Head Injury	**≤8**
Moderate Head Injury	**9-12**
Minor Head Injury	**13-15**

PEDIATRIC TRAUMA SCORE

The Pediatric Trauma Score was developed to address the special needs of the injured child. The tool is composed of six variables:

1. Size (weight in kilograms)
2. Airway status
3. Systolic blood pressure
4. Level of consciousness
5. Cutaneous integrity
6. Skeletal injury

The variables are assigned a grade of +2, +1, –1, indicating a range of minimal or no injury to major or life-threatening injury. The range of the score is –6 to +12 (see Table 53). Tepas et al reported that children with a score of 6 or below had an increased potential for mortality.[5]

Table 53

Component	Category		
	+2	**+1**	**−1**
Size	>20 kg	10 to 20 kg	<10 kg
Airway	Normal	Maintainable	Unmaintainable
Systolic BP	>90 mmHg	50 to 90 mmHg	<50 mmHg
CNS	Awake	Obtunded/LOC	Coma/decerebrate
Skeletal	None	Closed fracture	Open/multiple fractures
Cutaneous	None	Minor	Major/penetrating

SUM _____

If proper-sized BP cuff is not available, BP can be assessed by assigning
+2 Pulse: Palpable at wrist
+1 Pulse: Palpable at groin
−1 No pulse palpable

(Reprinted with permission of Tepas JJ, Molitt DL, Talbert JL, Bryant M. The pediatric trauma score as a predictor of injury severity in the injured child. *J Pediatr Surg*. 1987; 22:14-18.)

ABBREVIATED INJURY SCALE

Another important application of injury severity indices is to compare patients with varying case mix. Indices based on anatomical information are computed retrospectively. More definitive diagnostic information, such as CT scan, x-ray, and surgery or autopsy findings is used.

The Abbreviated Injury Scale (AIS) was originally developed by the American Medical Association Committee on Medical Aspects of Automotive Injury to provide a common language for motor vehicle crash-related injuries. The system was developed by physicians and engineers. The severity grades are based on energy dissipation, threat to life, permanent impairment, treatment period, and incidence.[6]

The AIS provides a numerical ranking of the severity of injuries and designates one score for each injury. Unlike a physiologic severity index, the AIS will not change as the patient status improves or deteriorates. The AIS does not account for the impact of multiple organ injuries.

Since its original publication in 1971, the AIS has undergone multiple revisions, the most recent in 1990. The Abbreviated Injury Scale dictionary contains injury descriptors including those for pediatric injury and brain injury. The AIS 90 dictionary contains more than 2,000 injury descriptors in terminology compatible with current language.[7] A scale of 1 through 6 is used to describe the severity of each injury descriptor. The levels of severity are: 1) minor, 2) moderate, 3) serious, 4) severe, 5) critical, and 6) maximum.[7]

INJURY SEVERITY SCORE

The Injury Severity Score (ISS) was developed to describe the multiply injured patient. The ISS, based on the AIS injury descriptors, describes the overall severity in persons who have injured more than one body region. The sum of the squares of the highest AIS grade in each of the three most severely injured body regions is equal to the ISS. As an example, a person with a basilar skull fracture (HEAD; AIS=3), a hemothorax (CHEST:AIS=3), and a minor liver laceration (ABDOMEN=2) would have an ISS of 22 (9+9+4=22). ISS scores range from 1 to 75; with the higher the score, the more severely injured the patient.[8] An ISS of 15 or greater is the most universally accepted definition of a major trauma patient.[8]

ORGAN INJURY SCALES

The American Association for the Surgery of Trauma appointed the Organ Injury Scaling (OIS) committee to develop individual organ injury scales corresponding to International Classification of Diseases (ICD-9) and AIS codes for various body regions[9-12] (see Tables 54-70).

Table 54

SPLENIC INJURY SCALE			
Grade*	**Injury Description†**	**ICD-9**	**AIS 90**
I. Hematoma:	• Subcapsular, nonexpanding <10% surface area	865.01 865.11	2
Laceration:	• Capsular tear, nonbleeding, <1 cm parenchymal depth	865.02 865.12	
II. Hematoma:	• Subcapsular, nonexpanding, 10-50% surface area; Intraparenchymal, nonexpanding, <2 cm in diameter	865.01 865.11	2
Laceration:	• Capsular tear, active bleeding; 1-3 cm parenchymal depth which does not involve a trabecular vessel	865.02 865.12	2
III. Hematoma:	• Subcapsular, >50% surface area or expanding; Ruptured subcapsular hematoma with active bleeding; Intraparenchymal hematoma >2 cm or expanding		3
Laceration:	• >3 cm parenchymal depth or involving trabecular vessels	865.03 865.13	3
IV. Hematoma:	• Ruptured intraparenchymal hematoma with active bleeding		4
Laceration:	• Laceration involving segmental or hilar vessels producing major devascularization (>25% of spleen)	865.04 865.14	4
V. Laceration:	• Completely shattered spleen	865.04 865.14	5
Vascular:	• Hilar vascular injury which devascularizes spleen		5
* Advance one grade for multiple injuries to the same organ.			
† Based on most accurate assessment at autopsy, laparotomy, or radiologic study.			

511

Table 55

LIVER INJURY SCALE			
Grade*	**Injury Description†**	**ICD-9**	**AIS 90**
I. Hematoma:	• Subcapsular, nonexpanding, <10% surface area	864.01 864.11	2
Laceration:	• Capsular tear, nonbleeding, <1 cm parenchymal depth	864.02 864.12	2
II. Hematoma:	• Subcapsular, nonexpanding, 10-50% surface area; Intraparenchymal, nonexpanding, <2 cm in diameter	864.01 864.11	2
Laceration:	• Capsular tear, active bleeding; 1-3 cm parenchymal depth, <10 cm in length	864.03 864.13	2
III. Hematoma:	• Subcapsular, >50% surface area or expanding; Ruptured subcapsular hematoma with active bleeding; Intraparenchymal hematoma >2 cm or expanding		3
Laceration:	• >3 cm parenchymal depth	864.04 864.14	3
IV. Hematoma:	• Ruptured intraparenchymal hematoma with active bleeding		4
Laceration:	• Parenchymal disruption involving 25-50% of hepatic lobe	864.04 864.14	4
			5
V. Laceration:	• Parenchymal disruption involving >50% of hepatic lobe		5
Vascular:	• Juxtahepatic venous injuries; i.e., retrohepatic vena cava/major hepatic veins		
			6
VI. Vascular:	• Hepatic avulsion		

* Advance one grade for multiple injuries to the same organ.
† Based on most accurate assessment at autopsy, laparotomy, or radiologic study.

Table 56

Grade*		Injury Description†	ICD-9	AIS 90
I.	Contusion:	• Microscopic or gross hematuria; urologic studies normal		2
	Hematoma:	• Subcapsular, nonexpanding without parenchymal laceration	866.01 866.11	2
II.	Hematoma:	• Nonexpanding perirenal hematoma confined to renal retroperitoneum	866.01 866.11	2
	Laceration:	• <1.0 cm parenchymal depth of renal cortex without urinary extravasation	866.02 866.12	2
III.	Laceration:	• >1.0 cm parenchymal depth of renal cortex without collecting system rupture or urinary extravasation	866.02 866.12	3
IV.	Laceration:	• Parenchymal laceration extending through the renal cortex, medulla and collecting system		4
	Vascular:	• Main renal artery or vein injury with contained hemorrhage		4
V.	Laceration:	• Completely shattered kidney	866.03	5
	Vascular:	• Avulsion of renal hilum which devascularizes kidney	866.13	5

* Advance one grade for multiple injuries to the same organ.
† Based on most accurate assessment at autopsy, laparotomy, or radiologic study.

(Tables 54-56 were adapted with permission of Moore EE, Shackford SR, Pachter HL, McAninch JW, Browner BD, Champion HR, Flint LM, Gennarelli TA, Malangoni MA, Ramenofsky ML, Trafton PG. Organ injury scaling: Spleen, liver, and kidney. *J Trauma*. 1989;29:1664-1666.)

Table 57

PANCREATIC ORGAN INJURY SCALE			
Grade*	**Injury Description†**	**ICD-9**	**AIS 90**
I. Hematoma:	• Minor contusion without duct injury	863.81-	2
Laceration:	• Superficial laceration without duct injury	863.84	2
II. Hematoma:	• Major contusion without duct injury or tissue loss		2
Laceration:	• Major laceration without duct injury or tissue loss	863.81- 863.84	3
III. Laceration:	• Distal transection or parenchymal injury with duct injury		3
IV. Laceration:	• Proximal+ transection or parenchymal injury involving ampulla	863.92- 863.94	4
V. Laceration:	• Massive disruption of pancreatic head	863.91	5
.81,.91 = Head; .82,.92 = Body; .83,.93 = Tail			

* Advance one grade for multiple injuries to the same organ.
† Based on the most accurate assessment at autopsy, laparotomy, or radiologic study.
+ Proximal pancreas is to the patient's right of the superior mesenteric vein.

Table 58

Grade*	Injury Description†		ICD-9	AIS 90
I. Hematoma	•	Involving single portion of duodenum	863.21	2
Laceration	•	Partial thickness, no perforation	863.21	3
II. Hematoma:	•	Involving more than one portion	863.21	2
Laceration:	•	Disruption <50% of circumference	863.31	4
III. Laceration:	•	Disruption 50-75% circumference of D2	863.31	4
	•	Disruption 50-100% circumference of D1, D3, D4		4
IV. Laceration:	•	Disruption >75% circumference of D2	863.31	5
	•	Involving ampulla or distal common bile duct		5
V. Laceration:	•	Massive disruption of duodenopancreatic complex	863.31	5
Vascular:	•	Devascularization of duodenum	863.31	5

D1 = 1st portion duodenum, D2 = 2nd portion duodenum,
D3 = 3rd portion duodenum, D4 = 4th portion duodenum.
* Advance one grade for multiple injuries to the same organ.
† Based on the most accurate assessment at autopsy, laparotomy, or radiologic study.

Table 59

SMALL BOWEL ORGAN INJURY SCALE

Grade*	Injury Description†		ICD-9	AIS 90
I. Hematoma:	•	Contusion or hematoma without devascularization	863.20	2
Laceration:	•	Partial thickness, no perforation	863.20	2
II. Laceration:	•	Laceration <50% of circumference	863.30	3
III. Laceration:	•	Laceration ≥50% of circumference without transection	863.30	3
IV. Laceration:	•	Transection of the small bowel	863.30	4
V. Laceration:	•	Transection of the small bowel with segmental tissue loss	863.30	4
Vascular:	•	Devascularized segment	863.30	4

* Advance one grade for multiple injuries to the same organ.
† Based on the most accurate assessment at autopsy, laparotomy, or radiologic study.

Table 60

COLON ORGAN INJURY SCALE			
Grade*	**Injury Description†**	**ICD-9**	**AIS 90**
I. Hematoma:	• Contusion or hematoma without devascularization	863.40-	2
Laceration:	• Partial thickness, no perforation	863.44	2
		863.40-	
II. Laceration:	• Laceration <50% of circumference	863.44	3
III. Laceration:	• Laceration ≥50% of circumference without transection	863.50- 863.54	3
IV. Laceration:	• Transection of the colon		
		863.50-	4
V. Laceration:	• Transection of the colon with segmental tissue loss	863.54	
Vascular:	• Devascularized segment		4
			4
		863.50- 863.54	
		863.50- 863.54 863.50- 863.54	

.41,.51 = Ascending; .42,.52 = Transverse; .43,.53 = Descending; .44,.54 = Rectum

*   Advance one grade for multiple injuries to the same organ.
†   Based on the most accurate assessment at autopsy, laparotomy, or radiologic study.

Table 61

RECTAL ORGAN INJURY SCALE			
Grade*	**Injury Description†**	**ICD-9**	**AIS 90**
I. Hematoma:	• Contusion or hematoma without devascularization	863.45	2
Laceration:	• Partial thickness laceration	863.45	2
II. Laceration:	• Laceration <50% of circumference	863.55	3
III. Laceration:	• Laceration ≥50% of circumference	863.55	4
IV. Laceration:	• Full-thickness laceration with extension into the perineum	863.55	5
V. Vascular:	• Devascularized segment	863.55	5

*   Advance one grade for multiple injuries to the same organ.
†   Based on the most accurate assessment at autopsy, laparotomy, or radiologic study.

(Tables 57-61 were adapted with permission of Moore EE, Cogbill TH, Malangoni MA, Jurkovich GJ, Champion HR, Gennarelli TA, McAninch JW, Pachter HL, Shackford SR, Trafton PG. Organ injury scaling, II: Pancreas, duodenum, small bowel, colon, and rectum. *J Trauma*. 1990;30:1427-1429.)

Table 62

ABDOMINAL VASCULAR ORGAN INJURY SCALE*		
Grade	**ICD-9**	**AIS 90**
I. Grade I†		
• Nonnamed superior mesenteric artery or superior mesenteric vein branches	902.20/902.39	NS
• Nonnamed inferior mesenteric artery or inferior mesenteric vein branches	902.27/902.32	NS
• Phrenic artery/vein	902.89	NS
• Lumbar artery/vein	902.89	NS
• Gonadal artery/vein	902.89	NS
• Ovarian artery/vein	902.81/902.82	NS
• Other nonnamed small arterial or venous structures requiring ligation	902.90	NS
II. Grade II†		
• Right, left or common hepatic artery	902.22	3
• Splenic artery/vein	902.23/902.34	3
• Right or left gastric arteries	902.21	3
• Gastroduodenal artery	902.24	3
• Inferior mesenteric artery, trunk or inferior mesenteric vein, trunk	902.27/902.32	3
• Primary named branches of mesenteric artery (e.g., ileocolic artery) or mesenteric vein	902.26/902.31	3
• Other named abdominal vessels requiring ligation/repair	902.89	3
III. Grade III†		
• Superior mesenteric artery, trunk	902.31	3
• Renal artery/vein	902.41/902.42	3
• Iliac artery/vein	902.53/902.54	3
• Hypogastric artery/vein	902.51/902.52	3
• Vena cava, infrarenal	902.10	3
IV. Grade IV†		
• Superior mesenteric vein, trunk	902.25	3
• Celiac axis proper	902.24	3
• Vena cava, suprarenal and infrahepatic	902.10	3
• Aorta, infrarenal	902.00	4
V. Grade V†		
• Portal vein	902.33	3
• Extra-parenchymal hepatic vein	902.11	3 (hepatic vein) 5 (liver + veins)
• Vena cava, retrohepatic or suprahepatic	902.19	5
• Aorta, suprarenal, subdiaphragmatic	902.00	4

* This classification system is applicable for extraparenchymal vascular injuries. If the vessel injury is within 2 cm of the organ parenchyma, refer to specific organ injury scale.

† Increase one grade for multiple grade III or IV injuries involving >50% vessel circumference. Downgrade one grade if <25% vessel circumference laceration for grades IV or V.

517

Table 63

Grade*	Injury Description	ICD-9	AIS 90
URETER ORGAN INJURY SCALE			
I. Hematoma:	● Contusion or hematoma without devascularization	867.2/86 7.3	2
II. Laceration:	● <50% transection	867.2/86 7.3	2
III. Laceration:	● >50% transection	867.2/86 7.3	3
IV. Laceration:	● Complete transection with 2 cm devascularization	867.2/86 7.3	3
V. Laceration:	● Avulsion with >2 cm of devascularization	867.2/86 7.3	3

* Advance one grade if multiple lesions exist.

Table 64

Grade*	Injury Description	ICD-9	AIS 90
BLADDER ORGAN INJURY SCALE			
I. Hematoma: Laceration:	● Contusion, intramural hematoma ● Partial thickness	867.0/86 7.1	2 3
II. Laceration:	● Extraperitoneal bladder wall laceration <2 cm	867.0/86 7.1	4
III. Laceration:	● Extraperitoneal (>2 cm) or intraperitoneal (<2 cm) bladder wall lacerations	867.0/86 7.1	4
IV. Laceration:	● Intraperitoneal bladder wall laceration >2 cm	867.0/86 7.1	4
V. Laceration:	● Intraperitoneal or extraperitoneal bladder wall laceration extending into the bladder neck or ureteral orifice (trigone)	867.0/86 7.1	4

* Advance one grade if multiple lesions exist.

Table 65

URETHRA ORGAN INJURY SCALE			
Grade*	Injury Description	ICD-9	AIS 90
I. Contusion:	● Blood at urethral meatus; urethrography normal	867.0/867.1	2
II. Stretch injury:	● Elongation of urethra without extravasation on urethrography	867.0/867.1	2
III. Partial disruption:	● Extravasation of urethrography contrast at injury site with contrast visualized in the bladder	867.0/867.1	2
IV. Complete disruption:	● Extravasation of urethrography contrast at injury site without visualization in the bladder; <2 cm of urethral separation	867.0/867.1	3
V. Complete disruption:	● Complete transection with >2 cm urethral separation or extension into the prostate or vagina	867.0/867.1	4
* Advance one grade if multiple lesions exist.			

Table 66

CHEST WALL ORGAN INJURY SCALE*			
Grade†	**Injury Description**	**ICD-9**	**AIS 90**
I. Contusion:	• Any size	911.0/92	1
Laceration:	• Skin and subcutaneous	2.1	1
Fracture:	• <3 ribs closed	875.0	1-2
	• Nondisplaced clavicle, closed	807.01/8 07.02	2
II. Laceration:	• Skin, subcutaneous and muscle	810.0-	1
Fracture:	• ≥3 adjacent ribs, closed	810.03	2-3
	• Open or displaced clavicle		2
	• Nondisplaced sternum, closed	875.1	2
	• Scapular body, open or closed	807.03- 807.09	2
III. Laceration:	• Full thickness including pleural penetration	810.10-	2
Fracture:	• Open or displaced sternum; flail sternum	810.13	2
	• Unilateral flail segment, (<3 ribs)	807.2 811.00-	3-4
IV. Laceration:	• Avulsion of chest wall tissues with underlying rib fractures	811.19	4
Fracture:	• Unilateral flail chest (≥3 ribs)	862.29 807.2/80	3-4
V. Fracture:	• Bilateral flail chest (≥3 ribs on both sides)	7.3 807.4 807.10- 807.19 807.4 807.4	5

* This scale is confined to the chest wall alone and does not reflect associated internal thoracic or abdominal injuries. Therefore, further delineation of upper versus lower or anterior versus posterior chest wall was not considered, and a grade VI was not warranted. Specifically, thoracic crush was not used as a descriptive term; instead, the geography and extent of fractures and soft tissue injury were used to define the grade.

† Upgrade by one grade for bilateral injuries.

(Tables 62-66 were adapted with permission of Moore EE, Cogbill TH, Jurkovich GJ, McAninch JW, Champion HR, Gennarelli TA, Malangoni MA, Shackford SR, Trafton PG. Organ injury scaling III: Chest wall, abdominal vascular, ureter, bladder, and urethra. *J Trauma*. 1992;33:337-339.)

Table 67

	THORACIC VASCULAR ORGAN INJURY SCALE		
Grade*	**Injury Description†**	**ICD-9**	**AIS 90**
I.	• Intercostal artery/vein	901.81	2-3
	• Internal mammary artery/vein	901.82	2-3
	• Bronchial artery/vein	901.89	2-3
	• Esophageal artery/vein	901.9	2-3
	• Hemizygous vein	901.89	2-3
	• Unnamed artery/vein	901.9	2-3
II.	• Azygous vein	901.89	2-3
	• Internal jugular vein	900.1	2-3
	• Subclavian vein	901.3	3-4
	• Innominate vein	901.3	3-4
III.	• Carotid artery	900.01	3-5
	• Innominate artery	901.1	3-4
	• Subclavian artery	901.1	3-4
IV.	• Thoracic aorta, descending	901.0	4-5
	• Inferior vena cava (intrathoracic)	902.10	3-4
	• Pulmonary artery, primary intraparenchymal branch	901.41	3
	• Pulmonary vein, primary intraparenchymal branch	901.42	3
V.	• Thoracic aorta, ascending and arch	901.0	5
	• Superior vena cava	901.2	3-4
	• Pulmonary artery, main trunk	901.41	4
	• Pulmonary vein, main trunk	901.42	4
VI.	• Uncontained total transection of thoracic aorta or pulmonary hilum	901.0 901.41 901.42	5 4

* Increase one grade for multiple grade III or IV injuries if >50% circumference, decrease one grade for grade IV and V injuries if <25% circumference.
† Based on most accurate assessment at autopsy, operation, or radiologic study.

Table 68

LUNG ORGAN INJURY SCALE			
Grade*	**Injury Description†**	**ICD-9**	**AIS 90**
I. Contusion:	• Unilateral, <1 lobe	861.12/8 61.31	3
II. Contusion:	• Unilateral, single lobe		3
Laceration:	• Simple pneumothorax	861.20/8 61.30 860.0/1	3
III. Contusion:	• Unilateral, >1 lobe	860.4/5	3
Laceration:	• Persistent (>72 hours), air leak from distal airway	861.20/8	3 to 4
Hematoma:	• Nonexpanding intraparenchymal	61.30 860.0/1	
IV. Laceration:	• Major (segmental or lobar) airway leak	860.4/5	
Hematoma:	• Expanding intraparenchymal	862.20/8	4 to 5
Vascular:	• Primary branch intrapulmonary vessel disruption	61.30	3 to 5
V. Vascular:	• Hilar vessel disruption	862.21/8 61.31	4
VI. Vascular:	• Total, uncontained transection of pulmonary hilum	901.40	4
		901.41/9 01.42	
		901.41/9 01.42	

* Advance one grade for bilateral injuries; hemothorax is graded according to the thoracic vascular scale.
† Based on most accurate assessment at autopsy, operation, or radiologic study.

Table 69

CARDIAC INJURY ORGAN SCALE			
Grade*	**Injury Description**	**ICD-9**	**AIS 90**
I.	• Blunt cardiac injury with minor ECG abnormality (nonspecific ST or T wave changes, premature atrial, ventricular contraction or persistent sinus tachycardia) • Blunt or penetrating pericardial wound without cardiac injury, cardiac tamponade or cardiac herniation	861.01	3
II.	• Blunt cardiac injury with heart block (right or left bundle branch, left anterior fascicular, or atrioventricular) or ischemic changes (ST depression or T wave inversion) without cardiac failure • Penetrating tangential myocardial wound up to, but not extending through endocardium, without tamponade	861.01 861.12 861.01	3 3 3 to 4
III.	• Blunt cardiac injury with sustained (≥5 beats/min) or multifocal ventricular contractions • Blunt or penetrating cardiac injury with septal rupture, pulmonary or tricuspid valvular incompetence, papillary muscle dysfunction, or distal coronary arterial occlusion without cardiac failure • Blunt pericardial laceration with cardiac herniation • Blunt cardiac injury with cardiac failure • Penetrating tangential myocardial wound up to, but not extending through endocardium, with tamponade	861.01 861.01 861.01 861.12 861.12	3 to 4 3 to 4 3 to 4 3 3
IV.	• Blunt or penetrating cardiac injury with septal rupture, pulmonary or tricuspid valvular incompetence, papillary muscle dysfunction or distal coronary arterial occlusion producing cardiac failure • Blunt or penetrating cardiac injury with aortic or mitral valve incompetence • Blunt or penetrating cardiac injury of the right ventricle, right atrium, or left atrium	861.03 861.13 861.03 861.13 861.03	5 5 5
V.	• Blunt or penetrating cardiac injury with proximal coronary arterial occlusion • Blunt or penetrating left ventricular perforation	861.13	
VI.	• Stellate injuries <50% tissue loss of the right ventricle, right atrium or left atrium • Blunt avulsion of the heart; penetrating wound producing >50% tissue loss of a chamber		6

* Advance one grade for multiple penetrating wounds to a single chamber or multiple chamber involvement.

Table 70

Grade*	Injury Description	ICD-9	AIS 90
DIAPHRAGM ORGAN INJURY SCALE			
I.	• Contusion	862.0	2
II.	• Laceration ≤2 cm	862.1	3
III.	• Laceration 2-10 cm	862.1	3
IV.	• Laceration >10 cm with tissue loss ≤25 cm²	862.1	3
V.	• Laceration with tissue loss >25 cm²	862.1	3

*   Advance one grade for multiple injuries to the same organ.
†   Based on the most accurate assessment at autopsy, laparotomy, or radiologic study.

(Tables 67-70 were adapted with permission of Moore EE, Cogbill TH, Shackford SR, Champion HR, Jurkovich GJ, McAninch JW, Trafton PG. Organ injury scaling IV: Thoracic vascular, lung, cardiac, and diaphragm. *J Trauma*. 1994;36:299-300.)

REFERENCES

1. Champion HR, Sacco WJ, Copes WS, Gann DS, Gennarelli TA, Flanagan ME. A revision of the trauma score. *J Trauma.* 1989;29:623-629.

2. Champion HR, Sacco WJ, Hannan OS, Lepper RL, Atxinger ES, Copes WS, Prall RH. Assessment of injury severity: the triage index. *Crit Care Med.* 1980;8:201-208.

3. Champion HR, Sacco WJ, Carnazzo AJ, Copes WS, Fouty WJ. Trauma score. *Crit Care Med.* 1981;9:672-676.

4. Teasdale G, Jennett B. Assessment of coma and impaired consciousness: a practical scale. *Lancet.* 1974;July 13:81-83.

5. Tepas JJ, Molitt DL, Talbert JL, Bryant M. The pediatric trauma score as a predictor of injury severity in the injured child. *J Pediatr Surg.* 1987;22:14-18.

6. Committee on Medical Aspects of Automotive Safety. Rating the severity of tissue damage. The abbreviated scale. *JAMA.* 1972;215:277-280.

7. Association for the Advancement of Automotive Medicine. *The Abbreviated Injury Scale 1990 Revision.* Des Plaines, Ill: Author; 1990.

8. Baker S, Oneill B, Hadden W, Long W. The injury severity score: a method for describing patients with multiple injuries and evaluating emergency care. *J Trauma.* 1974;14:187-196.

9. Moore EE, Shackford SR, Pachter HL, McAninch JW, Browner BD, Champion HR, Flint LM, Gennarelli TA, Malangoni MA, Ramenofsky ML, Trafton PG. Organ injury scaling: spleen, liver, and kidney. *J Trauma.* 1989;29:1664-1666.

10. Moore EE, Cogbill TH, Malangoni MA, Jurkovich GJ, Champion HR, Gennarelli TA, McAninch JW, Pachter HL, Shackford SR, Trafton PG. Organ injury scaling, II: pancreas, duodenum, small bowel, colon, and rectum. *J Trauma.* 1990;30:1427-1429.

11. Moore EE, Cogbill TH, Jurkovich GJ, McAninch JW, Champion HR, Gennarelli TA, Malangoni MA, Shackford SR, Trafton PG. Organ injury scaling, III: chest wall, abdominal vascular, ureter, bladder, and urethra. *J Trauma.* 1992;33:337-339.

12. Moore EE, Malangoni MA, Cogbill TH, Shackford SR, Champion HR, Jurkovich GJ, McAninch JW, Trafton PG. Organ injury scaling, IV: thoracic vascular, lung, cardiac, and diaphragm. *J Trauma.* 1994;36:299-300.

EYE TRAUMA

Preface

Prior to reading this optional chapter, it is strongly suggested that the learner read the initial section on "Anatomy and Physiology." Specific anatomic and physiologic concepts are presented to enhance the learner's ability to correlate such concepts with specific injuries. This material related to anatomy and physiology will not be covered during lectures, nor will it be evaluated by testing. However, knowledge of normal anatomy and physiology serves as the foundation for understanding the anatomic derangements and pathophysiologic compromises which may ensue as a result of trauma.

ANATOMY AND PHYSIOLOGY

Globe

The globe (eyeball) is composed of three concentric layers. The outermost layer is formed by the sclera and cornea (see Figure 45). The sclera is a white, opaque, fibrous coat which covers the majority of the globe. Its posterior portion is continuous with the outer sheath of the optic nerve,[1,2] and is the attachment surface for the extraocular muscles and tendons responsible for normal movement of the globe in the orbit. The sclera's anterior portion is continuous with the cornea. The cornea is a multilayered, convex, transparent structure covering the anterior segment of the globe.[1] The circular margin where the cornea and sclera are contiguous is called the limbus. The outermost corneal layer, the anterior corneal epithelium, is continuous with the bulbar conjunctiva.

The uvea is the middle layer of the globe. It is composed of the iris, ciliary body and choroid. The choroid is a thin, pigmented vascular sheath which underlies the optic portion of the retina. The innermost layer of the globe is the retina, which is continuous with the optic nerve (II), and lines the entire uveal layer of the globe. The segments of the retina that line the ciliary body and the posterior aspect of the iris are not involved in visual perception.

Segments and Chambers

The eye is divided into the anterior and posterior segment. The posterior segment includes the retina, choroid, and the vitreous humor. The vitreous humor is a transparent, colloidal gel. The anterior segment includes the cornea, iris, ciliary body, lens, and zonular fibers (suspensory ligaments of the lens). The anterior segment encloses the aqueous compartment and contains aqueous humor. The aqueous compartment is further subdivided (by the plane of the iris) into anterior and posterior chambers. The posterior chamber is bounded anteriorly by the posterior aspect of the iris, laterally by the ciliary body, and posteriorly by the lens and zonular fibers. The anterior chamber is bounded anteriorly by the endothelial layer (posterior aspect) of the cornea, and posteriorly by the anterior aspect of the iris. Aqueous humor is secreted continuously by special cells in the ciliary body (i.e., in the posterior chamber of the aqueous compartment). The aqueous humor flows through the pupil, and drains from the angle of the anterior chamber. The angle of the anterior chamber is the junction of the posterior surface of the cornea and outer margin of the iris.[3] Obstruction of the drainage of aqueous humor at this junction leads to an increase in intraocular pressure known as narrow-angle, or angle-closure glaucoma.

Lens and Pupil

The lens is a transparent disc, concave on both its anterior and posterior surfaces. It refracts and focuses light on the optic retina. The lens is supported by circumferentially-radiating ligamentous fibers that attach to the ciliary body. Contractions of the muscles of the ciliary body alter how light is focused on the retina by altering the thickness of the lens. The pupil is not a structure, it is the aperture in the center of the iris. The pupillary sphincter muscle is a muscular ring in the iris which constricts the pupil in response to parasympathetic stimulation.[1] It is innervated by the oculomotor nerve (III). Pupillary dilation occurs with sympathetic stimulation.[4]

Orbit

The orbit, which is a bony socket formed by the junction of seven facial bones, protects the globe. The orbital rim is formed by the zygoma (laterally), maxilla (inferiorly and medially), and the frontal bone (superiorly). The orbital surfaces of these three bones form, respectively, parts of the lateral wall, floor, and ceiling of the orbit. The more posterior surfaces of the orbit are formed by portions of the sphenoid, ethmoid, and lacrimal bones, and the orbital process of the palatine bone.[2] The orbit is large enough to accommodate the globe, the extraocular muscles and their vascular and cranial nerve supply (III, IV, and VI).

Eyelids

The anterior surface of the globe is protected by the eyelids (palpebra). Each lid contains a tarsal plate, and a band of cartilaginous connective tissue which gives the lids their shape. The eyelids have a rich blood supply, and can accommodate significant edema and/or hematoma formation when injured. The eyelids are lined by the palpebral conjunctiva, which are continuous with the bulbar conjunctiva of each eye. The conjunctiva are vascularized, transparent membranes which take on the color of the underlying tissue. Hence, the palpebral conjunctiva appear to be pink, and the bulbar conjunctiva white. The conjunctiva serve as a protective barrier to the surface of the globe and tarsal surface of the eyelids. Either or both conjunctival surfaces may be injured or inflamed causing bloodshot eyes or subconjunctival hemorrhage. Conjunctival edema (chemosis) frequently accompanies eye injuries. The eyelashes (cilia) also have a protective function in helping to screen the globe from small foreign bodies.

Lacrimal Glands

The lacrimal glands are in the upper lid, near the lateral canthus. Tears drain from the medial canthal region, via the small openings (puncta) of the canaliculi (lacrimal ducts). Therefore injury to either canthal region may disrupt normal lacrimal lubrication.

Figure 45
The Eye

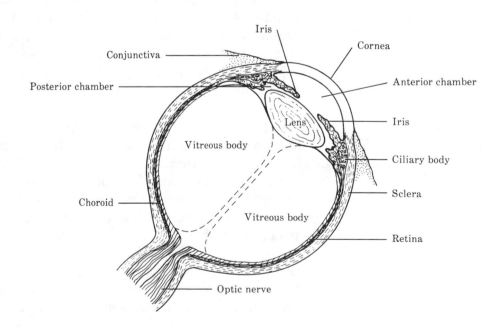

529

EYE TRAUMA

OBJECTIVES

Upon completion of this chapter/lecture, the learner should be able to:

1. Identify the common mechanisms of injury in eye trauma.
2. Analyze the pathophysiologic changes as a basis for signs and symptoms of eye injuries.
3. Discuss the nursing assessment of the patient with eye injuries.
4. Based on the assessment data, identify appropriate nursing diagnoses and expected outcomes.
5. Plan appropriate interventions for patients with eye injuries.
6. Evaluate the effectiveness of nursing interventions for patients with eye injuries.

INTRODUCTION

Epidemiology

An estimated 2.4 million eye injuries occur annually in the United States,[5] of which 20,000 to 68,000 are serious, vision-threatening injuries. These include open globe injuries, hyphemas, intraocular foreign bodies, or eye injury associated with facial or orbital fractures.[6] The average annual rate of hospital admission for a principal diagnosis of ocular trauma is estimated to be 13.2 per 100,000 population.[7] Among the most common causes of eye injuries requiring the patient to be admitted are injuries caused from: BB and air guns, motor vehicle collisions, interpersonal violence, falls, sports injuries, animal bites, intraocular or adnexal foreign bodies, or strikes to the eye from blunt or sharp objects.[7]

Males are at a greater risk for eye injury than females. The highest incidence of eye injury is among adult males between 15 and 34 years. Serious eye injuries occur in children less than 15 years old, and older adults, over 65 years.[7-9] Young children, particularly toddlers, are susceptible to eye injuries due to incoordination, lack of judgment about hazards, and the developmental need to explore.[10] Eye injuries associated with child treatment are due to direct blows and shaking.[11]

Older adults are susceptible to eye injury due to diminished visual and auditory acuity, and changes in coordination and reflexes.[12] The most common cause of ocular injury in older adults is falls.

A high proportion of serious eye injury is work-related, e.g., construction, auto repair, and agriculture.[7,8,13] Work-related eye injuries are preventable with proper protective eyewear.[8,13,14] It is estimated that fewer than 10% of persons with serious, work-related eye injuries were wearing proper protective gear at the time of injury. As many as 15% of persons with serious work-related eye injuries have a history of prior on-the-job eye injury.[8,13]

Recreational and sports activities are another common cause of serious eye injuries, e.g., hyphema and penetrating injuries. Approximately 35% of traumatic retinal detachments are sports-related. Most recreational and sports-related eye injuries are preventable with adequate protective equipment. There is an association between the use of alcohol and penetrating globe injuries resulting from vehicular collisions and intentional injuries.[5]

Mechanisms of Injury and Biomechanics

The most common mechanism of eye injury is associated with deceleration and acceleration forces to the surrounding structures. Penetrating eye injuries are caused by various projectiles and/or missiles, as in gunshot and knife wounds, fireworks, and broken glass. Blast forces can result in both blunt and penetrating injuries.

Chemical, Thermal, and Ultraviolet Radiation

Chemicals may cause injuries ranging from superficial inflammation to permanent blindness. Caustic chemicals, e.g., strong acids and bases, are the most devastating. Chemical burns can cause severe injury to the eyelids and other surrounding structures, as well as the eye. Thermal burns more commonly affect the eyelids and periorbital tissues, but if the heat is intense or the exposure protracted, the eyes themselves may be burned. Eye injuries from fireworks may result from both both thermal and chemical energy.

Injuries due to exposure to ultraviolet radiation (actinic), lead to a delayed onset of severe pain, diffuse corneal inflammation (keratitis), and anxiety. Examples of actinic injuries include welding burns, sunbathing, sunlamp exposure, and "snow blindness." Most actinic injuries are bilateral.

Foreign Bodies

The overwhelming majority of foreign bodies are superficial. Globe penetration must be suspected when the mechanism of injury was related to high-energy impact, such as with the use of a hammer power tool. Superficial corneal foreign bodies or abrasions are among the most common minor injuries of patients seen in any emergency department.

Types of Injuries

Eye injuries may be blunt or penetrating. It is important to remember that blunt mechanisms of injury can lead to a globe rupture, particularly in the elderly.

Usual Concurrent Injuries

Eye trauma is frequently associated with head or other facial injuries. Retinal hemorrhage is uncommon in pediatric head trauma patients, except related to maltreatment.[11] Intraocular hemorrhage is the most common finding in pediatric head trauma patients, often in association with a subdural hemorrhage. Brain injury may occur directly, due to comminuted fragments of orbital fractures, or indirectly due to accelerative or decelerative forces. Optic nerve injury may occur with an anterior fossa basilar skull fracture.

Blunt or penetrating injuries due to high energy forces can disrupt the architecture of the orbit, cause injury to the cranial nerves, or extraocular muscles and ligaments, disrupt the eyelids, or damage the lacrimal apparatus. On occasion, the optic nerve may be severed, causing permanent blindness. Patients with eye injuries may require ophthalmologic, maxillofacial, plastic surgery, or neurosurgical consultation.

PATHOPHYSIOLOGY AS A BASIS FOR SIGNS AND SYMPTOMS

Signs of Serious Eye Injury

Severe eye injury is associated with periorbital or midface fractures, no eye opening or eye opening only to painful stimuli, or abnormal pupillary reaction.[9,15] Specific pupillary abnormalities which correlate with serious eye injury include a nonreactive pupil or a pupil that paradoxically dilates when direct light is reflected on the uninjured eye.[9] Other predictors of serious injury include an initial visual acuity (corrected, if possible) of greater than 20/40, diplopia, and concomitant head injury with amnesia.[15] Patients with open globe injuries may only be able to visualize hand motion.[5]

Visual Disturbances

Loss of vision may be due to direct injury to the globe, or by the application of acceleration or deceleration forces to the eye region or to the brain. Causes of immediate or early onset blindness include:

- Posterior segment (vitreous) hemorrhage

- Prolapse or extrusion of globe contents

- A large intraocular foreign body

- Optic nerve laceration or avulsion

- Intracerebral hemorrhage, particularly in the occipital lobe

Causes of late-onset blindness or diminished acuity include:

- Retinal detachment

- Hemorrhage

- Cataract formation

- Glaucoma associated with a hyphema

- Open globe injuries may lead to sympathetic ophthalmia (bilateral panuveitis) weeks to years following the injury; the risk is greater if there has been traumatic extrusion of the contents of the lens or retained, intraocular foreign bodies.

Blurred vision may be due to injuries to the lens or posterior segment, but may also be due to tearing, or photophobia associated with more superficial injury. Diplopia (double vision) can be either unilateral or bilateral. Unilateral diplopia may be due to subluxation of the lens, orbital edema or hematoma, macular edema, or injury to the extra-ocular muscles. Bilateral diplopia can occur with orbital fractures with extraocular muscle entrapment, or from direct injury to the extraocular muscles or cranial nerves III, IV, or VI.

The degree of visual impairment due to hyphema is proportional to the degree of hemorrhage. A severe hyphema obscures the entire anterior chamber (eight-ball hemorrhage) and will diminish visual acuity severely or completely.

Pain

Eye pain varies depending on the depth of injury. Corneal injuries tend to be associated with intense, sharp, burning, or searing pain,[2] often with localized or diffuse redness. Pain from actinic injury is similar, but the redness is diffuse, and usually there is a history of gradual onset of pain six to 12 hours after welding, skiing or sunbathing. Corneal foreign bodies are immediately painful and provoke considerable tearing which may wash out the foreign body. A history of a foreign body sensation, with a hiatus when the pain seems to improve, followed by return of the pain, suggests a corneal abrasion. Pain from the uveal structures, as in iritis or hyphema, is a deep aching or boring pain, and may be accompanied by profuse tearing.[16] Photophobia is a painful response to bright light.[16] Photophobia may represent pain from a corneal injury, ciliary spasm, or posterior segment injury.

Pain associated with acute glaucoma may be severe and deep. Patients with acute glaucoma may also experience nausea and vomiting.

Redness and Ecchymosis of the Eye

Many eye injuries are associated with different patterns of redness from corneal or conjunctival inflammation or injury, to uveal inflammation or deeper injury. The redness from a superficial foreign body tends to be diffuse, but with localized intensity in the area of the foreign body or resulting abrasion(s). Redness from actinic or noncorrosive chemical injury is very diffuse. Redness from subconjunctival hemorrhage is bright to deep red, opaque, and may range from being localized to obscuring most of the sclera. In spite of its alarming appearance, subconjunctival hemorrhage does not threaten the patient's vision, although it may exist concomitantly with other injuries which are more serious. Iritis or acute angle closure glaucoma may cause diffuse redness, with increased intensity around the corneal limbus, known as a "ciliary flush."

Periorbital contusion and hematoma may cause a black eye. It is important to distinguish between a black eye and raccoon's sign, which is ecchymosis due to an anterior basilar skull fracture. Other facial injuries, e.g., nasal fractures, may lead to unilateral periorbital ecchymosis.

NURSING CARE OF PATIENTS WITH EYE TRAUMA

Assessment

History

Refer to Chapter 3, Initial Assessment, for a description of general information that should be collected regarding every trauma victim. Only pertinent questions specific to patients with eye injuries are described below.

- What was the mechanism of injury?

  Was the injury caused by a missile, shrapnel, or foreign body? Was the projectile metal, wood, glass, plastic, or mineral? Was the velocity of the projectile such that intraocular penetration might have occurred? Is there a periorbital entry wound with no obvious exit? Is a foreign body still present either superficially or intraocularly?

- Was protective eyewear used?

- What are the patients complaints?

  - Diminished visual acuity

  - Blurred or double vision in one or both eyes

  - Photophobia

  - Eye blinking (blepharospasm)

- Does the patient normally wear glasses or contact lenses? Was the patient wearing them at the time of injury? If the patient was wearing glasses, did they shatter? If the patient wears contact lenses, what type are they, and are they still in place?

- Does the patient have a history of eye problems or prior eye injuries?

- Has the patient ever had eye surgery such as cataract surgery, lens implants, or corneal surgery?

- Does the patient have visual or ocular changes associated with a chronic illness, e.g., hypertension, congestive heart failure, diabetes mellitus, glaucoma?

Physical Assessment

Refer to Chapter 3, Initial Assessment, for a description of the assessment of the patient's airway, effectiveness of breathing, and circulation.

Because of the potential for permanent visual impairment, and the consequences in terms of self-concept, work, and functional disability, eye injuries have a high priority for intervention. In terms of triage, serious eye injury takes priority over everything except life-threatening injuries. Deferred assessment of a badly swollen eye or failure to remove contact lenses can lead to serious eye injury, and can contribute to serious, permanent visual impairment.

INSPECTION

- Inspect the eye, periorbital tissues, and facial architecture

- Observe for symmetry, edema, ecchymosis, ptosis, lacerations. Determine if a lid laceration transects the lid margin or involves the lateral or medial canthus.

- Inspect the globe for:

  - Lacerations of the sclera, cornea, or iris

  - Large corneal abrasions, hyphema

  - Extrusion or prolapse of intraocular contents

  - Exophthalmos or enophthalmos

- Assess pupils for size, shape (roundness), equality, and reactivity to light

  - When testing the reaction to light of each pupil, assess the pupillary reaction in the eye being tested and in the opposite eye (consensual reaction).

  - The affected pupil is generally constricted in iritis, and dilated or midsize in acute glaucoma.

  - In patients with iritis, the pupil of the affected eye will be constricted relative to the opposite eye, but direct and consensual response to light will be intact.

- Assess for redness, eye watering, and blepharospasm

- Determine the presence of any foreign bodies or impaled objects

- Assess extraocular eye movements in all six directions to test function of cranial nerves III, IV, and VI

  Do not test extraocular eye movements if the patient is suspected of having an open globe injury.

- Assess for gaze defects such as crossed-eyes (estropia) or lateral strabismus

- Perform a visual acuity exam

  Use a Snellen or hand-held eye chart. Assess the uninjured eye first. Note visual acuity in each eye separately and then both eyes together. If the patient has corrective lenses and can wear them, it is best to measure visual acuity as corrected. If the patient is unable to participate in the examination due to the extent of injury, developmental stage, cognitive impairment, or intoxication, an assessment of finger-counting, hand-motion, and light perception should still be attempted.[17]

- Assess for blurred or double vision in the injured eye with the uninjured eye closed. Then, test with both eyes open.

PALPATION

- Palpate the periorbital area for:

  - Tenderness

  - Edema

  - Step-offs or depressions

  - Subcutaneous emphysema

- Do not palpate if an open globe injury is known or suspected, or if an object is impaled

- Assess sensory function of the infraorbital and supraorbital regions

Diagnostic Procedures

RADIOGRAPHIC STUDIES

- Eye radiographs to identify intraocular foreign bodies

- CT to determine small foreign bodies

- MRI to determine wood or vegetable foreign bodies

OTHER DIAGNOSTIC STUDIES

- Fluorescein staining

  Fluorescein staining and examination under cobalt blue lamp (Wood's light) or slit-lamp is conducted to identify surface defects, e.g., corneal abrasions, small conjunctival tears. The abraded areas absorb more dye and appear as punctate or larger areas of increased dye (green) intensity under fluorescent illumination. Single-use fluorescein strips should be stocked. Fluorescein drops are associated with increased infection rates.

- Slit-lamp examination

  Slit-lamp examination is used to identify a hyphema, or injury and inflammation of the cornea or anterior chamber. Removal of embedded corneal foreign bodies is generally performed under direct visualization with a slit-lamp.

- Tonometry (measures intraocular pressure)

Nursing Diagnoses and Outcome Identification

The following nursing diagnoses are potential problems for the patient with eye injuries. Once a patient has been assessed, diagnoses can be defined as either actual or risk. An actual nursing diagnosis is derived from a decision based on the patient's presenting signs and symptoms. A risk diagnosis is a judgment that the nurse makes based on a particular patient's risk and potential for developing certain problems.

POSSIBLE NURSING DIAGNOSES AND EXPECTED OUTCOMES	
Nursing Diagnosis	**Expected Outcome**
Sensory/perception, altered visual related to: • Visual impairment • Involvement of sensory receptors, CNS function • Direct trauma to the eye[18]	The patient will experience normal vision as evidenced by: • Normal responses to visual acuity examination
Pain related to: • Actual injury: puncture wounds, tissue destruction • Irritation and inflammation • Nonintact extraocular movement secondary to orbital edema, muscle entrapment, cranial nerve damage • Visible foreign body or substance • Chemical injury	The patient will experience relief of pain as evidenced by: • Diminishing or absent level of pain through patient's self-report using an objective measurement tool appropriate for developmental age • Absence of physiologic indicators of pain which include: tachycardia, tachypnea, pallor, diaphoretic skin, increasing blood pressure, restlessness. • Absence of nonverbal cues of pain: crying, grimacing, inability to assume position of comfort • Ability to cooperate with care as appropriate
Infection, risk related to: • Loss of skin or structural integrity secondary to actual injury • Foreign bodies • Introduction of organisms during invasive procedures	The patient will be free from infection as evidenced by: • Core temperature measurement of 36° - 37.5°C (98° - 99.5°F) • Absence of systemic signs of infection: fever, tachypnea, tachycardia • Wounds free from redness, swelling, purulent drainage or odor • Urinary output 1 ml/kg/hr • Negative blood cultures • WBC count within normal limits
Injury, risk related to: • Visual field defect • Impaired depth perception secondary to patching • Disruption of orbit architecture • Concomitant brain injury	The patient will have minimal complications of the injury as evidenced by: • No iatrogenic extension of the injury • Movement of eye is minimized with patching • Verbalizes and demonstrates understanding of need for no movement of eye • Absence of increase in extent of original injury

POSSIBLE NURSING DIAGNOSES AND EXPECTED OUTCOMES	
Nursing Diagnosis	**Expected Outcome**
Fear (patient, family) related to: • Actual or perceived threat of vision loss • Unfamiliar environment • Invasive procedures and therapeutic treatment • Separation from support systems	The patient/family will experience decreasing fear as evidenced by: • Absence of fear-related behavior, e.g., crying, shouting, agitated behavior, noncommunicative behavior, blank stare, facial expressions, voice tone, and body posture within normal for patient • Acknowledging fear and states decreasing fear • Absence of physiologic indicators of fear, e.g., palpations, increased blood pressure, diaphoresis, tachycardia • Absence of pain with coughing • Oriented to surroundings • Participating in decision-making regarding care when appropriate
Altered health maintenance, risk related to: • Insufficient knowledge of wound care, equipment, medications, prevention of injury • Restrictions to activity • Signs and symptoms of complications • Follow-up care	The patient is knowledgeable about self-care and follow-up as evidenced by: • Recognizing and promptly reporting signs and symptoms that indicate serious complications • Stating necessity and planning for ongoing medical care • Ability to describe and demonstrate proper administration of medications, means of preventing injury, wound care, restrictions on mobility and activity. • Accepting referrals to rehabilitative services, if appropriate

Planning and Implementation

Refer to Chapter 3, Initial Assessment, for a description of the specific nursing interventions for patients with compromises to airway, breathing, and/or circulation.

• Irrigate the eye if contaminated with any chemical (see chemical burns)

• Stabilize impaled objects without placing pressure on the globe

• Apply cool packs to decrease pain and periorbital swelling, as indicated

- Apply eye patch to the affected eye, as prescribed

  - Shield but do not patch the eye with a suspected open or ruptured globe. Use a metal or plastic eye shield or paper cup. Do not put pressure on the globe.

  - Patch the unaffected eye of a patient with an impaled object or ruptured globe.

  - Double-patch (two patches) the injured eye of a patient with a superficial corneal injury to reduce further corneal erosion and to facilitate corneal re-epithelization.

  - Do not double patch the eye of a patient who has hyphema, infection (corneal ulceration), or other anterior chamber injury (traumatic iritis).

  - Lightly patch or shield both eyes to reduce movement and photophobia in patients with retinal injuries.

  - Patch, shield, or cover with a cool pack, any injured eye that has been anesthetized.

- Elevate the head of the bed to minimize increases in intraocular pressure, especially in patients with a hyphema or open globe injury. If contraindicated, position the entire stretcher with the head higher than the feet.

- Instruct the patient not to bend forward, cough, or perform a Valsalva maneuver as these may raise intraocular pressure

- Instill prescribed topical anesthetic drops (ophthalmic tetracaine, proparacaine, etc.) for pain control and to facilitate eye examination

  - Topical anesthesia is contraindicated in open globe injuries.

  - An anesthetized eye should be patched, shielded, or covered with a cool pack to protect it from further injury.

  - Patients should not be discharged with topical anesthetic drops as continued use can lead to corneal breakdown and keratitis.

- Administer medications, as prescribed

  - Use a new tube or bottle of medication for each patient to prevent inadvertent cross-contamination.

541

- Topical steroids should only be used if ordered by a consulting ophthalmologist. For this reason, do not routinely stock steroids on an eye tray.

- Eye drops may be ordered to reduce ciliary spasm or dilate the pupillary sphincter, which may relieve pain and prevent formation of adhesions. Certain eye drops may be contraindicated if acute angle closure glaucoma is suspected.

- Admister tetanus prophylaxis, as prescribed.

- Admister topical antibiotics, as prescribed.

- Systemic, rather than topical antibiotics may be used preoperatively for patients with penetrating injury.

- Instill normal saline drops or artificial tears to keep the corneas moist, as indicated. Use a solution without preservatives. Cover the eyelids with a sterile, moist saline dressing to prevent corneal drying and ulceration.

● Obtain an ophthalmologic consult for patients with chemical burns, open globe injuries, impalements, intraocular foreign bodies, severe hyphema, prolapsed intraocular structures, optic nerve injury, retinal detachment, orbital blowouts, and complex lid lacerations.

● Provide psychosocial support

- Remember that eye injuries are associated with pain, fear, anxiety, and fright.

- Orient the patient to the surroundings.

- Explain responses and/or sensations to the injury or treatments.

● Prepare patient for operative intervention, hospital admission, or transfer, as indicated

● Provide discharge instructions

- Explain the nature of the injury, functional limitations, and time-frame for recovery.

- Provide self-care instructions including how to recognize the signs and symptoms of a worsening condition.

- Discuss the importance of protective eyewear.

- Instruct patient not to drive while wearing eye patches.

- Discourage patient from using the unpatched eye to read or watch TV since this will cause consensual movement of the affected eye.

- Instruct the patient not to squeeze the eyelids tightly to reduce pain and further tissue injury.

- Advise the patient to wear sunglasses to reduce photophobia and tearing, especially if eye patches are not indicated or pupil-dilating medications have been instilled.

Evaluation and Ongoing Assessment

Refer to Chapter 3, Initial Assessment, for a description of the ongoing evaluation of the patient's airway, effectiveness of breathing, and circulation. Additional evaluations include:

- Reassessing visual acuity at reasonable intervals.

- Reassessing pain, including the response to nonpharmacologic and pharmacologic interventions.

- Monitoring the appearance, position, and movements of the globe, and pupillary responses.

SELECTED EYE INJURIES

Refer to "Nursing Care of Patients with Eye Injuries" for a description of the phases of the trauma nursing process.

Hyphema

Hyphema is a collection of blood in the anterior chamber. It is generally caused by a direct blow to the globe resulting in hemorrhage from the blood vessels of the ciliary body. It may be accompanied by injury to the iris. Concomitant corneal injury is common, and some degree of iritis will generally develop. Corneoscleral (anterior chamber) rupture may occur near the limbus.[19] Hyphema injuries are graded as follows:

- Grade 1: A blood layer in the lower third of the anterior chamber

- Grade II: A blood layer between one third to one half of the anterior chamber

- Grade III: A blood layer one half or nearly filling the anterior chamber

- Grade IV: Blood filling the entire anterior chamber ("eight-ball")

Anterior chamber hemorrhage (hyphema) is usually easily diagnosed, but if there is severe periorbital swelling, it may be difficult to adequately visualize the anterior chamber. The classic, sharply demarcated fluid/blood level in the anterior chamber is also more difficult to appreciate in patients with dark irises or who are lying supine (e.g., due to spinal immobilization).

Signs and Symptoms

- Blood in the anterior chamber

  Because blood is more dense than aqueous humor, it will settle at the bottom of the anterior chamber.

- Deep, aching pain

- Mild to severe diminished visual acuity

- Increased intraocular pressure

- Somnolence

Interventions

- Shield with a metal or plastic eye shield. Bilateral patching and reading restrictions are unnecessary.[19]

- Position the patient in an examination chair or with the head of bed elevated

- Obtain ophthalmologic consult since there is a risk of rebleeding, particularly from the second to fifth day postinjury. Patients who have had a hyphema have an increased risk of glaucoma later in life.[19]

- Provide discharge instructions for those patients who are being sent home, especially to avoid taking salicylates or nonsteroidal anti-inflammatory drugs pending further instructions from their ophthalmologist.[19]

Penetrating Trauma/Open or Ruptured Globe

Penetrating ocular injury may be due to projectiles, missiles, foreign bodies, impalement, or stab wounds. Common causes of such injuries are BBs, broken glass, knives, bullets or metal shrapnel, knitting needles, and pencils. Intraocular foreign bodies may not be immediately obvious. The entry wound to the globe may be occult or very small. Suspect a globe injury if an eye-injured patient presents with substantial, acute, unilateral reduction in visual acuity. Consider a BB a high energy injury and the BB as a large intraocular foreign body.

An open globe injury may result from forces that penetrate the globe or cause a sudden rise in intraocular pressure. Acceleration and deceleration of ocular tissues can lead to rupture, especially where the globe is weak, i.e., the limbus or prior surgical site. Fragments from orbital fractures may lead to lacerations of the globe, extraocular muscles, nerves or vascular structures. On occasion, severe orbital fractures may communicate with the anterior cranial fossa, giving rise to direct brain injury, internal carotid injury, or intracranial infection (e.g., meningitis, cavernous sinus thrombosis, or brain abscess). Globe rupture from blunt trauma has a poor prognosis.[9,20] Other bad prognostic signs include an initial visual acuity worse than finger-counting, an afferent pupillary defect, a laceration of greater than 10 mm in length, a laceration to the posterior segment, and a large, intraocular foreign body.[20]

Signs and Symptoms

- Severe reduction in visual acuity or complete visual loss, most commonly unilateral

- Severe pain

- Obvious impalement or globe disruption

- Boggy or obviously asymmetrical globe

- Extrusion of aqueous or vitreous humor

- Extrusion of intraocular contents

- Bulging of the eye

- Grade IV hyphema

- Hemorrhage

- Decreased intraocular pressure

- Globe may not have any striking abnormalities if associated with high velocity intraocular foreign bodies or posterior segment lacerations.

Interventions

- Stabilize an impaled object

- Shield the injured globe and patch the unaffected eye

- Do not instill medications in an eye with an open globe injury

Chemical Burns

The most severe chemical eye injuries are caused by caustic, corrosive substances, particularly acids and alkalies. Alkali burns are more serious because they penetrate more deeply and can destroy the entire anterior chamber. Acids cause coagulation of surface proteins and can cause serious corneal and scleral injury, but the depth of injury tends to be limited to the surfaces directly exposed. Other common chemical exposures include petroleum distillates, organic solvents, pesticides, and perfumes.

The most common alkalis causing eye injuries include lye, caustic potash, ammonia, magnesium hydroxide (a constituent of some fireworks), and lime. Lye, e.g., oven cleaners and drain openers, and ammonia penetrate the most rapidly.[20] Lime, which is a constituent of concrete, mortar, and plaster, is the most common occupational alkali exposure. Because it is usually in powdered form, small particles can get embedded under the eyelids and cause a time-release effect.[20]

The most common acids producing eye injury include sulfuric, sulfurous, hydrochloric, hydrofluoric, and acetic. Sulfuric acid is found in automobile batteries and has a number of industrial uses. If the exposure was from an automotive battery, it is important to establish whether the exposure occurred as a splash, in a collision, or from a battery explosion. The latter two mechanisms of injury carry a higher risk for blast injury, foreign body injury, or chemical exposure. Sulfurous acid is found with an oil base in some refrigerants, leading to prolonged exposure and a greater depth of injury. Hydrochloric acid is a common constituent of drain openers. In spite of its low pH, it does not penetrate very deeply. Hydrofluoric acid is a weaker acid, but the fluoride ion can penetrate tissues more deeply than other acids. Acetic acid is usually not concentrated enough to cause serious injury, but in higher concentrations (greater than 10%), as in some laboratory and photo processing uses, it can cause severe burns.[20]

The prognosis for chemical burns depends on:

- Agent

- Concentration

- Length of exposure

- Adequacy of decontamination

- Degree of corneal involvement

- Presence of ischemia of the corneal limbus

If less than one third of the cornea and limbus is damaged, the prognosis for maintenance of some degree of useful vision is relatively good.[20]

Signs and Symptoms

- Pain

- Corneal opacification

- Coexisting chemical burn and swelling of lids

Interventions

- Irrigate the affected eye

  - Use an eye shower, as indicated, followed by ongoing irrigation.

  - Use eye irrigation equipment specifically designed for ophthalmic.

  - Irrigate acids and alkalis with any neutral solution (water, saline, lactated Ringer's solution) for at least 30 minutes, or until the conjunctival pH is normal (7.4).[20]

  - Be careful not to contaminate opposite eye; irrigate from inner to outer canthus.

- Assess visual acuity

  - Do not delay irrigation to assess visual acuity.

  - Reassess visual acuity before discharge or admission.

- Remove any foreign bodies

- Administer medications, as prescribed

- Patch as previously described

SUMMARY

The spectrum of eye injury ranges from minor to severe, such as those that produce blindness. The nursing process for eye-injured patients includes: maintaining a high index of suspicion for vision-threatening injury, careful assessment, and prompt intervention based on the mechanism of injury and specific condition. Pain relief and caring for the patient's and family's specific concerns will help to alleviate fear and anxiety. The goals of emergency care include prevention or limitation of further injury, prevention of infection and other complications, reduction of pain, fear, and anxiety, and facilitation of ophthalmologic consultation or follow-up. Since the majority of eye injuries are preventable, the trauma nurse should discuss prevention strategies with the patient.

REFERENCES

1. *Dorland's Illustrated Medical Dictionary*. 27th ed. Philadelphia, Pa: WB Saunders Co; 1988.

2. Netter FH. *Atlas of Human Anatomy*. Summit, NJ: Ciba-Geigy; 1989.

3. Ganong WF. *Review of Medical Physiology*. 16th ed. Norwalk, Conn: Appleton & Lange; 1993:132.

4. Karesh J, Keys BJ. Ocular trauma. In: Cardona VD, Hurn PD, Mason PJB, Scanlon AM, Veise-Berry SW, eds. *Trauma Nursing: From Resuscitation through Rehabilitation*. 2nd ed. Philadelphia, Pa: WB Saunders Co; 1994:616-638.

5. Parver LM, Dannenberg AL, Blacklow B, Fowler CJ, Brechner RJ, Tielsch JM. Characteristics and causes of penetrating eye injuries reported to the national eye trauma system registry, 1985-91. *Public Health Reports*. 1993;108:625-632.

6. Feist RM, Farber MD. Ocular trauma epidemiology. *Arch Ophthalmol*. 1989;107:503-504.

7. Klopfer J, Tielsch JM, Vitale S, See LC, Canner JK. Ocular trauma in the United States: eye injuries resulting in hospitalization, 1984 through 1987. *Arch Ophthalmol*. 1992;110:838-842.

8. Schein OD, Hibberd PL, Shingleton BJ, et al. The spectrum and burden of ocular injury. *Ophthalmology*. 1988;95:300-305.

9. Joseph E, Zak R, Smith S, Best WR, Gamelli RL, Dries DJ. Predictors of blinding or serious eye injury in blunt trauma. *J Trauma*. 1992;33:19-24.

10. Semonin-Holleran R. Trauma in childhood. In: Neff JA, Kidd PS, eds. *Trauma Nursing: The Art and Science*. St. Louis, Mo: Mosby-Year Book; 1993:527-553.

11. Hoover DL, Smith LEH. Evaluation and management strategies for the pediatric eye trauma patient. In: Shingleton BJ, Hersh PS, Kenyon KR, eds. *Eye Trauma*. St. Louis, Mo: Mosby-Year Book; 1991:55-60.

12. Newman R. Trauma in the elderly. In: Neff JA, Kidd PS, eds. *Trauma Nursing: The Art and Science*. St. Louis, Mo: Mosby-Year Book; 1993:555-558.

13. Schein OD, Vinger PF. Epidemiology and prevention. In: Shingleton BJ, Hersh PS, Kenyon KR, eds. *Eye Trauma*. St. Louis, Mo: Mosby-Year Book; 1991:395-402.

14. Dannenberg AL, Parver LM, Brechner RJ, Khoo L. Penetrating eye injuries in the workplace: the national eye trauma system registry. *Arch Ophthalmol*. 1992;110:843-848.

15. Dutton GN, al-Qurainy I, Stassen LF, Titterington DM, Moos KF, el-Attar A. Ophthalmic consequences of mid-facial trauma. *Eye*. 1992;6:86-89.

16. Hitchings R. Eye pain. In: Wall PD, Melzack R, eds. *Textbook of Pain*. 3rd ed. Edinburgh, Scotland: Churchill Livingstone; 1994:555-562.

17. Neff JA. Visual acuity testing. *JEN*. 1991;17:431-436.

18. McFarland GK, McFarlane EA, eds. *Nursing Diagnosis and Intervention*. 2nd ed. St. Louis, Mo: Mosby-Year Book; 1993:437-449.

19. Shingleton BJ, Hersh PS. Traumatic hyphema. In: Shingleton BJ, Hersh PS, Kenyon KR, eds. *Eye Trauma*. St. Louis, Mo: Mosby-Year Book; 1991:104-116.

20. Sternberg P. Prognosis and outcomes for penetrating ocular trauma. In: Shingleton BJ, Hersh PS, Kenyon KR, eds. *Eye Trauma*. St. Louis, Mo: Mosby-Year Book; 1991:238-241.

GERIATRIC TRAUMA

OBJECTIVES

Upon completion of this chapter/lecture, the learner should be able to:

1. Identify the mechanisms of injury associated with geriatric trauma.
2. Analyze the pathophysiologic changes as a basis for signs and symptoms.
3. Discuss the nursing assessment of the geriatric trauma patient.
4. Based on the assessment data, identify appropriate nursing diagnoses and expected outcomes.
5. Plan appropriate interventions for the geriatric trauma patient.
6. Evaluate the effectiveness of nursing interventions for geriatric patients with specific types of injuries.

INTRODUCTION

Epidemiology

The proportion of the population over age 65 is growing steadily as a result of a decline in the birth rate after 1964, and a longer life expectancy. Currently, approximately 12% of the US population is age 65 or older.[1,2] By the year 2020, it is estimated that the number of people over age 65 will total 51 million and comprise 14% of the population.[3] Although the age of 65 is frequently cited as being "old," chronological age is not the only determining factor of aging. The patient's functional ability is a major determinant in describing the elderly. There is a difference in the ability of the "healthy" old and the "infirmed" old to withstand the stress of injury. The infirmed elderly are a great challenge for the health care system.[1]

Many elderly people remain active, participating in leisure activities and driving, therefore increasing the risk of injury. Although the number of miles driven annually decreases after age 50, the elderly have a high incidence of collisions. The pattern of injury for the older driver differs in that collisions are more likely to occur during the day, during normal weather conditions, and at distances closer to the victims home.[4] Older persons are injured less frequently than younger individuals, but they are more likely to die from their injuries.[5,6]

551

Those between the ages of 55 and 64 have a death rate (30.6) from accidents and their adverse effects that is less than those from age 15 to 24. Yet the death rate for those between 65 and 74 is 44.2 and escalates to 96.3 for those from 75 to 84 years of age. The greatest death rate is for those over the age of 85 (254.8).[7] The elderly population has the highest rate of hospitalization from injuries, more complications, and poorer outcomes related to the quality of life after trauma.[2,5,8,9]

Mechanisms of Injury and Biomechanics

Motor vehicle crashes, followed by falls are the most common fatal mechanisms of injury in geriatric patients.[9] They have high death rates from pedestrian injuries, excessive cold exposure, farm machinery, and burns.[10] Six percent of elderly deaths are the result of thermal injuries due to diminished temperature sensations and decreased reaction time.

Traffic fatalities accounted for 6,624 deaths in 1983 in persons over age 64.[11] This population may be predisposed to injury due to a decreased ability to perceive and avoid hazards and diminished visual acuity. In addition, proprioceptive and musculoskeletal changes associated with aging may decrease the ability to react. Use of multiple medications or unanticipated drug interactions may interfere with driving ability.[9]

Falls are the leading cause of injury for those over 75 and the second most common cause of injury in the 65 to 74 age group. Thirty-three percent of elderly deaths are attributable to falls.[10,12] Thirty-two percent of the deaths from falls occur in the population over age 85.[10] Falls are related to diminished function of the special senses resulting in impaired vision, gait, and balance. Transient compromise of the cerebrovascular system may cause syncope. Other factors which may contribute to falls are alcohol ingestion and inappropriate medication use.[1,12]

Usual Concurrent Injuries

The risk of fractures in the elderly is increased in the presence of osteoporosis.[9] Although hip fractures are the most common fractures associated with falls, the elderly may sustain concomitant fractures to other bones, e.g., wrist.[8] The elderly population is predisposed to the serious sequelae that can result from trauma including complications from infection, multiple organ failure, and the increased incidence of wound-healing problems.[4]

ANATOMIC AND PHYSIOLOGIC DIFFERENCES IN THE ELDERLY AS A BASIS FOR SIGNS AND SYMPTOMS

Aging is a gradual process that affects the homeostatic integration of multiple body systems. Physiological changes and chronic disease place the elderly at higher risk for injury.[9,13] Due to these changes in body function, the elderly have a limited ability to respond to stress (see Table 71). These changes are well tolerated as activity level decreases, but the insult of trauma challenges the compensatory limits of the elderly person. This restricted capacity to respond to stress is known as a lack of physiologic reserve. Even minor mechanisms of injury may cause serious injury, due to underlying diseases.[5,8,13] Minor injuries to the elderly patient can lead to complications including respiratory infection, hypothermia, and hypovolemia.[8,12,13] There is a higher mortality rate in the elderly population due to:

- Age-related deterioration of body system functions

- Decreased stress tolerance and physiologic reserve

- Greater complication risk

- Pre-existing chronic disease, particularly pulmonary and cardiovascular disease

- Pre-existing nutritional deficits[4,13,14]

Neurologic

Aging results in decreased cerebral blood flow and loss of functioning neurons, which may further compromise the level of consciousness and neurologic status if the patient is in shock.[1,9,12] Brain mass shrinks with cerebral atrophy and the dura adheres more tightly to the skull. The bridging veins in the subdural space are stretched between the brain and dura, making them susceptible to injury. In addition, the elderly have a higher incidence of coagulopathies. For these reasons, a minor blow to the head may result in a subdural hematoma, which is three times more common than an epidural hematoma. The cerebral atrophy associated with aging allows hematomas to expand freely, masking early signs and symptoms of increased intracranial pressure.[6,9]

Deterioration of the special senses and cognitive function is frequently noted. The ability of the brain to rapidly process, coordinate, and react to stimuli is diminished. The velocity of neuronal conduction is slowed. These physiologic changes are exhibited as concentration difficulties, memory loss, distractibility, slowed reaction time, de-

553

creased speed of performance, distraction to irrelevant stimuli, and difficulty organizing information.

Respiratory

With a decreased ability to compensate for the stress of injury, any degree of hypoxia may be detrimental. Loss of pulmonary reserve due to aging, coupled with the stress of trauma, predisposes the elderly trauma patient to respiratory complications.[15] Reduced lung mass and decreased elasticity of the costal cartilages limits the expansion of the rib cage, reducing vital capacity. This may be accentuated by a long history of smoking.[15] The ribs are less resilient, increasing susceptibility to fractures and damage to underlying lung tissue.[6] A gradual decrease in the strength of respiratory muscles, especially the diaphragm, along with a reduced cough reflex may impair the elderly's ability to cough.[12,14,15]

Cardiovascular

Atherosclerosis may limit the ability of the vessels to respond to traumatic stress. Arterial elasticity decreases, increasing peripheral resistance and cardiac workload resulting in the development of hypertension. Since older adults frequently have a history of hypertension, an auscultated blood pressure in the range considered as normal may actually indicate hypotension.[12,14] Baroreceptors become less sensitive, and arterial and cardiac muscles are less responsive to beta-adrenergic stimulation.[9,14]

Changes in the myocardium due to fatty infiltration and fibrosis cause the heart to pump less effectively.[9,11,14] Cardiac output and stroke volume decrease with aging due to stiffness of the myocardium, a decreased conduction velocity, and a decrease in coronary artery blood flow.[16]

Elderly patients who have pre-existing anemia and then sustain trauma may have a decrease in oxygen transport to the tissues, precipitating angina or myocardial infarction. All of these cardiovascular changes may lead to a decreased cardiac output, hypoxemia, and hypoxia in the presence of blood loss.

Musculoskeletal

With aging, muscle cells atrophy and are replaced by fat. These changes result in progressive loss of muscular strength.[14] Osteoporosis, a decrease in bone density, results from an imbalance in bone formation and calcium reabsorption. Osteoporosis is common in both males and females. In general, the elderly have a brittle skeleton which is easily fractured.[14]

Pre-existing arthritis may limit mobility and joint flexibility. Dehydration of the intervertebral disks occurs and joint cartilages atrophy. These degenerative joint changes make radiographic diagnosis of vertebral fractures difficult.[6]

Renal

Renal changes due to aging include decreased renal mass, impaired water reabsorption, decreased bladder capacity, and decreased diluting ability. A diminished glomerular filtration rate is caused by a decrease in the number of nephrons and decreased renal blood flow.[9,17] The result of this diminished filtration rate may result in fluid and electrolyte imbalances.

Nutritional, Metabolic and Gastrointestinal

Inadequate nutrition can alter the body's capacity to respond to the trauma. A pre-existing malnutrition may exist related to decreased appetite, economic status, and inability to prepare food. Poor nutritional status may weaken respiratory muscle contraction, leading to ventilatory fatigue. Peristalsis and gastric motility slow with aging.

Decreased metabolic rate, hypothyroidism, and decreased muscle mass results in diminished heat production. The decrease in the thickness of subcutaneous tissue layer compromises the insulation capacity, making the elderly prone to hypothermia.[12] Although subcutaneous fat is lost with aging, the proportion of body fat to muscle mass increases. Because fat contains less water than muscle, the percentage of total body water decreases in the elderly. This decreased volume, coupled with a poor nutritional intake, can place the individual at risk for rapid development of hypovolemia and fluid volume deficits.

Integumentary

With increased age, the skin becomes more fragile and loses its elasticity. The elderly person is more susceptible to shearing-type injuries, such as abrasions, that may be caused by lying on backboards or stretchers. The subcutaneous layer of the skin becomes thinner and offers less protection to the body, particularly over bony prominences. Changes in the condition of the skin lead to prolonged healing time and increased incidence of infection in soft tissue injuries.[5,6,9]

Table 71

PHYSIOLOGIC CHANGES AS A RESULT OF AGING	
Body System	**Physiologic Change**
Neurologic	<ul><li>Reduced cerebral blood flow</li><li>Decreased number of functional neurons</li><li>Cerebral atrophy/loss of brain mass</li><li>Short-term memory loss</li><li>Increased reaction time/decreased cognition</li><li>Diminished hearing and visual acuity</li><li>Decreased proprioception</li></ul>
Respiratory	<ul><li>Decreased number of functioning alveoli</li><li>Decreased vital capacity</li><li>Decreased respiratory muscle expansion and strength</li><li>Diminished cough</li><li>Increased residual volume</li><li>Decreased rib resiliency</li></ul>
Cardiovascular	<ul><li>Myocardial thickening</li><li>Atherosclerotic changes</li><li>Decreased stroke volume/cardiac output</li><li>Increased systemic vascular resistance</li><li>Increased systolic blood pressure</li><li>Pre-existing anemia</li></ul>
Musculoskeletal	<ul><li>Muscle atrophy</li><li>Muscle replaced with fat</li><li>Loss of muscle strength</li><li>Decreased joint flexibility</li><li>Changes in bone density</li><li>Spinal degenerative joint disease</li></ul>
Renal	<ul><li>Decreased renal mass</li><li>Decreased glomerular filtration rate</li><li>Diminished urine concentrating ability</li></ul>
Nutritional/Metabolic/ Gastrointestinal	<ul><li>Pre-existing malnutrition</li><li>Decreased basal metabolic rate</li><li>Decreased heat production/conservation</li><li>Decreased subcutaneous fat</li><li>Decreased gastric motility</li></ul>
Integumentary	<ul><li>Increased skin fragility</li><li>Reduced tissue elasticity</li><li>Decreased layer of subcutaneous tissue</li></ul>

NURSING CARE OF THE
GERIATRIC TRAUMA PATIENT

Assessment

History

Refer to Chapter 3, Initial Assessment, for a description of general information that should be collected regarding every trauma victim. Only pertinent questions specific to geriatric patients with injuries are described below.

- Does the patient have any pre-existing medical conditions?

- What medications are currently prescribed for the patient?

- What was the patient's neurologic status prior to the injury?

- Is the patient living independently or is someone else responsible for the care of this patient?

- What was the patient's functional mobility level prior to the injury?

- Does the patient have any advance directives?

Physical Assessment

Refer to Chapter 3, Initial Assessment, for a description of the assessment of the patient's airway, and effectiveness of breathing and circulation.

INSPECTION

- Inspect for dentures that can obstruct the airway

- Observe chest excursion for any limited movement

- Inspect for obvious arthritic changes, muscle atrophy, or loss of skin integrity

AUSCULTATION

- Auscultate breath sounds and determine the presence of any adventitious sounds, e.g., rales, rhonchi or wheezes

- Auscultate heart sounds

- Auscultate blood pressure

Since hypertension is associated with aging, record a baseline blood pressure to monitor responses to shock.

PALPATION

Palpate the cervical spine

Any deformities felt may be due to the injury or pre-existing osteo-arthritic changes

Diagnostic Procedures

Refer to Chapter 3, Initial Assessment, for frequently-ordered radiographic and laboratory studies.

LABORATORY STUDIES

- Serum electrolytes

- Serum magnesium

- Serum calcium

- Cardiac isoenzymes

OTHER

Electrocardiogram

Nursing Diagnoses and Outcome Identification

The following nursing diagnoses are potential problems for the geriatric trauma patient. Once the patient has been assessed, diagnoses can be defined as either actual or risk. An actual nursing diagnosis is one derived from a decision based on the patient's presenting signs and symptoms. A risk nursing diagnosis is a judgment the nurse makes based on a particular patient's risk and potential for developing certain problems.

POSSIBLE NURSING DIAGNOSES AND EXPECTED OUTCOMES

Nursing Diagnosis	Expected Outcome
Airway clearance, ineffective related to: • Pain • Decreased level of consciousness • Secretions and debris in airway • Decreased strength of respiratory muscles	The patient will have a patent airway as evidenced by: • Clear, bilateral breath sounds • Regular rate, depth, and pattern of breathing • Effective cough reflex • Absence of pain with coughing • Appropriate use of splinting techniques with coughing • Clear sputum of normal amount without color or odor • Absence of signs and symptoms of retained secretions: fever, tachycardia, tachypnea

Aspiration, risk related to:
• Reduced level of consciousness secondary to injury, drug interactions from multiple medications
• Impaired cough and gag reflex
• Structural defect to head, face, and/or neck
• Secretions and debris in airway
	The patient will not experience aspiration as evidenced by:
	• A patent airway
	• Clear and equal bilateral breath sounds
	• Regular rate, depth, and pattern of breathing
	• ABG value within normal limits
	  ■ PaO_2 80 - 100 mmHg (10.0 - 13.3 KPa)
	  ■ SaO_2 >95%
	  ■ $PaCO_2$ 35 - 45 mmHg (4.7 - 6.0 KPa)
	  ■ pH between 7.35 - 7.45
	• Clear CXR without evidence of infiltrates
	• Ability to handle secretions independently

Gas exchange, impaired related to:
• Ineffective breathing pattern: loss of integrity of thoracic cage and impaired chest wall movement secondary to injury, deterioration of ventilatory efforts
• Ineffective airway clearance
• Aspiration
• Shock
	The patient will experience adequate gas exchange as evidenced by:
	• ABG values within normal limits:
	  ■ PaO_2 80 - 100 mmHg (10.0 - 13.3 KPa)
	  ■ SaO_2 >95%
	  ■ $PaCO_2$ 35 - 45 mmHg (4.7 - 6.0 KPa)
	  ■ pH between 7.35 - 7.45
	• Skin normal color, warm, and dry
	• Improved level of consciousness
	• Regular rate, depth, and pattern of breathing

559

POSSIBLE NURSING DIAGNOSES AND EXPECTED OUTCOMES

Nursing Diagnosis	Expected Outcome
Fluid volume deficit related to: • Hemorrhage • Fluid shifts • Alteration in capillary permeability • Alteration in vascular tone • Myocardial compromise • Decreased cardiopulmonary compensatory mechanisms secondary to aging process	The patient will have an effective circulating volume as evidenced by: • Stable vital signs • Urinary output of 1 ml/kg/hr • Strong, palpable peripheral pulses • Improved level of consciousness • Skin normal color, warm, and dry • Maintains HCT = 30 ml/dl or Hgb = 12 - 14 g/dl or greater, or at preinjury level • CVP reading of 5 - 10 cm H_2O • External hemorrhage is controlled
Hypothermia related to: • Rapid infusion of intravenous fluids • Decreased tissue perfusion • Exposure • Impaired thermoregulation and heat production secondary to aging	The patient will maintain a normal core body temperature as evidenced by: • Core temperature measurement of 36° - 37.5°C (98° - 99.5°F) • Absence of shivering, cool skin, pallor • Skin normal color, warm, and dry
Pain related to: • Soft tissue injury and edema • Fractures • Pleural irritation • Stimulation of nerve fibers • Invasive procedures	The patient will experience relief of pain as evidenced by: • Diminishing or absent level of pain through patient's self-report using an objective measurement tool • Absence of physiologic indicators of pain which include: tachycardia, tachypnea, pallor, diaphoretic skin, increasing blood pressure • Absence of nonverbal cues of pain: crying, grimacing, inability to assume position of comfort, and/or guarding • Ability to cooperate with care as appropriate

POSSIBLE NURSING DIAGNOSES AND EXPECTED OUTCOMES	
Nursing Diagnosis	**Expected Outcome**
Impaired skin integrity, risk related to: • Pressure, shear, friction, maceration forces on skin and tissue • Mechanical irritants: fixation devices • Impaired mobility • Urinary and bowel incontinence • Sensory and motor deficits • Altered peripheral perfusion • Pre-existing nutritional deficiencies • Pre-existing chronic diseases • Lack of physiologic reserve secondary to aging process	The patient will demonstrate absence or resolution of impaired skin integrity as evidenced by: • Absence of signs of irritation: redness, ulceration, blanching, itching • Signs of progressive healing of dermal layer • Understanding and willingness to participate in frequent movement to relieve pressure • Verbalizing an understanding of immobilization devices
Infection, risk related to: • Contact with contagious agents (community and nosocomial acquired) • Contamination of wounds from injury or instrumentation • Prolonged immobility • Lack of physiologic reserve secondary to aging process • Break in aseptic technique • Iatrogenic introduction of organisms during invasive procedures • Pre-existing nutritional deficiencies • Pre-existing chronic diseases	The patient will be free from infection as evidenced by: • Core temperature measurement of 36° - 37.5°C (98° - 99.5°F) • Absence of systemic signs of infection: fever, tachypnea, tachycardia • Wounds free from redness, swelling, purulent drainage or odor • Urinary output 1 ml/kg/hr • Negative blood cultures • WBC within normal limits

Planning and Implementation

Refer to Chapter 3, Initial Assessment, for a description of the specific nursing interventions for patients with compromises to airway, breathing, and/or circulation.

- Obtain and consider the patient's past medical history and current health status

- Assist with endotracheal intubation

   Carefully consider the need to intubate the patient as this increases the risk of pneumonia.[6,18]

- Stabilize and/or immobilize the cervical spine

   Since elderly patients may have pre-existing vertebral deformities, additional padding may be required.

- Pad bony prominences to protect the skin from pressure forces

- Remove splints, backboard, and cervical collar as soon as injuries are ruled out in order to increase the patient's comfort, decrease pressure forces on the skin, and monitor circulatory status

- Assist with the insertion of cardiovascular monitoring devices, if indicated, i.e., CVP, pulmonary artery catheter

   These monitoring devices can assist in determining fluid requirements and assessing cardiovascular responses.[6,12,18] It has been recommended that geriatric, blunt multiple trauma patients be admitted to intensive care as soon as possible for continued cardiovascular monitoring.[18]

- Keep the patient warm since the elderly are prone to hypothermia

- Administer analgesics and other medications in doses recommended for the elderly

- Provide psychosocial support

   Depression may have preceded or followed the injury event.

- Prepare patient for operative intervention, hospital admission, or transfer, as indicated

Evaluation and Ongoing Assessment

Refer to Chapter 3, Initial Assessment, for a description of the ongoing evaluation of the patient's airway, effectiveness of breathing, and circulation. Additional evaluations include:

- Assessing vital signs frequently to determine trends

- Monitoring cardiovascular and pulmonary response to intravenous therapy

- Monitoring temperature frequently

- Observing ventilatory status frequently

- Monitoring urinary output frequently to assess perfusion status

- Monitoring for pain

  Adequate pain management can assist in the improvement in pulmonary status, particularly in patients with chest injuries.[5,9]

SPECIAL CONSIDERATION IN THE ELDERLY

Maltreatment of the Elderly

Maltreatment of the elderly is defined as anything that endangers the life of an elderly person, including physical or emotional assault, intimidation, neglect, financial exploitation, and willful deprivation of medical care or food. It has been reported that patients with pre-existing medical illnesses constituted the largest portion of maltreated elderly patients.[19] Geriatric maltreatment may be difficult to identify because of the victim's fear of isolation and reluctance to report it.[19,20]

Signs and Symptoms

- Unexplained bruises or cigarette burns in various stages of healing on the torso or extremities[20]

- Signs of confinement including soft tissue injuries from restraints[20,21]

- Unexplained fractures[19]

- Head injuries

563

- Unexplained malnutrition or dehydration[1]

- Lack of medical attention to lacerations or open wounds[19,21]

- Caregiver disinterest in the patient's problems

- Unusual interaction between patient and caregiver including fear, withdrawal, verbal abuse, and harassment[1]

- Evidence of over-medication with sedatives[1]

Interventions

- Ask questions of the patient and caregivers in a nonjudgmental manner

- Utilize institutional protocols to screen for and report episodes of maltreatment

SUMMARY

Knowledge and understanding of the concepts of aging will enhance the trauma nurse's ability to deliver trauma care to the elderly. Injured older adults, due to their decreased physiologic reserve, may not have the ability to respond to the stress of injury. Psychologic as well as physiologic responses to the aging process will affect the patient's overall adaptation to the injury. Consider even a minor or moderate injury a major consequence to the elderly as it may pose a threat in his or her ability to perform the activities of daily living. All interventions for elderly trauma patients should be considered in relation to their pre-existing medical conditions, overall preinjury status, and initial response to the injury event. Discuss with the patient, family, and caregivers prevention measures that may help to reduce future injury.

REFERENCES

1. American Medical Association. White paper on elderly health. *Arch Internal Med.* 1990;150:2459-2472.

2. Randall T. Demographers ponder the aging of the aged and await unprecedented looming elder boom. *JAMA.* 1993;269: 2331.

3. Spencer G. Projections of the population of the United States by age, sex, and race: 1988 to 2080. *Current Population Reports.* US Bureau of the Census, Washington, DC; 1989: Series P-25 1018.

4. Dries DJ, Gamelli RL. Issues in geriatric trauma. In: Miles RH, Dries DJ, Gamelli RL, eds. *Trauma 2000: Strategies for the New Millennium.* Austin, Tex: RG Landes Co; 1992:191-197.

5. DeMaria EJ. Evaluation and treatment of the elderly trauma victim. *Clin Geri Med.* 1993;9:461-471.

6. Levy D, Hanlon D, Townsend R. Geriatric trauma injury. *Clin Geri Med.* 1993;9:601-617.

7. Advance report of final mortality statistics, 1992. *Monthly Vital Statistics Report.* National Center for Health Statistics, Hyattsville, Md; 1994;43:1-76.

8. Oreskovich MR, Howard JD, Copass MK, Carrico C. Geriatric trauma: injury patterns and outcome. *J Trauma.* 1984;24:565-572.

9. Schwab CW, Kauder DR. Trauma in the geriatric patient. *Arch Surg.* 1992;127:701-706.

10. Baker SP, O'Neill B, Ginsburg MJ, Guohua LM. *The Injury Fact Book.* 2nd ed. New York, NY: Oxford University Press; 1992:41-43.

11. National Highway Traffic Safety Administration. *Traffic Safety Facts 1994.* US Department of Transportation, Washington, DC; 1994:DOT HS 808 169.

12. Bobb JK. Trauma in the elderly. In: Cardona VD, Hurn PD, Mason PJB, Scanlon AM, Veise-Berry SW, eds. *Trauma Nursing: From Resuscitation through Rehabilitation.* 2nd ed. Philadelphia, Pa: WB Saunders Co; 1994:721-735.

13. Andrews JF. Trauma in the elderly. *Contemporary Perspectives in Trauma Nursing.* Berryville, Va: Forum Medicum, Inc; 1990:1-9.

14. Rebemson-Piano M, Forrest JM. Gerontologic alterations and management. In: Thelan LA, Davie JK, Urden LD, Lough ME, eds. *Critical Care Nursing.* 2nd ed. Chicago, Ill: Mosby-Year Book; 1994:906-927.

15. Timiras PS. Aging of respiration. In: Timiras PS, ed. *Physiological Basis of Geriatrics.* New York, NY: MacMillan & Co; 1988:303-314.

16. Osler TM, Demrest GB. Geriatric trauma. In: Moore EE, Mattox KL, Feliciano DV, eds. *Trauma.* Norwalk, Conn: Appleton & Lange; 1991:703-714.

17. Timiras ML. The kidney, the lower urinary tract, and body fluids. In: Timiras PS, ed. *Physiological Basis of Geriatrics.* New York, NY: MacMillan & Co; 1988:315-333.

18. Scalea TM, Simon HM, Duncan AO, et al. Geriatric blunt multiple trauma: improved survival with early invasive monitoring. *J Trauma.* 1990;30:129-136.

19. Jones J, Dougherty J, Scheible D, Cunningham W. Emergency department protocol for the diagnosis and evaluation of geriatric abuse. *Ann Emer Med.* 1988;17:1006-1015.

20. Rathbone-McCuan E, Voyles B. Case detection of abused elderly patients. *Am J Psychiatry.* 1982:189-192.

21. Mitchell FL, Metzler MH. Geriatric complications. In: Mattox KL, ed. *Complications of Trauma.* New York, NY: Churchill Livingstone; 1994:183-197.

GLOSSARY

A-Delta Fibers – one of two types of peripheral afferent fibers located in the skin that transmit information regarding pain to the spinal cord and brain; considered fast pain fibers since transmission velocity is 5 to 30 m/second; myelinated; respond usually to pressure and temperature; type of pain is sharp, stabbing, e.g., pinprick.

Abdomen – body cavity that extends from the diaphragm to the pelvis; bounded anteriorly by the abdominal wall and posteriorly by the vertebral column.

Abruptio Placentae – partial or total separation of the normally implanted placenta from the uterine wall.

Acceleration – any increase in speed or velocity.

Adaptation – the healthy response to stress.

Afterload – resistance or pressure in the aorta and pulmonary artery against which the heart must pump during systole; the arterial blood pressure is the source of the resistance.

Aldosterone – mineralocorticoid released by the adrenal cortex; release is stimulated by the presence of angiotensin II in the plasma; promotes the reabsorption of sodium and therefore the reabsorption of water to increase blood volume and blood pressure.

Amniocentesis – a procedure to obtain a sample of amniotic fluid from a pregnant woman; a needle is placed into the amniotic sac through the abdomen.

Anaerobic – in the absence of oxygen; anaerobic metabolism occurs in the cell's cytoplasm (vs. aerobic metabolism which occurs in the mitochondria) and liberates energy and pyruvic acid from glucose molecule.

Anemia of Pregnancy – in late pregnancy, a hematocrit of 31 to 34% is common; pregnant women have an increase in plasma volume without a proportional increase in red blood cell volume, therefore, the hematocrit is lower than normal.

Angiotensin – a substance in the plasma which is split from the substance angiotensinogen due to the enzymatic function of renin from the kidneys; angiotensin I is converted to angiotensin II with the help of angiotensin converting enzyme from the lungs; basic role is vasoconstriction.

Angiotensin Converting Enzyme – catalytic enzyme in the lungs that converts angiotensin I to angiotensin II.

Anterior Cord Syndrome – an incomplete spinal cord injury; loss of motor function, loss of pain, temperature, crude touch and crude pressure sensory functions; intact proprioception, vibration, fine touch and fine pressure.

Asphyxia – Decreased amount of oxygen and increased amount of carbon dioxide in the blood and body tissues.

Assaultive Violence – "assaultive violence includes both fatal and nonfatal interpersonal violence where physical force or other means is used by one person with the intent of causing harm, injury, or death to another." (Reference 14, Chapter 2).

Atelectasis – collapse or incomplete expansion of the lung; may be chronic or acute; may involve all or part of the lung; causes include airway obstruction, pneumothorax, loss of surfactant (surface tension inside alveoli increases, leading to collapse).

Atlas – the first cervical vertebra (C-1) that supports the weight of the head and articulates with the occipital condyles of the skull.

Autonomic Nervous System – a portion of the peripheral nervous system responsible for control of smooth muscle, cardiac muscle, and glands; two divisions: sympathetic system originating in spinal nerves T-1 through L-2, and parasympathetic nervous system originating in cranial nerves III, VII, IX, and X and S-2 through S-4.

Autotransfusion – a therapeutic method to transfuse the patient's own shed blood back to him/her after proper filtration.

AVPU – an acronym which stands for alert, verbal, painful, and unresponsive; used to classify the patient's level of consciousness.

Avulsion – a soft tissue wound in which the wound edges cannot be approximated; tearing away of a portion of the soft tissue.

Axial Loading – direct force transmitted along the length of the vertebral column or axial skeleton; force can be applied to the top of the head such as in a diving event or applied to the feet such as in a fall.

Axis – the second cervical vertebra (C-2) that articulates with C-1, the axis; has a perpendicular projection termed the odontoid process or dens where C-1 articulates.

Babinski Reflex – as the sole of the foot is stroked, the big toe dorsiflexes and the other four toes fan; a test for upper motor neuron lesions involving the motor pyramidal tracts; J. F. Babinski (1857-1932) born to Polish parents yet lived his whole life in France; known for his work with neurologic exam techniques, hysteria, and cerebellar disease; a great lover of theater, opera, ballet, and gourmet cooking.

Baroreceptors – specialized cells located in the carotid sinus, wall of the aortic arch and other major arteries; sensitive to changes in blood pressure; when blood pressure is high, baroreceptors are stimulated sending messages to the brainstem to decrease blood pressure through vasodilation; when blood pressure is low, baroreceptors are not stimulated causing vasoconstriction.

Base (basilar) Skull – bones which comprise the base of the skull forming three hollow depressions termed the anterior, posterior, and middle fossae.

Battle's Sign – ecchymosis behind the ear over the mastoid process; may indicate basilar skull fracture of the posterior fossa; W. Battle (1855-1936) was an English surgeon who was the surgical advisor to Lancet and was known for his work in obstetrics as well as surgery.

Benzodiazepines – a group of drugs with various effects depending on the particular benzodiazepine used and the mechanism of action; do not have a general CNS depressive effect; actions include anticonvulsant, antianxiety, muscle relaxation; commonly prescribed benzodazepines include diazepam (Valium), midazolam (Versed), lorazepam (Ativan).

Biomechanics – principles of action of forces and their effects.

Blood Alcohol Concentration (BAC) – the amount of alcohol isolated in a sample of blood serum; legal limits have been set by most states to determine the minimum BAC acceptable for driving a motor vehicle. The level varies in states between 0.08 g/dL to 0.1 g/dL.

Blood Pressure – arterial blood pressure is the result of cardiac output (stroke volume multiplied by heart rate) multiplied by total peripheral resistance.

Blood Urea Nitrogen (BUN) – byproduct of protein metabolism; formed in the liver from metabolism of amino acids and ammonia compounds; if not excreted in the urine, excess urea is found in the blood.

Bloodborne Pathogens – "pathogenic microorganisms that are present in human blood and can cause diseases in humans. These pathogens include, but are not limited to, hepatitis B virus (HBV) and human immunodeficiency virus (HIV)." (Reference 1, Appendix 3).

Blunt Trauma – injuries that do not cause disruption of the skin.

Bridging Veins – small veins extending from the cerebral cortex to the venous sinuses in the dura; these veins come from vessels in the pia mater, pass through the subarachroid space, arachnoid and dural meninges, then empty into the venous sinuses.

Brown-Sequard Syndrome – type of incomplete spinal cord lesion; transverse hemisection of the cord is affected; loss of motor function, proprioception, vibration on same side of injury; loss of pain and temperature opposite the side of injury; C. Brown-Sequard (1817-1894) was a French neurologist and physiologist who worked in the USA (Harvard) and England; known for his work related to the spinal cord, sensory function, and use of hormones.

Bruit – a sound heard during auscultation of a blood vessel; an auscultated murmur.

Bulla – a lesion that contains fluid such as a blister or a bleb.

C-Fibers – one of two types of peripheral afferent fibers that transmit information regarding pain to the spinal cord and brain, considered slow pain fibers since transmission velocity is 0.5 to 2.0 m/second, unmyelinated; respond usually to chemicals released from tissue damage; type of pain is burning, throbbing, or aching.

Cancellous Bone – spongy bone located in the interior of the bone; constructed in a lattice-like pattern; contains red marrow.

Carbon Monoxide – tasteless, odorless, and colorless gas present in the smoke released by the combustion of organic materials such as wood, coal, and gasoline; released when the available oxygen to support combustion is consumed and incomplete combustion occurs.

Carboxyhemoglobin – hemoglobin that has combined with carbon monoxide.

Cardiac Contractility – refers to "the ability of the heart to change its force of contraction without changing its resting (diastolic) length," e.g., sympathetic stimulation. Another factor that determines cardiac output is related to the actin and myosin filaments in heart muscle cells stretch to eject stroke volume during systole; the more the muscle fibers are stretched (to a point), the stronger the force of cardiac contraction according to the Frank-Starling Law of the Heart; the more preload, the more the stretch, the stronger the contraction, the greater the stroke volume; E. Starling (1866-1927) was a British physiologist known for his works in capillary fluid pressures and movement of fluids, discovery of secretin the duodenal precursor to bile secretion, glomerular reabsorption of glucose, water, and electrolytes, and he coined the word "hormone." Dr. Frank was another physiologist. (Reference 2, Chapter 4).

Cardiogenic Shock – shock syndrome caused by inadequate contractility of the cardiac muscle; causes include myocardial infarction, myocardial contusion, mitral valve insufficiency, dysrhythmias, and cardiac failure.

Cardiotocograph – instrument used in cardiotocography or the monitoring of the fetal heart rate and/or the mother's uterine contractions. An externally-placed Doppler ultrasound transducer sends sound waves onto the uterus and the waves are reflected to a monitor that calculates the fetal heart rate based on fetal movements. An externally-placed tocotransducer placed over the mother's fundus detects changes in the abdominal contour as a measure of uterine contractions and registers these changes as bell shapes on a monitor strip. The measure of uterine activity is related to frequency and duration but not necessarily intensity.

Carotid Bodies – located at the bifurcations of the common carotid arteries; chemoreceptors which are sensitive to low levels of oxygen and excess levels of carbon dioxide in arterial blood; when the blood pressure is low, the arterial flow that supplies the receptors becomes diminished, the receptors are stimulated, and the medulla is stimulated to cause vasoconstriction.

Case Fatality Rate – a calculated death rate where the numerator is the number of persons with a specific disease who die and the denominator is the number of persons with the specific disease.

Catecholamine – chemical substance such as epinephrine, norepinephrine, or dopamine which contains a catechol molecule; sympathomimetic substance released from adrenergic nerve endings or adrenal medulla; dopamine and epinephrine are precursors in the synthesis of norepinephrine.

Cavitation – a temporary cavity; refers to a localized area of blunt trauma along the bullet path; a stretch phenomenon.

Central Cord Syndrome – an incomplete spinal cord lesion; loss of motor and sensory function with greater loss in arms than in the legs.

Central Venous Pressure – pressure in the right atrium; normal 5 to 10 cm H_2O.

Cerebral Perfusion Pressure (CPP) – the difference between the mean arterial blood pressure and the intracranial pressure.

Cerebrospinal Fluid – formed in the choroid plexus of the brain's ventricles; circulates from the fourth ventricle down the central canal of the spinal cord and in the subarachnoid space; when a person is lying down, the normal cerebrospinal fluid pressure is 5 mmHg (100 mm H_2O); function is to cushion and protect the brain and spinal cord.

Cervical Dilation – opening of the cervix which occurs at the same time, but not at the same rate, as cervical effacement during labor; expressed in centimeters with 10 cm representing full dilation.

Cervical Effacement – thinning and shortening of the cervix during labor; uterine contractions pull the cervix upward at the same time they push the fetus downward. As the cervix is drawn over the fetus it becomes shorter and thinner losing its cylindrical shape. Effacement is designated as a percentage with 100% representing full effacement.

Cervical Stabilization – includes holding the head in a neutral position or placement of bilateral head support devices with tape and application of a rigid cervical collar (if available and if enough trauma team members are present) to secure the head and devices.

Chronotropy – rate; positive chronotropic effect increases the heart rate, negative chronotropic effect decreases the heart rate.

Citrate Phosphate Dextrose (CPD) – a solution of dextrose, citric acid, sodium citrate, and sodium biphosphate used as a 21-day anticoagulant in certain blood products.

Closed Fracture – skin integrity over or near a fracture site is intact.

Comminuted Fracture – splintering of the fractured bone into fragments or pieces.

Compact Bone – dense and rigid bone; forms the shaft of long bones and the exterior surface of other bones, i.e., short bones.

Compartment Syndrome – increased pressure in a fascial compartment due to either an internal source, such as hemorrhage or edema, or an external source, such as a cast; nerves, blood vessels and/or muscle can be compressed as pressure rises inside the compartment.

Compliance (pulmonary) – a compliant lung can be inflated with relative ease; a relationship between volume and pressure; a change in lung volume is related to a change in pressure; if lung tissue becomes stiff or loses elasticity, the lung becomes less compliant; if surfactant is lost or diminished, lung compliance decreases.

Concussion – transient loss of consciousness; no identifiable lesion; physiologic loss of the awake state due to transient disruption of the connection between the cerebral cortex and the brainstem center for wakefulness.

Conscious Sedation – medically-controlled state of altered consciousness that allows patients to maintain their protective reflexes, maintain an adequate airway, and respond appropriately to physical or verbal stimulation.

Continuous Positive Airway Pressure (CPAP) – used for spontaneously breathing patients who are receiving oxygen under positive pressure to keep the alveoli open until the end of expiration; similar to positive end expiratory pressure (PEEP) in patients who are receiving mechanical ventilation.

Contusion (brain) – focal brain injury in which brain tissue is bruised and damaged in a local area.

Cortex – surface or outer layer of an organ, such as cerebral cortex or adrenal cortex.

Corticospinal Tracts – descending, pyramidal, motor, and spinal nerve tracts that originate in the cerebral cortex, cross over in the medulla, and eventually innervate skeletal muscles; responsible for motor function.

Coup/Contrecoup Injury (brain) – applied force to the brain causes the brain to strike the interior skull on the same side as the applied force (coup), then the brain moves (accelerates) and strikes the opposite side of the skull (contrecoup).

Creatinine – formed in muscle as the byproduct of creatine metabolism; normally passes into the circulation and excreted in the urine.

Creatine Phosphokinase-Myocardial Bands (CPK-MB) – creatine phosphokinase; an enzyme found in the cells; CPK has three isoenzymes, CK1 found in the brain, CK2 found in the myocardium, CK3 found in the myocardium and skeletal muscle; can be released into the blood when these cells are injured; CK2 is the MB isoenzyme released when myocardial cells are injured, e.g., after a myocardial contusion.

Crepitus – dry, crackling sound (crepitant); bony crepitus is the sound heard when fractured bone ends rub together.

Cricothyroidotomy – a surgical procedure done to open a patient's airway; an incision through the skin and the cricothyroid membrane of the trachea to allow an opening into the trachea from the outside; also referred to as a cricothyrotomy.

Crisis – a state of disequilibrium that occurs when usual coping strategies are inadequate; it is not the event that constitutes the crisis, but how the person perceives the event.

Crisis Intervention – immediate help for a person to re-establish equilibrium; short-term goal is to solve immediate problems; long-term goal is to foster functional equilibrium higher than the precrisis level.

Critical Incident – any situation experienced by a trauma team member(s) that causes him/her to feel unusually strong emotional reactions with the potential to interfere with the ability to function.

Critical Incident Stress Management (CISM) Team – a team consisting of mental health professionals and peer support personnel; CISM teams prepare staff to manage their job-related stress, provide assistance for those staff who are experiencing the negative effects of stress, and provide education and prevention programs.

Cushing Response – significant cerebral ischemia initiates a central nervous system ischemic response; if the ischemia is due to a rise in intracranial pressure equal to or greater than arterial pressure, there is an increase in systolic pressure to maintain perfusion of the vasomotor center; there may be a concomitant reflex bradycardia; H. Cushing (1869-1939) was an American neurosurgeon known for his work related to pituitary gland physiology, the classification of brain tumors, and his neurosurgical skills that reduced neurosurgical mortality from 90% to 8%; he studied and worked at Johns Hopkins, the Massachusetts General Hospital, Yale, and was the Surgeon-in-chief at the Peter Bent Brigham Hospital in Boston for 20 years.

Deceleration Force or Drag – the force that stops or decreases the velocity of a moving victim.

Decerebrate Rigidity – extension and internal rotation of the upper extremities, wrist flexion, and extension, internal rotation and plantar flexion of the lower extremities; usually bilateral; may represent significant injury to the midbrain and\or pons.

Decorticate Rigidity – adduction of the shoulders, pronation and flexion of the elbows and wrists along with extremities; bilateral; may represent significant injury to the cerebrum or corticospinal motor tracts.

Deformation – bullet deformation refers to an increase in bullet diameter as a result of mushrooming or flattening of the bullet tip.

Depolarizing Neuromuscular Blocking Agents – cause peripheral skeletal muscle relaxation by depolarizing the postsynaptic membrane at the neuromuscular junction and then continuing to occupy the receptor site delaying repolarization and further depolarizations; cause an initial muscle contraction or fasciculation followed by flaccid paralysis; only agent used clinically is succinylcholine (Anectine).

Dermis – layer of skin under the epidermis; two-layered; contains collagen, elastic fibers, blood vessels, nerve endings, sweat glands, sebaceous glands, lymph vessels, and hair follicles; cannot regenerate if dermal cells are injured.

Diagnostic Peritoneal Lavage – a diagnostic procedure to detect blood or other contaminants in the abdomen.

Diaphysis – the compact bone that forms the shaft surrounding the medullary cavity.

Diffuse Axonal Injury (DAI) – diffuse, microscopic, hemorrhagic brain lesions due to acceleration and deceleration forces causing shearing of the axons of neurons; may affect the brain and/or brainstem.

Diplopia – double-vision or seeing a double image of one object.

Displaced Fracture – proximal and distal fracture sites are out of alignment.

Distributive Shock – syndrome resulting from either poor distribution (neurogenic shock) or poor blood flow (septic shock).

Doppler Ultrasonic Flowmeter – device used to measure blood flow through veins and arteries; transmits an audible sound which reflects velocity of blood flow; C. Doppler (1803-1853) was an Austrian physicist and mathematician.

Ductus Arteriosus – during fetal circulation blood bypasses the lungs; blood from the right ventricle leaves the heart via the pulmonary artery and then flows through the ductus arteriosus into the aorta bypassing the lungs; the fetal remnant of the ductus arteriosus is termed the ligamentum arteriosum.

Dysphagia – difficulty in swallowing.

Dysphonia – difficulty in speaking, e.g., hoarseness.

Dyspnea – difficult or labored breathing.

Ecchymosis – bluish areas of discoloration of the skin or mucous membranes; larger than petechiae.

Electromechanical Dissociation (EMD) – refers to one example of pulseless electrical activity, whereby, the patient has no pulse but narrow complexes indicating depolarization of the myocardium but no mechanical contraction.

Endocrine – relating to internal secretion of hormones directly into the circulation; examples of endocrine glands include the hypothalamus, thyroid, pituitary, and adrenal glands.

Endogenous – produced from factors within the body, such as the endogenous release of epinephrine from the adrenal gland during stimulation of the sympathetic nervous system.

Endorphins – two chemical substances (beta-endorphin and dynorphin) found in the amygdala, limbic system, and hypothalamus; when released have a morphine-like analgesic effect.

Enkephalins – two chemical substances (met-enkephalin and leu-enkephalin) found in the endogenous analgesia center or periaqueductal gray (PAG) region of the midbrain, limbic system, hypothalamus, and spinal cord; when released have a morphine-like analgesic effect; can be stimulated by hypotension.

Enophthalmos – the eye is sunken or displaced backward in the orbit.

Epidemiology – the study of the distribution of injuries in populations, the determinants of injury, and the associated causes and risk factors.

Epidermis – outermost layer of the skin; composed of five layers of which the deepest layer is a single layer of basal cells capable of producing new skin cells that move to the skin's surface to replace lost cells.

Epidural Hematoma – collection of blood between the dura mater and the skull; usually arterial in origin.

Epiphysis – located at each end of a bone; the end of the bone that is wider than the shaft; during times of bone growth, the epiphysis is separated from the end of the bone by cartilage.

Exocrine – relating to the external secretion of a substance via a duct, e.g. pancreatic secretions via the pancreatic duct to the ampula of Vater to the duodenum. The pancreas is an example of a gland with both endocrine (insulin) and exocrine (pancreatic secretions) functions.

Exogenous – produced from factors outside the body, e.g., microorganisms that produce a fever.

Expected Date of Confinement (EDC) – to determine an estimate of the birth of the baby of an expectant mother, count back three months from the date of the last menstrual period and add seven days.

Exposure Incident – "means a specific eye, mouth, other mucous membrane, nonintact skin, or parenteral contact with blood or other potentially infectious materials that result from the performance of an employee's duties." (Reference 1, Appendix 3).

Extraocular Eye Movements (EOMs) – movement of the globe in various directions; movements are under the control of cranial nerves III, IV, and VI which innervate the six eye muscles.

Extravasation – leak or escape of blood or fluid from a vessel or organ.

Facet – part of the vertebral arch which forms the enclosure, the vertebral foramen, for the passage of the spinal cord; four articular processes on a vertebral arch.

Family – an individual's support system; may include, but is not limited to, relatives, friends, and significant others.

Fascia – connective, fibrous tissue that covers or invests certain structures such as muscle; subcutaneous fascia lies beneath the skin; deep fascia is dense and gives off sheaths to certain muscles such as the fascia lata of the thigh.

Fascial Compartment – fascia, as described above, creates closed spaces or compartments where bones, nerves, muscles, and blood vessels are in close proximity. If the pressure rises in a closed tissue space, there is a possibility of compartment syndrome, a condition that could result in damage to contents of the space. The interosseus muscles of the foot and hand are compartments. The forearm has three osseofascial compartments, the deep flexor, extensor, and superfacial flexor. The lower leg has four compartments, the anterior, lateral, superficial posterior, and deep posterior. The thigh has three compartments corresponding to the quadriceps, hamstrings, and adductor muscles.

Fasciotomy – an incision into fascia usually to relieve pressure inside a fascial compartment.

Firearms – handguns, rifles, and shotguns.

Flail – abnormal movement; flail chest is two or more consecutive ribs broken in two or more places resulting in a portion of the rib cage becoming unstable and moving in a direction opposite the rest of the rib cage during inspiration and expiration; the sternum may also be fractured creating a flailed portion of the sternum.

Flank – the side of the body from the ribs to the ischium of the hip; similar in definition to loin which is the posterior area of the body from the chest to the pelvis.

Focal – adjective for the noun "focus," center of attention, or convergence.

Fontanelle – spaces at the junction of skull sutures; the anterior fontanelle is at the junction of the frontal and parietal bones and closes between the eighth and 15th month of life; the posterior fontanelle is at the junction of occipital and parietal bones and closes by the third to fourth month of life; referred to as "soft spots."

Fowler's Position – patient positioned with the head of the bed elevated, hips and knees flexed; high-Fowler's position is significant elevation of the head of the bed to assist with breathing (i.e., pulmonary edema) or drainage (i.e., facial bleeding); originally used to manage patients with peritonitis to relieve stretching of abdominal muscles and reduce pain; G. Fowler (1848-1906) American surgeon who practiced in New York and known for his work with adopting Lister's surgical aseptic techniques and for his operative management for appendicitis; he died of a myocardial infarction following surgery for a gangrenous appendix.

Fragmentation – bullet fragmentation refers to the breaking open or apart of a bullet into pieces; fragmentation causes the tissue to be multiply perforated before being subjected to the stretch of temporary cavitation.

Fundus – that portion of an organ furthest away from the mouth of the organ; the fundus of the uterus is that portion furthest away from the openings of the fallopian tubes.

Gestation – the time from fertilization of the egg to the birth; gestational age refers to the age of the fetus in utero at any given time.

Glasgow Coma Scale – a scoring system to measure the patient's level of consciousness; score ranges from 3 to 15; points correspond to responses in three areas: eye opening, verbal response to pain, and motor response to pain. The patient's best responses in each of three areas are added for a total score; developed by Drs. Jennett and Teasdale who are from Glasgow, Scotland.

Glycogen – stored form of glucose in the liver; can be converted to glucose as needed.

Glycogenolysis – process whereby stored glycogen is broken down into glucose by the hormones glucagon and epinephrine.

Glycosuria – glucose or sugar in the urine.

Greenstick Fracture – a buckle or bend in a bone; fracture does not go through the entire bone.

Grief – the physical, emotional, spiritual, cognitive, social, and behavioral response to loss.

Guarding – when an examiner palpates a patient's abdomen, the normal reaction of the patient is to tighten the abdominal muscles or guard the abdomen; when efforts to relax the patient fail to prevent guarding, the finding is termed involuntary guarding, meaning the patient is not voluntarily tensing the muscles, rather peritoneal irritation is causing the muscles to tense.

Hemiparesis – paralysis that is often incomplete on one side of the body.

Hemiplegia – paralysis of one side of the body.

Hemoptysis – blood coughed up from the respiratory tract.

Hemothorax – an injury resulting in blood accumulating in the pleural space.

Histamine – substance found in most cells, especially mast cells (connective tissue cells); released when body is exposed to an antigen or allergen; causes capillary dilation and increased permeability, decrease in blood pressure, bronchoconstriction, secretion of gastric acid, hives, and edema.

Hydrostatic Capillary Pressure – one of the forces that contribute to the outward movement of fluid from the capillary through the capillary membrane to the interstitium; hydrostatic pressure is approximately 30 mmHg at the arterial end of the capillary and 10 mmHg at the venule end; as blood flow increases to an area (hyperemia), the hydrostatic pressure increases.

Hyperbaric Oxygen (HBO) Therapy – hyperbaric refers to oxygen under greater pressure than atmospheric pressure; HBO therapy is the administration of 100% oxygen to a patient who is in an environment where the atmospheric pressure is high; reduces the half-life of carboxyhemoglobin; may also be used for cyanide, hydrogen sulfide, or tetrachloride poisoning.

Hyperemia – increased blood flow in an area.

Hypermetabolism – an increase in the metabolic rate; may occur after major trauma or burn.

Hyperosmotic Diuresis – hyperosmotic agent, such as mannitol, is administered to increase the capillary osmotic pressure pulling excess fluid from the brain into the vascular space and reducing cerebral edema and intracranial pressure.

Hyperresonance – increased resonance; resonance is a prolonged or intensified sound heard on percussion as the tap of the percussion is transmitted by vibration to a cavity; a more resonant sound is heard when more air is in the cavity.

Hyperthermia – an increase in body temperature that results in heat cramps, heat syncope, heat exhaustion, or heat stroke; a core temperature of greater than 40°C (104°F), unresponsiveness, and no diaphoresis is symptomatic of life-threatening heat stroke.

Hypnotics – chemical substances that induce sleep; the major difference between a sedative and hypnotic is the degree of CNS depression." (Reference 15, Appendix 4).

Hypothermia – low body temperature; mild hypothermia is 34 to 35°C (93.2 to 95°F); moderate is 30 to 34°C (86 to 93.2°F); severe is less than 30°C (86°F).

Hypovolemic Shock – shock due to inadequate blood volume; whole blood loss from hemorrhage, or plasma loss from burns may produce hypovolemic shock.

Hypoxemia – decreased oxygen in the blood; measured by arterial partial pressure of oxygen during blood gas analysis.

Hypoxia – decreased oxygen supply to tissues.

Immobilization – includes cervical stabilization as defined and the application of a backboard and straps.

Impacted Fracture – distal and proximal fracture sites are wedged into each other.

Incidence – the actual number of persons involved, e.g., the incidence of patients with gunshot wounds is the actual number of persons who sustained a gunshot wound; usually during a particular time period, e.g., in one year.

Initial Assessment – the content and process of conducting a complete primary and secondary examination of the patient; uses techniques of inspection, auscultation, palpation, and percussion.

Injury Severity Score (ISS) – measure of the anatomic severity of injuries; based on the abbreviated injury score (AIS) descriptors; equals the sum of the squares of the highest AIS grade (1 through 5) in each of three most severely injured body regions; injury severity scores range from 1 to 75; ISS of 15 or greater is considered a major trauma patient.

Inotropy – force of contraction; positive inotropic effect is to increase force of contraction, negative inotropic effect is to decrease force of contraction.

Intentional Injuries – injuries resulting from conscious intent such as those related to suicide, homicide, or maltreatment.

Intracranial Pressure (ICP) – pressure within the cranial cavity reflective of three volumes: brain (80%), blood (10%), and cerebrospinal fluid (10%); normal ICP is 10 to 15 mmHg.

Intrathecal – within a sheath or case, e.g., an intrathecal injection into the subarachnoid space is made through the theca of the spinal cord.

Journaling – writing notes in a diary or log, can be used as a method to learn about oneself or record reactions to specific experiences.

Kehr's Sign – referred left shoulder pain associated with splenic rupture due to blood irritating the phrenic nerve; H. Kehr (1862-1916) was a German surgeon known for his work related to bile duct surgery; extremely interested in the arts and died from septicemia due to an injury to his finger during an operation.

Kinematics – branch of mechanics that deals with the study of motion but does not consider the concepts of mass and force.

Kinetics – branch of mechanics that deals with the study of motion considering the concepts of mass and force; considers the rate of change in a factor.

KPa – unit of measurement to report arterial blood gas values in the UK. Conversion is the value in mmHg divided by 7.5 equals KPa.

Lactated Ringer's Solution – intravenous solution; isotonic electrolyte solution most similar to normal body extracellular fluid (near-physiologic); contains the following electrolytes (mEq/l): sodium 130, potassium 4, calcium 2.7, chloride 109, and bicarbonate 28; S. Ringer (1835-1910) was an English physician known for his outstanding clinical skills, a classic book on therapeutics, and the influence of calcium and other salts on body fluids and cardiac muscle.

LeFort Fracture – LeFort I is a transverse fracture of the maxilla; LeFort II is a pyramidal maxillary fracture involving the nose, lacrimal bone and ethmoid bone; LeFort III is craniofacial separation; named after a French pathologist, LeFort, who studied forces applied to the faces of cadavers.

Ligament – band of fibrous connective tissue that attaches bones to bones.

Ligamentum Arteriosum – the remnant of the fetal ductus arteriosus; relatively fixes the aortic arch to the pulmonary artery distal to the take-off of the left subclavian artery; acceleration-deceleration injuries to the aorta are most frequently found at this location.

Logroll – turning the patient as a unit; requires a team leader at the head of the patient who directs the turn and stabilizes the patient's head and cervical spine; other team members are positioned at the patient's side, usually one at the hips and one at the knees.

Lysosomes – organelles inside cells which contain enzymes responsible for ridding the cell of foreign substances.

Magnetic Resonance Imaging (MRI) – nuclear noninvasive diagnostic procedure especially useful for imaging body tissues composed of fat and/or water; distinguishes tissue types, i.e, malignant, traumatized, or athlerosclerotic.

Maxilla – the upper jaw; inferior borders support the upper teeth; form the floor of the orbits, as well as portions of the nasal cavities and the hard palate; each maxillary bone forms an air space termed the maxillary sinus.

Mean Arterial Pressure (MAP) – one third of the pulse pressure (difference between the systolic and diastolic pressures) added to the diastolic pressure; a measure of tissue perfusion.

Mechanism of Injury – refers to the mechanisms whereby the force or energy is transferred from the environment to the person; examples include motor vehicle crashes, gunshots, stabbings, burns.

Mediastinum – space between the two lungs containing the heart, great vessels, esophagus trachea, vagus and phrenic nerves.

Meninges – Three layers of connective tissue that form a protective covering for the brain and spinal cord; the layer closest to the skull is the dura mater, the middle layer is the arachnoid, and the layer closest to the brain is the pia mater.

Metabolic Acidosis – an acidotic body state resulting from excess acids; causes include excess acids from fat metabolism (keto acids), lactic acidosis, or inadequate bicarbonate ions.

Methemoglobin – injury or toxic substances may cause the iron molecule to convert from the ferrous to the ferric state leading to methemoglobin; methemoglobin cannot transport oxygen.

Microcirculation – refers to the capillaries, venules, arterioles, metarterioles and the arterio-venous anastomoses; functions in the exchange of gases, nutrients, and byproducts of metabolism; controls total peripheral resistance.

Mitochondria – structures inside cells which, through an oxidative process, utilize stored enzymes to extract energy from nutrients to produce more energy in the form of adenosine triphosphate or ATP.

MIVT – a mnemonic representing mechanism of injury, injuries, vital signs, and treatment; used by prehospital personnel to communicate to hospital personnel.

Modified Trendelenburg Position – patient position whereby legs are elevated and rest of body is flat and supine; see Trendelenburg Position.

Monro-Kellie Hypothesis – a slight increase in any one of the three volumes of the cranial cavity (brain, blood, cerebrospinal fluid) causes a decrease in another volume without a significant change in intracranial pressure.

Mortality Rate – computed by dividing the number of deaths being studied by the total number in the population. Adjusted death rates are computed by using only those people who have a chance to be in the numerator as well as the denominator. Example, if calculating the death rate for people who are female, the numerator would be all female deaths and the denominator would include the population of only females, not the whole population.

Myoglobinuria – myoglobin in the urine; myoglobin is a protein pigment in both cardiac and skeletal muscle that transports oxygen.

NANDA – the North American Nursing Diagnosis Association.

Needle Thoracentesis – an emergency procedure to relieve a tension pneumothorax; a needle is inserted into the chest in the second intercostal space at the midclavicular line or the fifth intercostal space in the midaxillary line on the injured side.

Negative Intrapleural Pressure – the pressure inside the pleural space is slightly negative, –4 mmHg, in relation to atmospheric pressure; keeps the two pleural membranes together so the lungs do not collapse; the negative pressure increases (becomes more negative) during inspiration facilitating air movement into the lungs.

Neurogenic Shock – distributive-type shock; etiology can be trauma, reactions to spinal anesthesia, insulin shock, damage to the vasomotor center in the medulla, or drug overdose; can be a consequence of cervical or high thoracic spinal cord injury whereby sympathetic nervous system activity is disturbed, resulting in a poor distribution of blood volume from venous dilation; heart rate does not accelerate; NOT synonymous with spinal shock.

Neuromuscular Blocking Agents – skeletal muscle relaxants that peripherally induce muscle relaxation by interfering with the cholinergic (acetylcholine) transmission at the neuromuscular junction; classified as nondepolarizing or depolarizing; result in muscle paralysis.

Nociceptors – one of five types of sensory receptors (mechanoreceptors, thermoreceptors, electromagnetic receptors, chemoreceptors, and nociceptors); free nerve endings distributed throughout skin, dural extensions, dental pulp, and some internal organs; receptors for pain from physical or chemical tissue damage.

Nondepolarizing Neuromuscular Blocking Agents – cause peripheral muscle relaxation of skeletal muscles by competing with acetylcholine for the receptor site, blocking acetylcholine's function of depolarizing the postsynaptic membrane, and preventing contraction of the muscle; common drugs in this class are atracurium (Tracrium), pancuronium (Pavulon), and vecuronium (Norcuron).

Nonrebreather Oxygen Mask – an oxygen delivery device with one outlet of the face mask covered to prohibit inflow of room air during inspiration and allow outflow of expired air during exhalation. An additional flap, located over the inlet to the attached reservoir system, prohibits inflow of expired air to the reservoir system during exhalation.

Normal Saline – intravenous solution that is a 0.9% isotonic solution of sodium chloride; has more sodium and chloride than plasma; contains 154 mOsm/L of sodium and 154 mOsm/L of chloride; normal plasma has 143 mOsm/L of sodium and 108 mOsm/L of chloride.

Nursing – a discipline that has seven central concepts: patient, environment, interaction, nursing process, interventions, transition, and health.

Nursing Diagnosis – classification system or taxonomy that labels or conceptualizes the patient's problems as actual or risk; diagnoses are derived from diagnostic reasoning.

Nursing Process – based on the standards of clinical nursing practice; assessment, diagnosis, outcome identification, planning, implementation, and evaluation.

Obstructive Shock – results from an inadequate circulating blood volume due to an obstruction or compression of the great veins, aorta, pulmonary arteries, or the heart; cardiac tamponade, tension pneumothorax or pulmonary embolus may lead to obstructive shock.

Open Fracture – skin integrity over or near a fracture site is disrupted.

Otorrhea – discharge from the ear; in trauma victims, the discharge may be cerebrospinal fluid.

Oxygen Saturation – the percentage of hemoglobin saturated with oxygen, as measured by pulse oximetry (SpO_2) or arterial blood gas sample (SaO_2); the normal percentage is 98%.

Pain – "an unpleasant sensory and emotional experience arising from actual or potential tissue damage or described in terms of such damage." (Reference 1, Appendix 5); sources of pain are: cutaneous (skin and subcutaneous tissues), deep somatic (periosteum, joints, muscles, tendons, and blood vessels), visceral or splanchnic (organs), functional or psychogenic (physical pain sensation is present but source of pain in unknown); pain is a dynamic experience; can be fast or slow, acute or chronic, or referred (perception of pain in a different location than the origin).

Paradoxical – opposite.

Parasympathetic Nervous System – portion of the autonomic nervous system that controls smooth muscle, cardiac muscle, and glands; nerve cell bodies originate in cranial nerves III, VII, IX, and X and sacral spinal cord segments S-2 to S-4; chemical mediator is acetylcholine; predominate number of fibers are found in the vagus nerves that maintain normal heart rate and cardiac contractility; referred to as the "feed and breed" system.

Parenchyma – is the functional portion or substance of an organ, e.g., lung parenchyma, kidney parenchyma; as opposed to the stroma or framework of an organ.

Paresthesia – abnormal sensation such as burning, prickling, or numbness.

Partial Pressure of Carbon Dioxide (PaCO₂) – pressure exerted by carbon dioxide in the arterial blood; represents the level of dissolved carbon dioxide in the plasma; normal is between 35 to 45 mmHg (4.7 to 6.0 KPa) or 35 to 45 Torr.

Partial Pressure of Oxygen (PaO₂) – pressure exerted by oxygen in the arterial blood; represents the level of dissolved oxygen in plasma; normal is above 80 mmHg (13.3 KPa) or 80 Torr.

Partial Thromboplastin Time (PTT) – a serum blood test that measures the body's intrinsic pathway of the coagulation system.

Pattern of Injury – a combination of the patient's age, anatomic structures involved, mechanism of injury, and pre-existing factors, e.g., alcohol ingestion, restraint systems.

Penetrating Trauma – injuries that cause penetration or disruption of the skin.

Pericardiocentesis – an emergency procedure to relieve a cardiac or pericardial tamponade; blood in the pleural sac is removed via an over-the-needle catheter inserted lateral to the left side of the xiphoid.

Pericardium – also called pericardial sac; double layered sac that surrounds the heart composed of a tough, outer fibrous layer and a thinner, serous layer referred to as the epicardium; between the two layers is 30 to 50 ml of lubricating fluid.

Periosteum – vascular layer that covers the bone except at articular surfaces; tendons and ligaments are continuous with the periosteum.

Peritoneum – complex, serous, double-layered membrane; parietal layer lines the abdominal wall; the visceral layer surrounds certain organs of the abdomen.

Personal Protective Equipment (PPE) – gloves, mask in combination with eye protection devices, gowns, aprons, surgical caps, and shoe covers worn as part of universal precautions as an infection control method. (Appendix 3).

Petechiae – small, round, purple/blue/reddish spots due to intradermal or submucosal hemorrhage.

Plasma Colloid Osmotic Pressure – the pressure inside the capillary that pulls fluid into the capillary; usually plasma proteins are not semipermeable and stay in the plasma to exert a force termed the plasma or capillary colloid osmotic pressure; approximate measure of this pressure is 28 mmHg throughout the capillary.

Pleural Space (cavity) – a potential space between two pleural layers; the parietal layer lines the thoracic cavity and the visceral layer is around the outside of the lungs; contains between 5 to 10 ml fluid.

Plexus – interlacing network of vessels or nerves; four major nerve plexuses are the cervical, brachial, lumbar, and sacral.

Pneumatic Antishock Garment (PASG) – inflatable, three compartmentalized garment which fits around the lower extremities and the abdomen; when inflated, causes an increase in tissue pressure with a subsequent increase in total peripheral resistance in those vessels it surrounds; used to increase blood pressure and can be used as a splint for suspected pelvic fractures.

Pneumothorax – injury to the lung leading to accumulation of air in the pleural space with a subsequent loss of intrapleural pressure; may be partial or complete; open pneumothorax is a wound through the chest wall leading to a pneumothorax.

Poikilothermy – patient's body temperature becomes the same as the enviromental temperature.

Positive End Expiratory Pressure (PEEP) – during mechanical ventilation, pressure keeps the alveoli open until the end of expiration; continuous positive airway pressure (CPAP) does the same thing in patients who are breathing spontaneously and receiving oxygen under positive pressure.

Posterior Cord Syndrome – an incomplete spinal cord syndrome; loss of proprioception, vibration, fine touch, and fine pressure; intact motor function, pain, temperature, crude touch and crude pressure.

Posterior Spinal Nerve Tracts – dorsal, sensory, spinal nerve tracts that originate in sensory receptors located throughout the body, cross over in the medulla, and end in the cerebral cortex; responsible for sensations of proprioception, vibration, fine touch, and fine pressure.

Potentially Infectious Materials – (1) the following body fluids: semen, vaginal secretions, cerebrospinal fluid, synovial fluid, pleural fluid, pericardial fluid, peritoneal fluid, amniotic fluid, saliva in dental procedures, any body fluid that is visibly contaminated with blood, and all body fluids in situations where it is difficult or impossible to differentiate between body fluids; (2) any unfixed tissue or organ (other than intact skin) from a human (living or dead); and (3) "HIV-containing cell or tissue cultures, organ cultures, and HIV or HBV-containing culture medium or other solutions; and blood, organs, or other tissues from experimental animals infected with HIV or HBV." (Reference 1, Appendix 3).

Pregnancy Induced Hypertension (PIH) – hypertension associated with pregnancy; protein in the urine, edema, and PIH is termed pre-eclampsia; etiology unknown; when seizures occur, the condition is termed eclampsia and can be life-threatening; delivery of the fetus reverses the condition.

Pregnancy Safety Categories – The Food and Drug Administration designates a pregnancy safety category to certain drugs as follows: Category A = "Studies indicate no risk to the fetus." Category B = "Animal reproductive studies no risk to the fetus; adequate and well-controlled studies in pregnant women are unavailable." Category C = "Animal reproductive studies indicate an adverse effect on the fetus, but adequate and well-controlled studies in pregnant women are not available. Potential benefit to risk must be evaluated, as it may be warranted to use drug in selected pregnant women at risk." Category D = "Human data or studies exhibit positive evidence of human fetal risk, but potential benefit to risk may warrant the use of the drug in pregnant women." Category X = "Fetal abnormalities and positive evidence of fetal risk in humans are available from animal or human studies or from marketing reports. The risks of using this drug far outweigh the benefits; thus such drugs should not be used in pregnant women." (McHenry LM, Salerno E. *Mosby's Pharmacology in Nursing. 18th ed. Mosby-Year Book: St. Louis, Mo; 1992.*)

Preload – refers to the volume in the left and right ventricles at the end of diastole; in the left ventricle, referred to as left ventricular end-diastolic volume (LVEDV); affected by blood volume and intrathoracic pressure; increases in intrathoracic pressure reduce preload.

Priapism – Abnormal and persistent erection of penis which can be due to loss of sympathetic autonomic nervous system function due to spinal cord injury; erection is maintained by intact parasympathetic function.

Primary Assessment – assessment of airway, breathing, circulation, and disability (level of consciousness).

Proprioception – the perception of where a body part is or has been moved; requires sensory proprioceptors.

Prostaglandins – nine different fatty acids located in certain body cells; actions include uterine contraction, platelet aggregation, smooth muscle contraction, additional roles in temperature regulation, inflammation, and blood pressure.

Prothrombin Time (PT) – a serum blood test that measures the extrinsic pathway of the body's coagulation system; measures the activity of factor I, II, V, VII, and X; used routinely to monitor oral anticoagulation.

Protoplasm – internal substance of a cell composed of 70 to 85% water and 15 to 30% lipids, carbohydrates, proteins, and electrolytes.

Pseudo-electromechanical Dissociation – form of pulseless electrical activity in a patient with no blood pressure by auscultation but some degree of myocardial muscle contraction.

Pulse Oximetry – a method to measure oxygen saturation; uses a light sensor usually attached to the finger.

Pulse Pressure – the difference between systolic and diastolic blood pressure; narrows when patient is in shock.

Raccoon's Eyes – ecchymosis around the eyes; may indicate basilar skull fracture of the anterior fossa.

Range – distance between the barrel of a weapon and the victim; affects the velocity at which the bullet strikes the body tissues.

Rapid Sequence Induction (RSI) – an anesthesia phrase relating to the use of certain drugs to induce anesthesia; induction relates to Stage 1 (analgesia and consciousness) and Stage 2 (unconscious yet no skeletal muscle relaxation); RSI is a method to facilitate the insertion of an endotracheal tube in a trauma patient.

Reflex Arc – stimulus-response mechanism that does not require consciousness to function; automatic response of the nervous system; examples include knee jerk, muscle stretch, anal reflex, and deep tendon reflex.

Renin – enzyme stored in the kidneys' juxtaglomerular cells; released during renal ischemia; causes angiotensinogen to release angiotensin I which is converted to angiotensin II; promotes arteriolar vasoconstriction, further stimulation of the sympathetic nervous system, and stimulation of the release of aldosterone.

Residual Capacity (functional) – refers to the volume of air remaining in the lungs at the end of expiration; it is the sum of the residual volume (volume of air in the lungs after maximal expiration) and expiratory reserve volume (maximum volume of air exhaled from the resting end-expiratory level).

Respiration – the physiologic process of oxygen transport to and the removal of carbon dioxide from cells; consists of (1) pulmonary ventilation or the mechanics of moving air in and out of the lungs, (2) diffusion or the movement of oxygen and carbon dioxide between the alveoli and the pulmonary capillaries, (3) the transport of oxygen to the peripheral tissues at the cellular level, and (4) the regulation of respiration.

Reticular Activating Systsm (RAS) – complex system found in the reticular formation of the midbrain and pons; connects to the cerebral cortex; system maintains wakefulness.

Retroperitoneum – space behind the peritoneum to the posterior abdominal wall; organs in the retroperitoneum are only partially covered by peritoneum.

Revised Trauma Score – measures the patient's physiologic response to injuries; measurements include a score for the Glasgow Coma Scale, systolic blood pressure, and respiratory rate. Coded values are used to represent ranges in each of three measured areas; total score ranges from 0 to 12.

Rhabdomyolysis – destruction of striated muscle fibers; as a result myoglobin, the protein in muscle that transports oxygen and gives the muscle its color, may be released and excreted in the urine (myoglobinuria).

Rhinorrhea – discharge from the nose; in trauma victims, the discharge may be cerebrospinal fluid if an anterior basilar fracture of the cribriform plate of the ethmoid bone exists.

Sacral Sparing – in the presence of an incomplete spinal cord injury, the patient still has perianal sensation, anal sphincter tone, and great toe flexor activity.

SaO$_2$ – oxygen saturation as measured and calculated by a sample of arterial blood.

Scalp – protective covering of cranium; composed of five layers (skin, subcutaneous tissue, galea aponeurotica, areolar tissue, and periosteum).

Secondary Assessment – assessment of the patient from head-to-toe to identify all injuries.

Sedatives – "chemical substances that reduce nervousness, excitability, or irritability by producing a calming or soothing effect." (Reference 15, Appendix 4).

Sellick Maneuver – a maneuver, used during endotracheal intubation, whereby the thumb and forefinger of someone's hand exerts downward pressure compressing the patient's cricoid cartilage onto C-6 and occluding the esophagus; a maneuver used when the patient being intubated has a full stomach and the risk of regurgitation and aspiration is high; the pressure is not relieved until the endotracheal tube is properly placed in the patient's trachea.

Serotonin – vasoactive hormone that leads to vasoconstriction; found in platelets, stomach, brain, and lungs; also considered a neurotransmitter; inhibits release of gastric acids.

Shock – syndrome, resulting from inadequate perfusion of tissues, leading to a decrease in the supply of oxygen and nutrients required to maintain the metabolic needs of cells.

Skull – bones of the cranium and face; composed of eight cranial bones (frontal, temporal [2], parietal [2], occipital, ethmoid, sphenoid) and 14 facial bones (two each maxilla, nasal, palatine, zygoma, lacrimal, inferior nasal concha, and one vomer and mandible).

Smoke – mixture of gases and particulate matter produced during the decomposition and combustion of natural or synthetic material; composition depends on substance burning, temperature and rate at which it is being generated, and amount of oxygen present in the burning environment.

Spinal Nerves – 31 pair each with a motor and sensory root; exit from the spinal cord; eight cervical, 12 thoracic, five lumbar, five sacral, and one coccygeal.

Spinal Shock – usually occurs shortly after a spinal cord injury; results in temporary loss of motor, sensory, and reflex functions below the level of the lesion; may last days or weeks; patient presents with flaccid paralysis that turns to spastic paralysis when spinal shock is resolved; NOT synonymous with neurogenic shock.

Spinothalamic Sensory Tracts – ascending, sensory, spinal nerve tracts that originate in the sensory receptors located throughout the body, cross over at the level they enter the spinal cord (anterolateral), and end in the cerebral cortex; responsible for sensations of pain, temperature, crude touch, and crude pressure.

Splanchive – related to organs or viscera.

SpO$_2$ – oxygen saturation as measured by pulse oximetry.

Straddle Trauma – injuries sustained when the perineum is the point of impact; may lead to bilateral disruption of the superior and inferior pubic rami and subsequent hemorrhage.

Strain – Tissue damage or deformation that results from stress; dependent on the properties of the particular tissue involved.

Stress (biomechanical term) – "the forces applied to deform the body or the equal and opposite forces with which the body resists." (Reference 19, Chapter 2). Stress can be tensile, compressive, or shearing.

Stress (mental health term) – "the body's arousal response to any demand, change, or perceived threat." (Reference 1, Chapter 13).

Stressor – "the circumstance or event that elicits this [stress] response." (Reference 1, Chapter 13).

Subcutaneous Emphysema – air beneath the subcutaneous tissue of the chest in the interstitial spaces; results from an air leak following disruption of the larynx, trachea, or bronchi.

Subdural Hematoma – collection of blood between the dura mater and the arachnoid in the subdural space; can be chronic or acute; usually venous in origin.

Supine – a position in which a person is lying on his or her dorsal (back) surface with the head facing up.

Surfactant – a lipoprotein that contains lecithin; produced in the lung by the alveolar Type II cells; reduces the surface tension inside alveoli and contributes to pulmonary compliance; keeps the alveoli dry; because a surfactant molecule has one end that is water-soluble and one end that is water-insoluble, it can interrupt the intermolecular tension caused by water and gas molecules and reduce surface tension.

Sympathetic Nervous System – thoracolumbar portion of the autonomic nervous system which innervates smooth muscle, cardiac muscle, and glands; activated during physiologic and psychologic stress; chemical mediator is norepinephrine; causes increase in heart rate, increase in force of cardiac contraction, vasoconstriction, and bronchodilation; referred to as the "fight or flight" system.

Tachypnea – increased number of respirations per minute above normal.

Tendon – thick, white fibrous connective tissue that attaches muscles to bones.

Tension Pneumothorax – life-threatening injury to the lung which allows air to enter the pleural space on inspiration but the air cannot escape on expiration; rising intrathoracic pressure collapses the lung causing a mediastinal shift, compressing the heart and great vessels.

Tentorium Cerebelli – dural extension which extends from the occipital bone to the center of the cranium; divides the cranial cavity into supratentorial and infratentorial compartments; cerebral hemispheres are in the supratentorium; the brainstem and cerebellum are in the infratentorium.

Tetanus – serious often fatal disease caused by the bacillus, Clostridium tetani; leads to convulsions, muscle spasms, stiffness of the jaw, coma, and death; bacilli are found in the intestines of animals and humans; the spore can be found in the soil and dust and is spread by animal and human feces; organism enters the human host through an open wound often caused by a nail, splinter, insect bite, or gunshot.

Thoracentesis – a puncture with a needle into the thorax to evacuate air (tension pneumothorax).

Thoracic Cavity – extends from the top of the sternum to the diaphragm.

Thoracostomy – an incision into the chest wall, e.g., chest tube thoracostomy.

Tidal Volume – amount of air moved in and out of the lungs with each breath; approximately 500 ml at rest.

Tissue – cells that are similar and are grouped together to perform a specific function; four types of tissues are epithelial, connective, muscle, and nervous.

Toxoid – an agent for active immunity; derived from the actual microorganisms that have been detoxified usually with formaldehyde; organisms are no longer toxic but are capable of stimulating antibody production, e.g., tetanus-diphtheria toxoid.

Trauma – a Greek word meaning wound; used interchangeably with injury; damage to human tissue and/or organs resulting from the transfer of some form of energy from the environment to a human host; an injury occurs when the energy is beyond the body's resilience.

Trauma Center – Level I trauma center is a regional tertiary trauma center with full capabilities to manage trauma patients from time of injury through rehabilitation; Level II trauma center is a facility with partial capability to manage trauma victims and can provide initial definitive trauma care; Level III trauma center is in an area where a Level I or II is not available, yet initial definitive care is available, and the patient with severe injuries will most likely need to be transferred to a Level I or II center; Level IV trauma center provides initial advanced life support in remote areas, may be a clinic, and usually does not have the inpatient services needed for trauma victims.

Trauma Nursing – the nursing knowledge and knowledge from other disciplines that forms the process and content of all the roles nurses have in the care of trauma patients.

Trendelenburg's Position – patient is supine on a surface, e.g., bed that is tilted 45 degrees so the head is lower and legs are over the edge. In a Modified Trendelenburg position, the patient is supine with the legs elevated 45 degrees to facilitate venous return; F. Trendelenburg (1844-1924) was a German surgeon who introduced operations for varicose veins, esophageal stricture, and suturing of the patella; founded the German Surgical Society.

Trismus – difficulty in opening the mouth; can be due to injury to the motor function of the trigeminal nerve or associated with mandibular fractures.

Type-specific – blood used for transfusion that is the same type as the recipient's; based on the ABO blood groups and Rh system; persons with Type A blood have A-type antigens on their red blood cells, persons with Type B have B-type antigens, persons with both A and B-type antigens are Type AB, and those persons with neither A or B-type antigens are Type O; Rh positive persons have the D antigen and those who do not are considered Rh negative.

Uncal Herniation – uncus (lateral portion) of the temporal lobe is forced medially and downward over the tentorium into the posterior fossa; causes compression of the diencephalon, midbrain, and the oculomotor cranial nerve causing a fixed pupil.

Unintentional Injuries – injuries not intentional; 10 leading causes are motor vehicle crashes, falls, poisonings, fires and burns, drowning, aspiration (nonfood), aspiration (food), firearm-related, machinery-related, and aircraft-related.

Universal Donor – O-negative blood type; no A, B, or D antigens on the red blood cells; if O-negative blood is transfused into a person with another type of blood, a transfusion reaction is unlikely since there are no antigens to react with antibodies in the recipient's plasma.

Universal Precautions – "is an approach to infection control. According to the concept of Univeral Precautions, all human blood and certain human body fluids are treated as if known to be infectious for HIV, HBV, and other bloodborne pathogens." (Reference 1, Appendix 3).

Urea – nitrogenous byproduct of protein metabolism; found in the urine; levels may increase in the blood if urea is not filtered properly into the urine; plasma urea is measured by the blood urea nitrogen or BUN.

Uric Acid – byproduct of purine metabolism which is normally excreted in the urine.

Viscosity (blood) – blood is a liquid substance made up of molecules that, due to the movement of blood, must move and cause friction leading to increased resistance to flow; the greater the friction, the greater the resistance to flow and the greater the viscosity.

Vital Capacity – maximum amount of air exhaled from point of maximum inspiration; approximately 4,600 ml.

Waddell's Triad – a description of possible injuries when a child is struck by a motor vehicle; injuries include those to the head, trunk, and extremities.

Xiphoid – sword-shaped; xiphoid process is the tip of the sternum surrounded by cartilage.

Yaw – deviation of the bullet from a straight path, within the tissue, up to a 90-degree angle.

Zones of a Burn – the zone of coagulation is the center of a burn where the tissue is not viable; zone of stasis surrounds the zone of coagulation and is the area where capillary occlusion, diminished perfusion, and edema occurs 24 to 48 hours after the burn; zone of hyperemia is the area around the zone of stasis with increased blood flow.

Zones of the Neck – three anatomic regions; zone I extends from the level of the cricoid cartilage down to the clavicles; zone II extends from the angle of the mandible to the area above the cricoid cartilage; zone III extends from the base of the skull to the angle of the mandible.